Yogurt: Roles in Nutrition and Impacts on Health

Yogurt: Roles in Nutrition and Impacts on Health

By
André Marette
Éliane Picard-Deland
Melissa Anne Fernandez

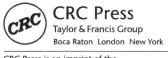
CRC Press
Taylor & Francis Group
Boca Raton London New York

CRC Press is an imprint of the
Taylor & Francis Group, an **informa** business

CRC Press
Taylor & Francis Group
6000 Broken Sound Parkway NW, Suite 300
Boca Raton, FL 33487-2742

© 2017 by Taylor & Francis Group, LLC
CRC Press is an imprint of Taylor & Francis Group, an Informa business

No claim to original U.S. Government works

Printed at CPI on sustainably sourced paper

International Standard Book Number-13: 978-1-138-03255-2 (Hardback)

This book contains information obtained from authentic and highly regarded sources. Reasonable efforts have been made to publish reliable data and information, but the author and publisher cannot assume responsibility for the validity of all materials or the consequences of their use. The authors and publishers have attempted to trace the copyright holders of all material reproduced in this publication and apologize to copyright holders if permission to publish in this form has not been obtained. If any copyright material has not been acknowledged, please write and let us know so we may rectify in any future reprint.

Except as permitted under U.S. Copyright Law, no part of this book may be reprinted, reproduced, transmitted, or utilized in any form by any electronic, mechanical, or other means, now known or hereafter invented, including photocopying, microfilming, and recording, or in any information storage or retrieval system, without written permission from the publishers.

For permission to photocopy or use material electronically from this work, please access www.copyright.com (http://www.copyright.com/) or contact the Copyright Clearance Center, Inc. (CCC), 222 Rosewood Drive, Danvers, MA 01923, 978-750-8400. CCC is a not-for-profit organization that provides licenses and registration for a variety of users. For organizations that have been granted a photocopy license by the CCC, a separate system of payment has been arranged.

Trademark Notice: Product or corporate names may be trademarks or registered trademarks, and are used only for identification and explanation without intent to infringe.

Library of Congress Cataloging-in-Publication Data

Names: Marette, André, author. | Picard-Deland, Éliane, author. | Fernandez, Melissa Anne, author.
Title: Yogurt : roles in nutrition and impacts on health / authors, André Marette, Éliane Picard-Deland, Melissa Anne Fernandez.
Description: Boca Raton : Taylor & Francis, 2017. | Includes bibliographical references and index.
Identifiers: LCCN 2016044962 | ISBN 9781138032552 (hardback : alk. paper)
Subjects: | MESH: Yogurt | Chronic Disease--prevention & control
Classification: LCC SF275.Y6 | NLM WB 428 | DDC 637/.1476--dc23
LC record available at https://lccn.loc.gov/2016044962

Visit the Taylor & Francis Web site at
http://www.taylorandfrancis.com

and the CRC Press Web site at
http://www.crcpress.com

Contents

Foreword xi
Acknowledgments xvii
Authors xix
Introduction xxi

SECTION I Yogurt Composition and Consumption

Chapter 1 Yogurt Composition 3

    1.1 Carbohydrates 3
    1.2 Proteins 5
        1.2.1 Biological Quality 5
        1.2.2 Casein and Whey 5
        1.2.3 Effect of Food Processing and Lactic Fermentation 7
            1.2.3.1 Digestion and Generation of Bioactive Peptides 7
            1.2.3.2 Interaction with Minerals 8
    1.3 Lipids 9
        1.3.1 Effect of Food Processing and Lactic Fermentation 10
    1.4 Minerals 10
        1.4.1 Effect of Food Processing and Lactic Fermentation 11
        1.4.2 Bioavailability 12
    1.5 Vitamins 13
        1.5.1 Effect of Food Processing and Lactic Fermentation ... 14
    1.6 Starter Cultures 14
    1.7 Yogurt Matrix 15
    1.8 Conclusions 16
    References 17

Chapter 2 Yogurt Consumption 23

    2.1 Food-Based Dietary Guidelines for Dairy and Yogurt 23
    2.2 Dairy and Yogurt Consumption 26
    2.3 Nutrient Density 28
    2.4 Nutrient Adequacy 30
    2.5 Dietary Patterns, Lifestyle, and Sociodemographic Factors 34
        2.5.1 Dietary Patterns 34
        2.5.2 Lifestyle and Sociodemographic Factors 35
    2.6 Conclusions 36
    References 37

SECTION II Yogurt and Cardiometabolic Health

Chapter 3 Weight Management and Obesity 45
    3.1   Studies in Children and Adolescents 46
    3.2   Studies in Adults 51
           3.2.1   Cross-Sectional Studies 51
           3.2.2   Prospective Studies 52
           3.2.3   Clinical Studies 55
           3.2.4   Reviews 55
    3.3   Mechanisms of Action 56
           3.3.1   Studies on Satiety 56
           3.3.2   Micro- and Macronutrients and Their Physiological Effects 56
           3.3.3   Viscosity 58
           3.3.4   Gut Microbiota 58
    3.4   Conclusions 58
    References 59

Chapter 4 Type 2 Diabetes 65
    4.1   Studies in Children and Adolescents 68
    4.2   Studies in Adults 68
           4.2.1   Cross-Sectional Studies 68
           4.2.2   Prospective Cohort Studies 68
           4.2.3   Meta-Analyses and Systematic Reviews 70
    4.3   Mechanisms of Action 71
           4.3.1   Vitamins and Minerals 72
           4.3.2   Glycemic Load 72
           4.3.3   Proteins 73
           4.3.4   Fatty Acids 73
           4.3.5   Fermentation and Ferments 75
    4.4   Conclusions 75
    References 76

Chapter 5 Hypertension 81
    5.1   Studies in Adults 81
           5.1.1   Cross-Sectional Studies 81
           5.1.2   Prospective Studies 82
           5.1.3   Meta-Analyses and Reviews 83
    5.2   Mechanisms of Action 84
           5.2.1   Effect of Dairy Proteins and Peptides 84
           5.2.2   Effect of Ca, K, Mg, and Lipids 85
    5.3   Conclusions 86
    References 86

Contents

Chapter 6 Cardiovascular Diseases 89
    6.1 Studies in Adolescents.. 91
    6.2 Studies in Adults.. 91
        6.2.1 Cross-Sectional Studies... 91
        6.2.2 Prospective Studies 92
        6.2.3 Clinical Studies 93
        6.2.4 Meta-Analyses and Systematic Reviews.................... 94
    6.3 Mechanisms of Action.. 95
        6.3.1 Effect of Lipids and Other Nutrients......................... 95
        6.3.2 Effect of Bacteria on Cholesterol 96
    6.4 Conclusions.. 97
    References 97

Chapter 7 Metabolic Syndrome 103
    7.1 Studies in Adolescents.. 104
    7.2 Studies in Adults.. 105
        7.2.1 Cross-Sectional Studies... 105
        7.2.2 Prospective Cohort Studies 106
    7.3 Mechanisms of Action.. 108
    7.4 Conclusions.. 108
    References 109

SECTION III *Yogurt and Other Health Conditions*

Chapter 8 Yogurt and Gut Health 113
    8.1 Lactose Deficiency, Malabsorption, and Intolerance 113
        8.1.1 Studies in Children.. 117
        8.1.2 Studies in Adults 118
        8.1.3 Mechanisms of Action.. 120
            8.1.3.1 Activity of Yogurt Bacteria 120
            8.1.3.2 Colonic Processing of Lactose and
                        Adaptation.. 121
            8.1.3.3 Physical Properties 121
        8.1.4 Conclusions 122
    8.2 Treatment of Diarrhea 122
        8.2.1 Treatment of Acute Diarrhea..................................... 123
        8.2.2 Treatment of Persistent Diarrhea............................... 124
        8.2.3 Antibiotic-Associated Diarrhea................................. 125
            8.2.3.1 Studies in Children 125
            8.2.3.2 Studies in Adults...................................... 126
        8.2.4 Mechanisms of Action 126
        8.2.5 Conclusions 127

	8.3	The Microbiota	128
		8.3.1 Conclusions	128
	8.4	Viability of Yogurt Bacteria	128
		8.4.1 Conclusions	131
	References		131

Chapter 9 Immune Responses 139

    9.1 Human Studies 139
        9.1.1 Cytokine Production 139
        9.1.2 Natural Killer Cell Activity...................................... 140
        9.1.3 T and B Lymphocyte Function 140
        9.1.4 Phagocytic Activity 141
    9.2 Mechanisms of Action... 141
    9.3 Conclusions.. 142
    References 143

Chapter 10 Cancer 145

    10.1 Colorectal Cancer 145
        10.1.1 Observational Studies... 146
            10.1.1.1 Case-Control Studies 146
            10.1.1.2 Prospective Cohort Studies..................... 147
            10.1.1.3 Meta-Analyses 149
        10.1.2 Clinical Studies 149
        10.1.3 Mechanisms of Action.. 149
        10.1.4 Conclusions 150
    10.2 Breast Cancer 150
        10.2.1 Case-Control Studies.. 151
        10.2.2 Prospective Cohort Studies 152
        10.2.3 Reviews 152
        10.2.4 Mechanisms of Action.. 152
        10.2.5 Conclusions 153
    10.3 Prostate Cancer 153
        10.3.1 Case-Control Studies.. 153
        10.3.2 Prospective Cohort Studies 154
        10.3.3 Meta-Analyses 154
        10.3.4 Mechanisms of Action.. 154
        10.3.5 Conclusions 155
    References 155

Chapter 11 Allergy and Atopic Diseases 159

    11.1 Eczema and Atopic Dermatitis.. 159
    11.2 Allergic Rhinitis 160
    11.3 Allergic Asthma 161

	11.4 Mechanisms of Action	162
	11.5 Conclusions	163
	References	163

Chapter 12 Bone Mineralization and Osteoporosis ... 167

    12.1 Studies in Children and Adolescents ... 169
    12.2 Studies in Older Adults ... 170
        12.2.1 Cross-Sectional and Case-Control Studies ... 170
        12.2.2 Prospective Studies ... 171
        12.2.3 Clinical Studies ... 172
        12.2.4 Systematic Reviews ... 172
    12.3 Mechanisms of Action ... 172
    12.4 Conclusions ... 173
    References ... 174

General Conclusion ... 179
Index ... 183

Foreword

Yogurt and Other Fermented Milks: Historical and Cultural Approach

Written by Éric Birlouez, agricultural engineer and sociologist specializing in food history

YOGURT: AN ORIGIN WHICH REMAINS MYSTERIOUS

Who invented yogurt? No one knows, even though many cultures—foremost among them the Turks and the Bulgarians—fiercely claim the paternity of the "true" yogurt. Yogurt, coexisting with several hundreds of other fermented milks, has appeared over thousands of years in numerous regions of the world. The true yogurt, however, is distinguished from its innumerable cousins by its distinctive microbial composition. According to Codex Alimentarius (FAO), two specific bacteria, and only these bacteria, must be present so that the product can claim the denomination of *yoghurt* or *yogurt*.* These two cultures are *Lactobacillus delbrueckii* subsp. *bulgaricus* and *Streptococcus thermophilus*. Yet, one cannot say if the ancestral yogurt of the Bulgarians and the Turks contained these two bacteria, which have only been identified since the beginning of the twentieth century.

The origin of "real" yogurt, therefore, remains uncertain. What is certain, though, is that *yoğurt* is legitimately a word from the Turkish language, appearing for the first time in a text written in 1072. But it was only at the beginning of the twentieth century that the word *yoghourt*, *yogurt*, or even *yaourt* appeared in the West.

ALL BEGAN WITH MILK, A HIGHLY SYMBOLIC BEVERAGE

Man began to drink milk other than that of human origin once they managed to domesticate certain species of wild mammals. This process of domestication was initiated 10,500 years ago in the Middle East, first with goats and then sheep and several centuries later with cattle. For a long period, the milk produced by these

---

* The Codex Alimentarius (Codex Stan A-11(a)—1975) defines yogurt thus: "Yoghurt is a coagulated milk product obtained by lactic acid fermentation through the action of *Lactobacillus bulgaricus* and *Streptococcus thermophilus* from fresh milk as well as that of pasteurized milk (or concentrated, partly skimmed, enriched with dry solids) with or without optional additions (milk powder, skim milk powder, etc.). The micro-organisms in the final product must be viable and abundant." Source: http://www.fao.org/docrep/t4280f/T4280F0d.htm.

animals was not consumed in its liquid form but was transformed into fermented milk curd or cheese. Indeed, several thousands of years were necessary for genetic mutation to disperse among certain human cultures, thereby allowing the persistence of lactase activity at an adult age. Lactase activity is the ability to digest the lactose content in milk.

Because it is exclusively the food of newborns, very early in history milk acquired a powerful symbolic weight; reinforced by its white color, it became synonymous with life, with fertility, with purity, and also with abundance. Moses promises to lead the captive Hebrew people in Egypt toward a land "where milk and honey flow." Mythologies of the ancient world are plentiful with tales in which young children with a promised exceptional destiny are fed animal milk from birth.

This is the case in the story of Zeus, breastfed by the goat, Amalthea, or twin orphans Remus and Romulus, the future founders of Rome, suckled by the milk of a she-wolf. A Greek myth recounts that one day the young Hercules threw himself with such greed on the breast of the goddess Hera that a stream of milk burst in gushes, crossing the heavens to form the Milky Way Galaxy (from the Greek *gala*: milk). For Hindus, the world was born from an ocean of milk churned by the Gods, while the Fulani herdsmen of the Sahel conjure up the universe from a drop of milk. The curd image is also prominent in many legendary tales. In the eighth century BC, the Greek Homer adds that according to custom, the Cyclops Polyphemus "race," their sheep, and their bleating goats engaged in cheese making: "then leaving half of the milk to curdle, he carefully set it aside in wicker strainers" (*The Odyssey*, Canto VI). Similarly, the curd appears repeatedly in biblical texts.

Yogurt, Fermented Milk

As soon as human cultures had milk at their disposal, they did not fail to observe the appearance of spontaneous fermentations. Under certain conditions, these were transforming lactose, poorly digested by the first milk drinkers, into galactose and glucose, easily absorbed molecules. These lactic fermentations equally allowed the preservation of milk for longer times. Such advantages enticed the first breeders and, gradually, they developed and perfected techniques to master the fermentation of the precious liquid. Traces of fermented milk have recently been identified on pottery surfaced in Libya, aged at 9,000 years old. Over thousands of years, certain cultures of breeders had become masters in the art of producing these fermented milks.

IN THE SIXTEENTH CENTURY, YOGURT MADE A SHORT-LIVED APPEARANCE IN WESTERN EUROPE

Milk and dairy products were denigrated by the French and European elites of the Middle Ages and the Renaissance. Very conscious of social distinction, the "powerful" saw in milk a food of the peasant, unworthy of their noble status. Yogurt made its first (but short-lived) incursion into the kingdom of France at the beginning of the sixteenth century. King François I was suffering from intestinal disorders and, in an attempt to relieve the king, a Turkish doctor from Constantinople was sought out. His remedy, fermented sheep milk, was apparently a marvel. The sovereign was cured and the doctor returned to the East, taking with him his sheep and the manufacturing secret of his "yogurt."

YOGURT AND HEALTH: THE GREAT DISCOVERERS

In the nineteenth century, the acceleration in the progress of knowledge in yogurt created new perspectives. In the 1850s, Louis Pasteur examined the process, which until then was seemingly mysterious fermentation. He demonstrated that this transformation of living material was the result of the activity of microscopic organisms. At the end of the century, a researcher of Ukrainian origin, Elie Metchnikoff (1845–1916), led work in Paris demonstrating the positive effects of yogurt on the intestinal disorders of newborns. In 1905, Stamen Grigorov, a young Bulgarian scientist, was interested and focused his studies on the sour milk product fermented in his country. He highlighted evidence of the presence of many bacteria; in particular, one which transformed the lactose in milk into lactic acid and which would be later referred to as *Lactobacillus bulgaricus*.

THE ROAD TO SUCCESS IS OPEN

At the beginning of the twentieth century, Aram Deukmedjian, an Armenian native of Constantinople, established a creamery in Paris, which he named *Cure de Yaourt*. He then contacted Professor Metchnikoff and obtained from him the following text: "I have eaten and analyzed the Aram yoghurt. It is not harmful to health. On the contrary, it contains lactic cultures which are useful for our body." Equipped with this scientific approval, the Armenian entrepreneur created a yogurt manufacturing factory. Some years later, a Catalonian industrialist, Isaac Carasso, followed in his footsteps. In 1929, his son Daniel founded the *Société parisienne du Yaourt Danone*. The name of the brand makes reference to the first name of the enterprise's founder: *Danon* is a derivative of the Catalan name *Daniel*.

MORE THAN 400 NAMES OF FERMENTED MILKS!*

An exact count of fermented milks is not easy because the same type of fermented milk can have different names according to the language of the people who consume it. For instance, the Turks call *ayran* a drink consisting of fermented milk diluted in water and slightly salted. The same name is used in Bulgaria, Greece, and Macedonia. But in the Middle East, the beverage takes the name of *leben aryân*. The Armenians call it *tahn*, Iraqis *shinena*, and Iranians *doogh*, the Afghans and Pakistani *dugh*, the Nepali *mohi*, and so on. In contrast, a similar designation can regroup products by their different textures and tastes: the traditional yogurt consumed in Bulgaria, firm

---

* Puniya, 2016. p. 10.

and gelatinous like a flan, is not uncommon with the "yoghurt brewed in Bulgarian taste" of our superstores!

In France, the Bretons are well acquainted with *Lait Ribot*. It is manufactured by souring skimmed milk that has been previously lightly salted and pasteurized. Among the Anglo-Saxons, this type of fermented milk is known as buttermilk. In the Maghreb, this corresponds to *leben*.

For centuries, the breeders of the Central Asian steppes have been manufacturing a sparkling and slightly alcoholic beverage from milk from their mares: the *koumiss* (called *airag* in Mongolia and China). The milk of camels is used by the Kazakh for the manufacture of *shubat*, while the Mongols of the Gobi Desert make *khormog* and the Turkish *chal*. For their part, the Uzbeks ferment yak milk to obtain *kourout*.

Like *koumys*, *kefir* of the Caucasus is a fermented milk liquid, very rich in carbonic gas (therefore very fizzy) and slightly alcoholic. However, it is never manufactured from mare's milk but from that of a cow, sheep, or goat. Traditionally, milk was put to ferment in a skin bag that was shaken regularly and in which fresh milk replaced the coagulated milk as soon as the latter was extracted. After a number of batches, the whitish sediment that had dried on the inner wall of the skin bag was collected. Thus, one obtained the "kefir grains," small agglomerates of proteins and polysaccharides containing bacteria and living yeasts. These kefir grains allowed the inoculation of new quantities of milk and they were passed down from one generation to the next.

In India, *dahi* is the fermented milk of the cow or zebu. When it is diluted, *dahi* becomes *lassi*, a refreshing drink. Indians add cumin and mustard seed to *dahi* to prepare the famous *raita* sauce. Another Indian yogurt sauce that is famous is *korma* sauce.

Laban is very present in the Lebanese kitchen. By leaving it to strain, one produces *labne*; seasoned with oil and consumed with olives, it constitutes the breakfast of numerous Lebanese. The Syrians strain the *laban* longer and flavor it with cumin, thyme, pepper, and chili peppers: this is *shenglish*.

The inhabitants of the Nordic countries have also created numerous fermented milk products; Swedish *filmjölk*, milk of cow; *längfil* and *piimä* (a reindeer milk) from Sami; Finnish *viili*; Danish *ymer*; Icelandic *skyr*; and even *fillebunke*, *kjadermilk*, and *tättmjölk* (a liquid yogurt derived from a milk that has been curdled with *Pinguicula* or butterwort; a carnivorous marsh plant). Finally, the African continent also produces many fermented milks, from that of the camel (Mauritania) or zebu.

YOGURT TODAY

The global consumption of yogurt began to grow strongly in the 1950s. Estimated at 62 billion euros in 2013, the market could exceed 78 billion euros in 2018, having a 26% growth in 5 years (source: Euromonitor, AC Nielsen, 2013). But this demand is still characterized by large geographic disparities. According to a study conducted in 2014 by Euromonitor/AC Nielsen, the greatest consumers of yogurt were the Dutch, the Turks, the French, and the Germans, with, respectively, 286, 282, 280, and 277 pots (125 g) per person. They were followed by the Saudis (221 pots), the South Africans (221), and the Spanish (202). Far behind were the

Russians (122), the Japanese, the British, the Canadians, the Americans, and the Italians (only 53 pots).

A survey conducted in 2014 by the enzyme producer DSM Food Specialities* highlights other differences. While the Chinese prefer probiotic fermented milks, the Turks prefer natural yogurt, the Americans prefer Greek yogurt, and the Polish, French, and Brazilians prefer flavored yogurt. The Brazilians and the Americans consume yogurt primarily at breakfast, the Turks eat it with hot dishes, and the French prefer it as a dessert. Health awareness—both bone and digestive—is the primary motivation of respondents to buy more yogurt; it is cited by nearly 7 out of 10 interviewed (more than 8 out of 10 in Turkey and China). In North America, the success of Greek yogurt is due, according to the authors of the study, to the actual desire of many consumers to increase the protein content of their diet.

Eugène Ionesco, the Nobel Prize winner for Literature, praised the benefits of yogurt in his play *The Bald Soprano* (1950): Ionesco tells Mrs Smith, "Yogurt is excellent for the stomach, kidneys, appendicitis and the apotheosis."

REFERENCES

Euromonitor, AC Nielsen. 2013. Global yogurt consumption per capita and per year. Palaiseau, France: Danone Nutriticia Research. Accessed July 12, 2016. http://nutrijournal.danone.com/en/articles/stories/global-yoghurt-consumption-per-capita-and-per-year.

Puniya, A. K. 2016. *Fermented Milk and Dairy Products*. Boca Raton, FL: CRC Press.

---

* Online survey conducted in April and May 2014 among 6000 people aged 25 years and more in Brazil, China, France, Poland, Turkey, and the United States.

Acknowledgments

The authors would like to thank Danone Nutricia Research for commissioning through a research grant the review of the literature that served as the foundation for the writing of this book.

Authors

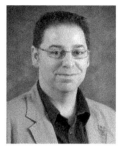

André Marette is professor of medicine at the Quebec Heart and Lung Institute, Laval Hospital, and scientific director of the Institute of Nutrition and Functional Foods at Laval University, Quebec City, Québec, Canada. He also holds a research chair on the pathogenesis of insulin resistance and cardiovascular diseases. Dr. Marette is an internationally renowned expert on the pathogenesis of insulin resistance and cardiometabolic diseases, and his research has advanced our understanding of the physiological and molecular mechanisms of inflammation and opened new possibilities for the prevention and treatment of type 2 diabetes and CVD. He is also studying how nutrition and food ingredients can modulate the gut microbiota to protect against obesity-linked intestinal inflammation, fatty liver disease, and type 2 diabetes. Dr. Marette has been invited to many international conferences in the last 20 years and is the author of more than 180 peer-reviewed papers, reviews, book chapters, and editorials in the field of metabolism, nutrition, and cardiometabolic diseases. He has been on the editorial boards of several journals and currently serves as editor-in-chief for the *American Journal of Physiology-Endocrinology and Metabolism*. Dr. Marette has received several awards for his work, including the prestigious Young Scientist Award of the Canadian Diabetes Association and the Charles Best Award from the University of Toronto for his overall contribution to the advancement of scientific knowledge in the field of diabetes.

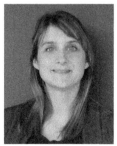

Éliane Picard-Deland is a registered dietitian and obtained a master's degree in nutrition in 2010 at the Institute of Nutrition and Functional Foods (INAF), Laval University. Through her work as a research assistant in the laboratory of Dr. André Marette, she contributes to the advancement of knowledge and valorization of science in the field of nutrition and related diseases, particularly type 2 diabetes, obesity, and cardiometabolic diseases. She works closely with researchers and partners on the development and coordination of international scientific projects.

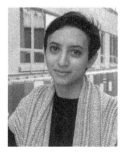

Melissa Anne Fernandez is a registered dietitian and a PhD candidate at the School of Nutrition at Laval University, specializing in public health nutrition. She has a background in molecular biology and physiology, which complements her current work as a research assistant in Dr. Marette's lab at the Quebec Heart and Lung Institute. Under Dr. Marette's guidance, she has contributed to several articles and book chapters, reviewing different aspects of yogurt consumption, its role in the diet, and its effects on health.

Introduction

Yogurt's unique combination of nutritive components and live microorganisms make it an interesting food from a nutritional standpoint that can be easily incorporated into a healthy diet (German 2014). Historically, fermentation has been used as a traditional method of preserving food, and yogurt has been one of the most commonly consumed fermented foods globally (Marsh et al. 2014). In the early 1900s, particular microorganisms were used to ferment milk, and yogurt developed a specific identity based on the type of milk and microbial species used to produce it at an industrial scale (Tamime et al. 2006). Figure I.1 provides a brief timeline of yogurt's history and commercialization as a commonly consumed fermented milk product. The last decades have been marked by the appearance of an increasing number of commercial yogurts with different flavors, textures, and nutritional compositions targeting specific consumers. In countries like the United States, the per capita yogurt consumption has increased from approximately 0.9 kg (2 lbs) in 1975 to 6.8 kg (14.9 lbs) in 2013 (U.S. Department of Agriculture 2016), which demonstrates the increased popularity of this product. Moreover, the keen interest in the consumption of yogurt is, at least in part, attributed to its reported beneficial effects on health. Even though there has been a marked increase in yogurt consumption over the last several decades in the United States, per capita annual consumption has been considerably higher in many European countries. For example, in 2013, the French consumed 70 L of yogurt per capita compared with Americans, who consumed 15.4 L.

The Codex standard for fermented milks characterizes them by the specific starter cultures used for fermentation. Figure I.2 describes traditional fermented milks consumed in different regions around the world. Yogurt is specifically defined as the product of milk fermented with *Lactobacillus delbrueckii* subsp. *bulgaricus* and *Streptococcus thermophilus*. However, alternate yogurt cultures may be used and can include a combination of *S. thermophilus* and any *Lactobacillus* species. Yogurt composition standards are also defined in the Codex Alimentarius: yogurt must contain at least 10^7 cfu/g microorganisms in the starter culture, a minimum of 2.7% of milk protein (% mass/mass), less than 15% of milk fat (% mass/mass), and a minimum of 0.6% of titratable acidity, expressed as the percentage of lactic acid (% mass/mass). However, the regulations vary from one country to another, and there are processing differences with regard to additives, the analytical criteria, the required quantity of living bacteria, and so on (Joint FAO/WHO Codex Alimentarius Commission 2010).

In addition to international variability in nutritional composition, there is no consensus regarding yogurt's potential benefits for health (German 2014). The objective of this book is to explore the state of knowledge on the effects of yogurt and its nutrients on health and compile the scientific literature to date into a reference document. While there are many varieties of novel yogurt currently available on the market, the focus of this book is commercialized cow-milk yogurt. Furthermore, the primary focus of this book is yogurt that has been inoculated with traditional cultures, *S. thermophilus* and *L. delbrueckii* ssp. *bulgaricus*, and not specific probiotic

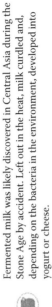

FIGURE I.1 History of yogurt development and commercialization. (Reprinted with permission from Danone Nutricia Research.)

- **10,000 B.C.** — Fermented milk was likely discovered in Central Asia during the Stone Age by accident. Left out in the heat, milk curdled and, depending on the bacteria in the environment, developed into yogurt or cheese.
- **2,000 B.C.** — It was estimated that half of the population was eating and drinking dairy products. Yogurt had evolved as a way to preserve milk from domestic animals through fermentation.
- **800 B.C.** — It has been reported that the secrets of fermented milk were revealed by an angel to Abraham, who then lived to be 175 years old—perhaps with the help of this healthful elixir.
- **1070** — The word yogurt is thought to be derived from a Turkish word that means "to curdle" or "to thicken." The first written description of yogurt was printed in Diwanul-Lugat al-Turk, a Turkish dictionary in 1070–1073.
- **1211** — Genghis Khan reportedly fed his army "kumis," a fermented milk that was a staple in the Mongolian diet; the conqueror believed this food made his warriors brave.
- **1542** — Yogurt became known in France when King Francis I was suffering from severe depression and a doctor from Constantinople brought the king a concoction made from fermented sheep's milk.
- **1670** — Turkish immigrants brought yogurt to the United States in the eighteenth century.
- **1905** — Stamen Grigorov, a Bulgarian scientist, discovered that yogurt was made from a specific strain of bacillus. The strain was named *Lactobacillus bulgaricus* in his honor. Grigorov's subsequent research on yogurt found that yogurt may help treat various conditions.
- **1919** — Industrialized production of yogurt, led by Isaac Carasso, began in Barcelona. Carasso built a factory and named his company "Danone" after his son, little Daniel.
- **1933** — The first patent for yogurt with fruit was granted to a company in Prague.
- **1950 to date** — Yogurt's popularity soared in the 1950s and 1960s due to its reputation as a health food. Today, yogurt is consumed in many countries around the world.

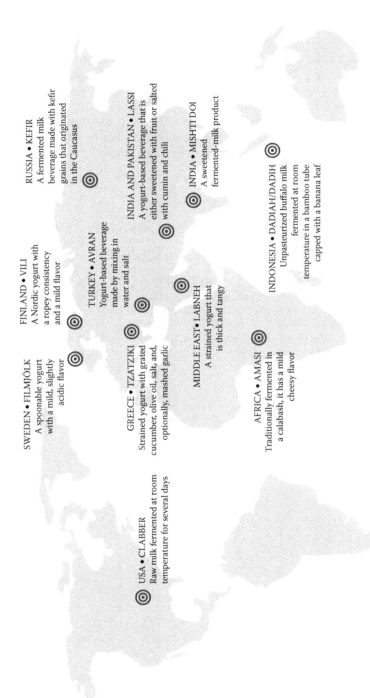

FIGURE I.2 Fermented milks and yogurts consumed around the world. (Source: Danone Nutricia Research.)

cultures added to yogurt. The information that will be presented in this book was identified by querying multiple search engines to primarily identify clinical and epidemiological studies on yogurt involving different populations and age groups. Furthermore, additional key studies, systematic analyses, and prominent reviews on yogurt and its components will be discussed. The choice of material covered in this book is primarily based on present-day research interests on yogurt and health (e.g., diabetes), the existent body of literature of commonly studied health conditions related to yogurt (e.g., lactose intolerance), and some particular research interests (e.g., yogurt and immunity). This book will also provide an overview of yogurt's role in the diet, and individual yogurt nutrients and their impacts on health, as well as potential mechanisms explaining these impacts.

REFERENCES

German, J. B. 2014. The future of yogurt: Scientific and regulatory needs. *Am J Clin Nutr* 99 (5 Suppl):1271S–78S.

Joint FAO/WHO Codex Alimentarius Commission. 2010. Standard for fermented milk. In *Codex Alimentarius*. Edited by FAO/WHO. Rome: Food and Agriculture Organization.

Marsh, A. J., C. Hill, R. P. Ross, and P. D. Cotter. 2014. Fermented beverages with health-promoting potential: Past and future perspectives. *Trends Food Sci Tech* 38 (2):113–24.

Tamime, A.Y., A. Skriver, and L. M. Nilsson. 2006. Historical background. In *Fermented Milks*. Edited by Tamime A.Y. Oxford: Blackwell Science.

U.S. Department of Agriculture, Economic Research Service. 2016. Dairy data. USDA. Accessed May 27. http://www.ers.usda.gov/data-products/dairy-data.aspx.

Section I

Yogurt Composition and Consumption

1 Yogurt Composition

Given that dairy products have a high concentration of major nutrients in comparison with the energy that they provide, they are considered as nutrient-dense foods. The macronutient distribution of different dairy products is described in Table 1.1. The nutrient composition of yogurt is based on the the milk from which it is derived. The composition of milk varies with the diet, energy balance, health status, stage of lactation, breed, and age of the cow (Haug et al. 2007).

Yogurt composition can be modified by the source and type of milk, as well as ingredients (e.g., fruit, sweeteners, stabilizers, colors, flavors, texturizers, and preservatives) that may be added during manufacturing (Tamime et al. 2006). Additionally, the composition of yogurt can also be modified by other factors such as the species and strains of bacteria used for fermentation, the temperature, the duration of the fermentation process, and the storage time (Adolfsson et al. 2004). Furthermore, heat and acidic, and alkaline environments can disrupt the integrity of the nutrients, altering the yogurt's final composition (Vignola 2002). The final composition of the product may vary from one country to another and within a country depending on the source of the ingredients and the types of additives used. Despite minor variations in nutritional composition, yogurt consumption contributes to intakes of important nutrients, as described in Table 1.1.

1.1 CARBOHYDRATES

Yogurt contains three types of carbohydrates: available, unavailable, and exopolysaccharides (Tamime and Robinson 2007). In plain yogurt, lactose is the dominant available carbohydrate, accounting for around 98% of total carbohydrates and 54% of total nonfat milk solids, although there are also small amounts of galactose, glucose, and oligosaccharides (Yildiz 2010). Lactose provides a fermentation substrate for lactic acid bacteria (LAB). The lactose content in yogurt is around 6% before lactic fermentation (Chandan and Shahani 1993). During milk fermentation, 20%–30% of lactose is partially hydrolyzed into glucose and galactose and, depending on other ingredients contained in the yogurt, it could have a lower lactose concentration than milk (Bourlioux and Pochart 1988, Adolfsson et al. 2004). Yogurt bacteria utilize lactose as a source of energy and produce lactic acid; this decreases the pH value of milk, creating a more acidic dairy product. The pH change produces the typical acidic flavor of yogurt and protects the product against microbial agents (Haug et al. 2007). After ingesting yogurt, lactose is hydrolyzed by the intestinal brush border ß-galactosidase (lactase) into glucose and galactose. The monosaccharides are absorbed into the bloodstream via active transport mechanisms (Chandan and Shahani 1993).

In addition to naturally found carbohydrates, sweetened yogurts contain simple sugars (Table 1.1), which can contribute to the intake of added sugars in the diet.

TABLE 1.1
Comparison of the Nutrient Composition of Different Types of French Dairy Products

	Milk (Whole-Fat) 100 mL	Milk (Skimmed) 100 mL	Plain Yogurt (Whole-Fat) 100 g	Plain Yogurt (Low-Fat) 100 g	Fresh Cheese (Whole-Fat) 100 g	Sweetened Fruit Yogurt (Low-Fat) 100 g
Energy (kcal)	64	31	65	42	116	94
Protein (g)	3.2	3.3	4.0	4.3	6.8	4.3
Carbohydrates (g)	4.7	4.3	2.6	5.1	3.5	15
Fats (g)	3.7	0.15	3.9	0.31	8.1	1.7
Saturated fats (g)	2.3	0.11	2.0	0.16	5.6	0.86
Sodium (mg)	42	42	52	54	33	58
Cholesterol (mg)	14	2.5	10	2.5	8.6	11
Calcium (mg)	112	113	138	149	113	114
Phosphorus (mg)	87	89	95	113	102	88
Zinc (mg)	0.38	0.41	0.44	0.46	0.41	0.47
Iodine (µg)	11	12.7	19	19	19	<5
Retinol (µg)	47	0.50	30	<8	68	24
Beta-carotene (µg)	20	Trace	14	2	29	2
Vitamin D (µg)	0.03	Trace	0.04	0.005	<0.2	0.07
Vitamin B2 (mg)	0.18	0.17	0.24	0.25	0.24	0.16
Vitamin B12 (µg)	0.20	0.27	0.2	0.25	0.34	0.15

Source: Data from French Ciqual (2013) nutrition composition tables.
Note: Nutrient composition may be different in other countries.

Sweetened yogurt as a source of added sugars should be monitored in certain populations, such as very young children who have little dietary diversity (Williams et al. 2015). In fruit-containing yogurt, stabilizers are added to minimize syneresis, many of which are complex carbohydrates that are hydrocolloidal in nature and cannot be degraded by the digestive system (i.e., unavailable carbohydrates). Although nonenergetic, these molecules may contribute to the digestion of nutrients by providing a source of added bulk in the intestine, delaying the diffusion of simple sugars through the intestinal wall and decreasing the orocecal transit time of lactose. Exopolysaccharides, produced by some LAB (e.g., *Streptococcus thermophilus*), can improve the texture of yogurt and are suspected to remain intact during their passage through the digestive system (Tamime and Robinson 2007).

1.2 PROTEINS

1.2.1 BIOLOGICAL QUALITY

Dairy products represent a major source of dietary protein. The protein content of yogurt is generally higher than that of milk, because of protein standardization and enrichment during processing via the addition of nonfat dry milk and milk protein, which are used to develop or improve texture (Hewitt and Bancroft 1985). American yogurts often contain added milk powder and are likely to be more concentrated in protein and calcium than milk (Rozenberg et al. 2016). Depending on the ingredients used during manufacturing, yogurt can be a good or even an excellent source of bioavailable proteins. Given that yogurt proteins are derived from milk proteins, they have very high biological quality. Indeed, animal proteins such as those found in milk, cheese, yogurt, meat, fish, and eggs provide all nine essential amino acids (lysine, threonine, valine, isoleucine, leucine, methionine, phenylalanine, tryptophan, and histidine) and have a more complete amino acid profile than most plant proteins (Tome 2012). Milk and yogurt proteins are not only recognized for their quality, but also for their physiological properties, which include ion carriers, growth factors, hormones, precursors for bioactive peptides, immunoregulation, and protection, as well as anticarcinogen, antiviral, and antioxidative agents (Yildiz 2010, Haug et al. 2007). The digestion of milk protein and the release of its amino acids, which are essential for growth and development, are efficient in humans and will be discussed in the next sections. Furthermore, the availability of free amino acids may be greater in yogurt than in milk because of fermentation and/or the addition of bacterial cultures, which can result in a higher concentration of free amino acids (Yildiz 2010).

1.2.2 CASEIN AND WHEY

Milk proteins are composed of a casein fraction (around 80%) and a whey fraction (around 20%). The primary biological function of the casein fraction is calcium and phosphate transport, which is facilitated by a supramolecular structure; the casein micelle is a large colloidal complex of particles accounting for 95% of the casein found in milk. They are composed of submicelles, molecules containing four different caseins ($\alpha s1$-casein, $\alpha s2$-casein, β-casein, and κ-casein) bound to calcium phosphate. The particular structure of the micelle imparts biological and functional processing properties—casein micelles remain stable during dairy processing (Chandan and Kilara 2011). The structure of the casein micelle is very flexible and amphiphilic (hydrophobic and hydrophilic residues), which permits its polymerization in aqueous solutions (Chandan and Kilara 2013). The high level of phosphorylation and a sensitivity of 84% of the caseins (αs1-casein, αs2-casein, and β-casein) to calcium precipitation allow the micelle to strongly bind calcium at milk pH, which stabilizes the supramolecular structure. Colloidal stability is provided by κ-caseins, which are located at the surface of the micelle, creating repulsive charges. In yogurt manufacturing, LAB produce lactic acid during the fermentation of lactose and the pH of milk drops to 4.6. This acidic medium results in the removal of the κ-caseins' repulsive charges on the surface, allowing micelles to aggregate and a dense gel to form (Chandan and Kilara 2011). In addition to calcium transport, casein is known to form a clot in the stomach, facilitating protein digestion (Haug et al. 2007). The clot or gel is able to provide a sustained slow release of amino acids into the bloodstream.

Compared with the flexible conformation and limited structural elements of casein, whey proteins are more water soluble than caseins (Haug et al. 2007), but their globular structure makes them susceptible to denaturation when heated (Chandan and Kilara 2013). The principal whey fractions are β-lactoglobin (approximately half the total whey proteins), α-lactalbumin, bovine serum albumin, and immunoglobulins (Vasbinder 2002). In addition, whey contains small proportions of lactoferrin, proteose-peptone, and numerous enzymes. Whey protein is an excellent source of amino acids, which are effective in stimulating muscle protein synthesis and enhancing fat loss. The high content of branched-chain amino acids and sulfhydryl-containing amino acids (cysteine and glutathione) also make whey an important protein for promoting immune function and quenching free radicals. Furthermore, whey is a precursor for bioactive peptides that may play a role in body weight management, satiety, and angiotensin converting enzyme (ACE) inhibition (Chandan and Kilara 2011).

Due to their distinct structures, casein and whey exhibit different digestion kinetics. The high solubility of whey protein bestows it with a reputation as a "fast" or rapidly digested protein. In contrast, the characteristic clots formed following casein ingestion delay its absorption and make it a slowly digested protein (Boirie et al. 1997). A "fast" whey protein might be more beneficial than a "slow" casein one to limit protein losses during aging by increasing amino acid availability (Dangin et al. 2003). Whey proteins have been shown to stimulate amino acid oxidation and postprandial protein synthesis without modifying proteolysis. On the other hand, casein, which is considered a "slow" protein, has a modest effect on whole-body protein synthesis, but inhibits whole-body protein breakdown (Bos et al. 2003, Boirie et al. 1997).

The high leucine content of whey protein is of particular interest for elderly populations since leucine may act as an active modulator of protein synthesis (Dangin et al. 2003). However, there is little evidence to support the differences in digestion and absorption kinetics on the muscle protein synthetic response after intake of protein between young and older individuals (Koopman et al. 2009). Ingestion of "fast" protein (whey or free amino acids) has been shown to be useful in stimulating insulin secretion in diabetic individuals by providing a greater postprandial amino concentration and a higher beta-cell response than the ingestion of casein (Tessari et al. 2007).

1.2.3 Effect of Food Processing and Lactic Fermentation

Whey proteins are heat sensitive and heat treatment leads to structural changes that are important for yogurt texture. The degree of denaturation of heat treatment depends on processing parameters (pasteurization temperature and holding time). It has been shown that, compared with milk, the nutritional value of yogurt proteins is well preserved during the fermentation process (Hewitt and Bancroft 1985). It has been suggested that fermentation during yogurt manufacturing results in a product with low pH, liberating protein from its associated calcium and thereby making it more digestible (Park and Haenlein 2013).

1.2.3.1 Digestion and Generation of Bioactive Peptides

The intestinal availability of nitrogen in milk proteins is reported as high (Gaudichon et al. 1994, 1995). A small percentage (1%–2%) of protein in yogurt undergoes pre-digestion with proteolytic bacteria, which may result in a slightly higher free amino acid content than that found in milk (Tamime and Robinson 2007). Thus, some authors have argued that yogurt protein is more easily digested than milk protein (Shahani and Chandan 1979). However, other studies have shown that fermentation modifies the gastric emptying rate of nitrogen, but does not affect the digestion rate in humans (Gaudichon et al. 1995, Rychen et al. 2002). It is actually possible that the digestion kinetics are influenced by the food structure, as presented by Dupont et al. (2014) in their study of two different dairy gels with similar compositions but showing different digestion kinetics.

The proteolytic enzyme and peptidase activity is preserved throughout the shelf life of yogurt, so the concentration of free amino acids increases. Interestingly, *Lactobacillus bulgaricus* has been shown to have a much higher proteolytic activity during storage and milk fermentation than *S. thermophilus* (Adolfsson et al. 2004). Some amino acids, such as glutamic acid, proline, alanine, and serine, are presumably not required by *S. thermophilus* and *L. bulgaricus* and so they are more available than the remaining amino acids that are utilized by the bacteria during growth and/or fermentation (Tamime and Robinson 2007). The quantity of active peptides present in milk and dairy products is low; however, peptides can be detected in the intestinal lumen after consumption of dairy products (Bos et al. 2000). Moreover, numerous active peptides are present in the casein sequences and could affect the immune system, as well as the digestive, cardiovascular, and nervous systems (Korhonen and Pihlanto 2006, Beermann and Hartung 2013, Nagpal et al. 2011).

Examples of bioactive peptides derived from casein in milk are shown in Figure 1.1.

Lactoferrin is also a precursor of different active peptides with biological activities (Bos et al. 2000), including antimicrobial activity. The bioactivity of peptides will depend on their interaction and synergistic activity with nonpeptide milk components, such as oligosaccharides, glycolipids, and fats (Schanbacher et al. 1997).

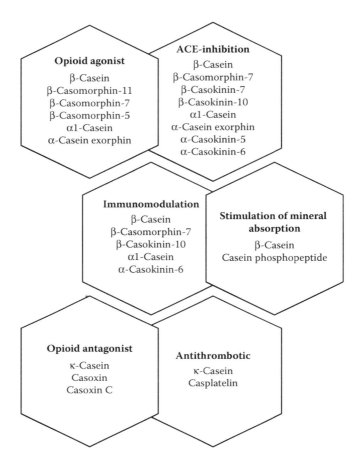

FIGURE 1.1 Examples of biological activity of peptides derived from milk casein. (Modified from Nagpal, R. et al. *Food Funct*, 2 (1), 18–27, 2011.)

The structure and biological function of many milk and yogurt peptides are not yet known. The biological activity of some dairy proteins and peptides explaining, in part, the beneficial effects of yogurt on health and some diseases will be discussed in Section II of this book (under mechanisms of action).

1.2.3.2 Interaction with Minerals

In dairy products, casein phosphopeptides may enhance the bioavailability of minerals such as calcium, phosphorus, and magnesium. Furthermore, the α-lactalbumin fraction of whey are calcium-binding proteins that enhance calcium absorption (Chandan and Kilara 2011). Folate-binding protein in milk could increase folate absorption; however, the daily intake of dairy folate–binding protein is so low that its role in folate absorption may be negligible in the majority of adults (Nygren-Babol and Jagerstad 2012). As an iron-binding protein, lactoferrin is believed to improve iron absorption. However, few studies have investigated the digestion of this protein *in vivo*. Nevertheless, there has been an indication that phosphopeptides play a positive role in iron absorption (Peres et al. 1997). Whey proteins, vitamin B12–binding protein, β-lactoglobulin, and α-lactalbumin could also interact with mineral and vitamin absorption (Bos et al. 2000, Vegarud et al. 2000).

1.3 LIPIDS

Milk fat is mainly composed of triglycerides (around 98%), phospholipids, cholesterol, and β-carotene and has great fatty acid diversity. Traditional full-fat yogurt contains 3–4 g of lipids/100 g of which 65% are saturated fatty acids (SFA). The remaining fractions are made up of 31% monounsaturated fatty acids (MUFA) and 4% polyunsaturated fatty acids (PUFA) (Legrand 2008). The fatty acid profile of plain yogurt is described in Table 1.2. All fatty acids contribute to the proper functioning of the body. About 50% of SFA in milk are myristic and palmitic acid, whereas the remainder consists of short-chain and medium-chain fatty acids. SFAs have generally been labeled as detrimental for cardiovascular health (Visioli and Strata 2014). Generally, SFAs contribute to a pro-inflammatory state (Da Silva and Rudkowska 2015), which can lead to the systemic inflammation that underlies cardiometabolic abnormalities (Da Silva and Rudkowska 2014). However, SFAs should not be considered as one unique group, because individually they exert multiple and different effects on health depending on the amount and type consumed. For example, short- and medium-chain SFAs (C4–C12) do not contribute to increasing plasma cholesterol levels and some can be

TABLE 1.2
Fatty Acid Profile of Plain Whole-Milk French Yogurt

Type of Fatty Acid	Average Content
Total fat (g/100 g)	3.9
Cholesterol (mg/100 g)	9.96
Saturated (g/100 g)	2
Monounsatured (g/100 g)	0.924
Polyunsatured (g/100 g)	0.16
4:0, Butyric (g/100 g)	0.101
6:0, Caproic (g/100 g)	0.0658
8:0, Caprylic (g/100 g)	0.0409
10:0, Capric (g/100 g)	0.0886
12:0, Lauric (g/100 g)	0.133
14:0, Myristic (g/100 g)	0.355
16:0, Palmitic (g/100 g)	0.908
18:0, Stearic (g/100 g)	0.304
18:1 n-9 cis, Oleic (g/100 g)	0.627
18:2 9c,12c (n-6), Linoleic (g/100 g)	0.0599
18:3 c9,c12,c15 (n-3), Alpha-linolenic (g/100 g)	0.0242

Source: Data from French Ciqual (2013) nutrition composition tables.
Note: Nutrient composition may be different in other countries.

used directly for energy by the liver as they are easily hydrolyzed, absorbed through the intestinal wall, and transported via the portal vein (Chandan and Kilara 2011). Some SFAs can increase the risk of cardiovascular diseases (CVD) when consumed in excess, whereas others are essential to basic cellular functions (e.g., lignoceric acid and myristic acid) (Legrand 2008). Emerging evidence about the differing health profiles of individual SFA is indeed creating conjecture over the long-standing dietary recommendations to indiscriminately reduce SFA intakes for CVD and mortality prevention (Astrup 2014). Dairy also contains unsaturated fatty acids and trans-fatty acids that are thought to be beneficial to health. One of the most abundant fatty acids in milk, oleic acid, and the PUFA linoleic acid, likely impart anti-inflammatory properties to yogurt (Da Silva and Rudkowska 2014). Conjugated linoleic acid (CLA), a trans-fatty acid occurring naturally in milk, has many reported health properties, including anti-inflammatory, immune-modulatory, antibiotic, anticarcinogenic, and antiobesogenic properties (Chandan and Kilara 2013, Bhattacharya et al. 2006, Wang and Jones 2004).

There are seasonal and regional differences in milk fat composition, most likely because of local differences in cow feed (Palmquist et al. 1993). The cow's food source influences milk fat composition, such as the omega 3/omega 6 ratio and the content of CLA (Kalač and Samková 2010). Although many studies have evaluated the effect of cow's feeding on milk and dairy nutrient content, there is need for an in-depth evaluation into different feeding strategies that could change the nutritional, sensorial, and technological aspects of milk fat quality (Chilliard and Ferlay 2004). Interestingly, Benchaar et al. (2012) demonstrated that linseed oil can be safely supplemented (up to 4%) in dairy cows' diet to enrich milk with fatty acids with potential health benefits such as n-3 PUFA. No detrimental effects of this diet were seen on rumen function, digestion, or milk production (Benchaar et al. 2012). The indispensable lipophilic vitamins (A, D, E, and K) and carotenoids are found only in the fat phase of the milk. Consequently, these vitamins are found in whole milk, cream, butter and cheese. Skimming the milk results in a loss of these vitamins and the concentration of the hydrophilic vitamins' nutrients (e.g., riboflavin, vitamin B12) (Gaucheron 2011).

1.3.1 Effect of Food Processing and Lactic Fermentation

Changes undergone by milk during fermentation depend greatly on the origin of the milk and the bacterial strains used. Yogurt has been shown to have a higher concentration of CLA, a long-chain biohydrogenated derivative of linoleic acid, than milk (Aneja and Murthi 1990, Shantha et al. 1995). Interestingly, lactobacilli and *S. thermophilus* strains have been shown to produce CLA from linoleic acid using two conversion pathways. Fermentation also changes the level of free, esterified, and volatile fatty acids (Tamime and Robinson 2007). Moreover, the fermentation of milk by *S. thermophilus* and *L. bulgaricus* has been shown to lead to the reduction of cholesterol content in milk (see Chapter 3.6.2).

1.4 MINERALS

The mineral fraction of milk and dairy products is composed of macroelements (Ca, Mg, Na, K, P, and Cl) and oligoelements (Fe, Cu, Zn, and Se). The average content of different minerals found in whole-milk plain yogurt is described in Table 1.3. Minerals

TABLE 1.3
Mineral Content of Plain Whole-Milk French Yogurt

Mineral	Average Content
Magnesium (mg/100 g)	12
Phosphorus (mg/100 g)	95
Potassium (mg/100 g)	180
Calcium (mg/100 g)	138
Manganese (mg/100 g)	<0.0121
Iron (mg/100 g)	0.1
Copper (mg/100 g)	<0.0087
Zinc (mg/100 g)	0.441
Selenium (µg/100 g)	<2.2
Iodide (µg/100 g)	18.8
Sodium (mg/100 g)	51.6

Source: Data from French Ciqual (2013) nutrition composition tables.

Note: Nutrient composition may be different in other countries.

are present in different forms in dairy products. For example, calcium could be free or associated with citrate, phosphates, and free fatty acids (Gaucheron 2011). It is recognized that yogurt and dairy products are a rich source of calcium and phosphorus per unit of energy compared with other typical foods in an adult diet (e.g., plain whole-milk American yogurt contains approximately 138 mg of Ca and 95 mg of P per 100 g or 65 Kcal of yogurt) (Heaney 2000). The Ca:P ratio in plain yogurt is around 1.5 and those minerals are essential to the structural integrity of bones. Furthermore, the calcium available for intestinal absorption in yogurt is equivalent gram for gram to milk. Calcium absorption of dairy is reported to be partly facilitated by its high lactose and casein content (Rozenberg et al. 2016) and may possibly be further facilitated in a fermented medium (Trinidad et al. 1996) such as yogurt. During yogurt production, the fermentation process decreases the pH of milk, which is thought to enhance the solubility of calcium and phosphorus (Fisberg and Machado 2015).

The magnesium, zinc, and calcium concentrations in cow's milk are relatively constant, with little variation during lactation (Haug et al. 2007). However, the concentration of selenium and iodine in bovine milk is dependent on the concentration of the nutrients in the feed and there is great variation within any given country and between seasons (Casey et al. 1995). For example, feed is more often enriched with iodine during the winter season and 25% of the iodine intake could be excreted in cow's milk (Haug et al. 2007, Crout and Voigt 1996).

1.4.1 Effect of Food Processing and Lactic Fermentation

The mineral content of yogurt is not only influenced by the composition of milk from which it is produced, but also by the dairy ingredients added for protein standardization (skim milk powder, milk protein concentrate, etc.). Some commercial yogurts may be a more concentrated source of minerals such as calcium than milk due to milk proteins added during processing. For example, fortified yogurts containing 400 mg of Ca and 200 IU of vitamin D per portion are a commercially available and affordable source of calcium in Belgium (Ethgen et al. 2016). This fact is of particular interest in populations where there are low intakes of calcium and where yogurt (and other dairy products) can be a source of additional nutrients such as protein, potassium, and magnesium (Rozenberg et al. 2016). Moreover, during yogurt production, a decrease in pH changes the ionic equilibria of milk, leading to the micellar solubilization of calcium phosphate (Mekmene et al. 2010). Indeed, yogurt is a result of milk acidification by bacteria and therefore calcium and magnesium are present in yogurt mostly in their ionic forms (Adolfsson et al. 2004). The composition of minerals in milk is not altered by fermentation.

1.4.2 BIOAVAILABILITY

Yogurt is an excellent source of many essential minerals that are highly available (Buttriss 1997). Indeed, dairy products are the primary source of bioavailable calcium in the typical Western diet (Adolfsson et al. 2004). Different factors could affect mineral bioavailability in yogurt. Heat treatment could adversely affect the absorption of some minerals, including calcium, iron, and zinc, through the denaturation of proteins that facilitate their uptake in the intestine (Ebringer et al. 2008). Moreover, acidity found in yogurt may also influence the absorption of minerals (Allen 1982). For example, calcium uptake may be enhanced by the low pH of yogurt, which ionizes calcium (Bronner and Pansu 1999). Phosphopeptides also help to keep calcium in solution, thereby facilitating its absorption by passive diffusion (Gueguen and Pointillart 2000), but the biological significance of this effect is controversial (Teucher et al. 2006). Increased solubilization may play a minor role in calcium bioavailability (Bronner and Pansu 1999). Indeed, calcium absorbability and bioavailability also depend on physiological factors such as hormones, calcium reserves, and interactions between the nutrients and foods ingested (Gueguen and Pointillart 2000). Interestingly, Unal et al. (2005) evaluated the calcium bioavailability of different dairy products (milk, yogurt, cheese, and infant formulas) using an *in vitro* method simulating gastrointestinal digestion. With the exception of cheese, no statistical difference was found within each group (e.g., different kinds of yogurt) in terms of calcium bioavailability. However, when different dairy products were compared, yogurt had the highest calcium bioavailability compared with the other dairy products and acidity was shown to have a significant effect on calcium bioavailability. The high viscosity of yogurt compared with milk could also contribute to improved mineral absorption by increasing orocecal transit time, which may imply an increase in the time available for mineral absorption (Heaney 1998, Parra et al. 2007).

It has been shown in rats that lactose could enhance the absorption of some minerals, including calcium (Schaafsma et al. 1988). Lactose is a slowly absorbed disaccharide that prolongs the passive absorption of calcium in the ileum (Gueguen and Pointillart 2000). However, there is only a net effect on the passive absorption of calcium with high doses of lactose (>50 g lactose/day) (Cochet et al. 1983). No effect has been shown at normal doses, except if Ca intake is high, especially in infants and the elderly; for whom solubility is a limiting factor and passive absorption is the main route (Schuette et al. 1991). Given that the lactose content of yogurt could be lower than that of milk, the bioavailability of these minerals may be negatively affected, but the effect seems to be negligible (Adolfsson et al. 2004). Vitamin D plays an important role in intestinal Ca absorption. Indeed, active calcium transport during absorption is proportionally dependent on calbindin-D9k in the intestinal cell, the biosynthesis of which is vitamin D dependent (Bronner and Pansu 1999).

1.5 VITAMINS

The vitamin fraction of milk and dairy products is composed of lipophilic and hydrophilic vitamins. The list of vitamins found in plain yogurt is given in Table 1.4. Whole-milk yogurt can contain a significant amount of vitamin A, complex B vitamins, and vitamin D (when yogurt is made from milk fortified in vitamin D). The vitamin D fortification of dairy products is a significant dietary source of a nutrient that is often deficient in many populations across the globe due to lack of sun exposure (Al-Daghri et al. 2015). While yogurt is fortified along with milk in the United States, it is not universally fortified in other countries and the level of fortification can also vary greatly from country to country (Cashman and Kiely 2016). A theoretical model of vitamin D supplementation in an Iranian population estimated that the percentage of the population that would reach the recommended daily allowance for vitamin D would increase from 1.1% to 77.4% and 1.4% to 80% in men and women, respectively, when both calcium and vitamin D were fortified in yogurt (Ejtahed

TABLE 1.4
Vitamin Content of Plain Whole-Milk French Yogurt

Vitamins	Average Content
Retinol (μg/100 g)	29.5
Beta-carotene (μg/100 g)	14
Vitamin D (μg/100 g)	0.04
Vitamin E (mg/100 g)	0.065
Vitamin K (μg/100 g)	–
Vitamin C (mg/100 g)	<1
Vitamin B1 or thiamin (mg/100 g)	0.049
Vitamin B2 or riboflavin (mg/100 g)	0.24
Vitamin B3 or niacin (mg/100 g)	0.165
Vitamin B5 or pantothenic acid (mg/100 g)	0.435
Vitamin B6 (mg/100 g)	0.0775
Vitamin B9 or folate (μg/100 g)	20
Vitamin B12 (μg/100 g)	0.2

Source: Data from French Ciqual (2013) nutrition composition tables.
Note: Nutrient composition may be different in other countries.

et al. 2016). Similarly, in Canada, fortifying yogurt and cheese with vitamin D, in addition to the current fortification of milk and margarine, would see the rates of vitamin D deficiency decrease from over 80% to under 50% across age groups and in both sexes (Shakur et al. 2014). Because of their hydrophobic properties, the lipophilic vitamins are mainly in the fat fraction, whereas the hydrophilic vitamins are in the aqueous phase.

1.5.1 Effect of Food Processing and Lactic Fermentation

Animal feeding, physicochemical conditions (heat, light, oxygen, and oxidants), and the analytical methods used influence the reporting of the vitamin content in yogurt (Gaucheron 2011, Bourlioux and Pochart 1988). A much greater loss of vitamins than minerals can occur during the processing of yogurt because vitamins are more sensitive to changes in environmental factors. Moderate heat treatment and an excess of dissolved oxygen are known to have adverse effects on the vitamin content of dairy products. They can significantly reduce the vitamin content and the most susceptible vitamins are C, B6, B12, and folic acid (Ebringer et al. 2008, Tamime and Robinson 2007). The concentration of certain vitamins, such as vitamin B12, may also decrease during yogurt storage at 4°C (Adolfsson et al. 2004).

Dairy sources of vitamin B12, a nutrient of concern in older populations, are strongly associated with serum levels in Dutch older adults, indicating that dairy foods such as yogurt are excellent sources of this nutrient (Brouwer-Brolsma et al. 2015). On the other hand, in populations with lower intakes of dairy products, milk and yogurt consumption were not associated with vitamin B12 status (Christian et al. 2015). Bacteria also affect the vitamin content of the final product. LAB require B vitamins for growth, but some of them are capable of synthesizing B vitamins (Buttriss 1997). During fermentation, the consumption of vitamins B12 and C as well as the production of folic acid are the main changes observed and they differ with the strains used (Bourlioux and Pochart 1988). For example, folate-enriched yogurt can be developed by combining specific strains of *L. delbrueckii* ssp. *bulgaricus* and *S. thermophilus* (Emiliano Laino et al. 2013). It has been shown that vitamin D content was unaffected during milk acidification (Kazmi et al. 2007). However, acid production may have a small effect on the stability of vitamin D3 in yogurt, but this requires further investigation (Kazmi et al. 2007).

1.6 STARTER CULTURES

The primary roles of starter cultures in dairy food preparation are (1) bio preservation through fermentation, (2) production of bacteriocins, (3) enhancement of sensory properties, (4) improvement of rheological properties, and (5) improvement of the nutritional and functional properties of milk. Both of the traditional yogurt genera, *Lactobacillus* and *Streptococcus*, belong to a group of microorganisms called LAB (Tamime et al. 2006). *L. delbrueckii* ssp. *bulgaricus* and *S. thermophilus* are traditional starter cultures used to manufacture yogurt. When they are grown in milk, the bacteria interact synergistically, allowing milk to be completely fermented within

3–4 hours. These cultures impart a characteristic flavor to yogurt and specific strains can also produce metabolites that contribute to enhancing the viscosity of the final product. LAB exert different roles in dairy fermentation. They preserve the milk by the generation of lactic acid, produce different compounds (e.g., flavor compounds like acetaldehyde in yogurt, polysaccharides, and lactase) and modify the nutritional value of food (e.g., the synthesis or consumption of vitamins or the release of free amino acids). Moreover, they can exert beneficial health effects (Parvez et al. 2006). Indeed, yogurt and individual LAB species have shown promising health effects via the intestinal tract, particularly on lactose intolerance, the immune system, allergies, constipation, diarrheal diseases, inflammatory bowel disease, *Helicobacter pylori* infection and colon cancer (Adolfsson et al. 2004, Parvez et al. 2006). The lactic acid fermentation of yogurt also creates various peptides with ACE-inhibitory properties depending on the yogurt culture (Rai et al. 2015). The benefits of traditional yogurt cultures on lactose intolerance in humans are well established, while other probiotic features are still being debated (Guarner et al. 2005). Alternative cultures may be considered to be probiotic and are now commonly used in commercial yogurt manufacturing for their purported health benefits. These nontraditional cultures include *Lactobacillus* spp. (*acidophilus*, *gasseri*, *helveticus*, *johnsonii*, *casei*, *reuteri*, *plantarum*, and *rhamnosus*) and *Bifidobacterium* spp. (*adolescentis*, *animalis*, *bifidum*, *breve*, *infantis*, *lactis*, and *longum*).

1.7 YOGURT MATRIX

The food matrix hypothesis, suggesting that the sum of each component within a food contributes to a greater nutritive capacity than would be possible if each nutrient were consumed individually, is a relative emergent and poorly understood concept (Lecerf and Legrand 2015). It does, however, explain the differences in effects that can be seen when nutrients are consumed in their pure form versus in whole-food formats. For example, probiotics administered in a yogurt matrix had a significant effect on reducing gut permeability, which was not possible when the same probiotics were administered in capsule form (Agostini et al. 2012). Similarly, in a randomized control trial on calcium and weight loss, a high dairy diet (1400 mg dairy calcium) was more effective than a high calcium treatment (1400 mg calcium) in supressing calcitriol (Zemel et al. 2009). The matrix effect would also help to explain differences in health outcomes seen between foods with equivalent nutrient composition. For example, the consistent inverse association observed between type 2 diabetes and yogurt, but not milk or cheese, in a robust meta-analysis of prospective cohort studies (Chen et al. 2014). Figure 1.2 illustrates how the yogurt matrix may exert beneficial health effects. The texture, microstructure, unique nutrient interactions, and enhanced nutrient bioavailability in yogurt contribute to promoting a dairy matrix with synergistic properties (Marette and Picard-Deland 2014). Ingredients added during yogurt manufacturing can have a profound effect on the matrix and even change its metabolic activity. For example, the addition of skim milk powder and whey protein concentrate during manufacturing to a test yogurt increased the buffering capacity of their matrix, which affected their organic acid profiles and lactic acid content (Ines Venica et al. 2014). An *in vitro* model examined

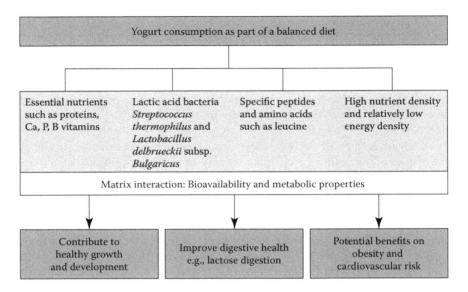

FIGURE 1.2 Proposed mechanisms by which yogurt consumption as a part of a balanced diet exerts beneficial health effects. (Reprinted with permission from Marette, A. and Picard-Deland, E., *Am J Clin Nutr*, 99, supplement 1, 1243S–47S, 2014.)

the effects of adding green tea extract to a dairy matrix and observed that there was an increase in antioxidant activity in the presence of a dairy matrix compared with a control. The increased antioxidant activity was attributed to the ability of the dairy matrix to maintain the integrity of polyphenols during digestion via the formation of polyphenol–protein complexes (Lamothe et al. 2014). The food matrix confuses the ability to isolate the beneficial effects of yogurt cultures from those linked to the food itself (Hill et al. 2014) and further study of the intricate interactions between different food components is warranted.

1.8 CONCLUSIONS

- The nutrient composition of yogurt is similar to the milk from which it is derived, but can be modified by adding milk solids, different bacterial species and strains, and by other ingredients such as fruits that can be added to some types of yogurt.
- Lactose is by far the predominant carbohydrate of plain yogurt and provides the fermentation substrate for LAB.
- The high digestibility and essential amino acid concentration make yogurt an excellent source of high-quality protein. The bioactivity of peptides depends on their interaction and synergic activity with nonpeptidic milk components, such as oligosaccharides, glycolipids, and fats.
- Yogurt contains a wide range of fatty acids. The fatty acid composition of yogurt depends greatly on the origin of the milk and ferment strains

used, but proportions of saturated, unsaturated, and polyunsaturated fats are similar to that of milk. Also, there is growing evidence of the beneficial effects of fats from dairy sources, possibly in relation to their fatty acid composition and structure.
- Yogurt and dairy products contain several micronutrients essential for health: calcium, zinc, phosphorus, potassium, magnesium, iodine, vitamin A, vitamin B2, vitamin B5, and vitamin B12. Not only are the concentrations of micronutrients significant, but they are also highly bioavailable (i.e., a high proportion are available for absorption and utilization within the body).
- Yogurt and dairy products are excellent sources of calcium and phosphorus, which are the main constituents of bone mineral.
- The impact of the food matrix and fermentation with specific bacterial strains on nutrient content and bioavailability still requires investigation.

REFERENCES

Adolfsson, O., S. N. Meydani, and R. M. Russell. 2004. Yogurt and gut function. *Am J Clin Nutr* 80 (2):245–56.

Agostini, S., M. Goubern, V. Tondereau, C. Salvador-Cartier, V. Bezirard, M. Lévèque, H. Keränen, et al. 2012. A marketed fermented dairy product containing bifidobacterium lactis CNCM I-2494 suppresses gut hypersensitivity and colonic barrier disruption induced by acute stress in rats. *Neurogastroenterol. Motil* 24:376-e172.

Al-Daghri, N. M., N. Aljohani, O. S. Al-Attas, S. Krishnaswamy, H. Alfawaz, A. Al-Ajlan, and M. S. Alokail. 2015. Dairy products consumption and serum 25-hydroxyvitamin D level in Saudi children and adults. *Int J Clin Exp Pathol* 8 (7):8480–86.

Allen, L. H. 1982. Calcium bioavailability and absorption: A review. *Am J Clin Nutr* 35 (4):783–808.

Aneja, R. P., and T. N. Murthi. 1990. Conjugated linoleic acid contents of Indian curds and ghee. *Indian J Dairy Sci* 43:231–38.

Astrup, A. 2014. A changing view on saturated fatty acids and dairy: From enemy to friend. *Am J Clin Nutr* 100 (6):1407–8.

Beermann, C., and J. Hartung. 2013. Physiological properties of milk ingredients released by fermentation. *Food Funct* 4 (2):185–99.

Benchaar, C., G. A. Romero-Perez, P. Y. Chouinard, F. Hassanat, M. Eugene, H. V. Petit, and C. Cortes. 2012. Supplementation of increasing amounts of linseed oil to dairy cows fed total mixed rations: Effects on digestion, ruminal fermentation characteristics, protozoal populations, and milk fatty acid composition. *J Dairy Sci* 95 (8):4578–90.

Bhattacharya, A., J. Banu, M. Rahman, J. Causey, and G. Fernandes. 2006. Biological effects of conjugated linoleic acids in health and disease. *J Nutr Biochem* 17 (12):789–810.

Boirie, Y., M. Dangin, P. Gachon, M. P. Vasson, J. L. Maubois, and B. Beaufrere. 1997. Slow and fast dietary proteins differently modulate postprandial protein accretion. *Proc Natl Acad Sci USA* 94 (26):14930–35.

Bos, C., C. Gaudichon, and D. Tome. 2000. Nutritional and physiological criteria in the assessment of milk protein quality for humans. *J Am Coll Nutr* 19 (2 Suppl):191S–205S.

Bos, C., C. C. Metges, C. Gaudichon, K. J. Petzke, M. E. Pueyo, C. Morens, J. Everwand, R. Benamouzig, and D. Tome. 2003. Postprandial kinetics of dietary amino acids are the main determinant of their metabolism after soy or milk protein ingestion in humans. *J Nutr* 133 (5):1308–15.

Bourlioux, P., and P. Pochart. 1988. Nutritional and health properties of yogurt. *World Rev Nutr Diet* 56:217–58.

Bronner, F., and D. Pansu. 1999. Nutritional aspects of calcium absorption. *J Nutr* 129 (1):9–12.
Brouwer-Brolsma, E. M., R. A. Dhonukshe-Rutten, J. P. van Wijngaarden, N. L. Zwaluw, N. Velde, and L. C. de Groot. 2015. Dietary sources of vitamin B-12 and their association with vitamin B-12 status markers in healthy older adults in the B-proof study. *Nutrients* 7 (9):7781–97.
Buttriss, J. 1997. Nutritional properties of fermented milk products. *Int J Dairy* 50 (1):21–17.
Casey, C. E., A. Smith, and P. Zhang. 1995. Microminerals in human and animal milk. Edited by Jensen RG, *Handbook of Milk Composition*, 622–42. San Diego, CA: Academic Press.
Cashman, K. D., and M. Kiely. 2016. Tackling inadequate vitamin D intakes within the population: Fortification of dairy products with vitamin D may not be enough. *Endocrine* 51 (1):38–46.
Chandan, R. C., and A. Kilara. 2011. *Dairy Ingredients for Food Processing*. Hoboken, NJ: Wiley-Blackwell.
Chandan, R. C., and A. Kilara. 2013. *Manufacturing Yogurt and Fermented Milks*. Hoboken, NJ: Wiley-Blackwell.
Chandan, R. C., and K. M. Shahani. 1993. Yogurt. Edited by Hui YH, *Dairy Science and Technology Handbook*. New York: VCH Publishers.
Chen, M., Q. Sun, E. Giovannucci, D. Mozaffarian, J. E. Manson, W. C. Willett, and F. B. Hu. 2014. Dairy consumption and risk of type 2 diabetes: 3 cohorts of U.S. adults and an updated meta-analysis. *BMC Med* 12:215.
Chilliard, Y., and A. Ferlay. 2004. Dietary lipids and forages interactions on cow and goat milk fatty acid composition and sensory properties. *Reprod Nutr Dev* 44 (5):467–92.
Christian, A. M., G. V. Krishnaveni, S. H. Kehoe, S. R. Veena, R. Khanum, E. Marley-Zagar, P. Edwards, B. M. Margetts, and C. H. Fall. 2015. Contribution of food sources to the vitamin B12 status of south Indian children from a birth cohort recruited in the city of Mysore. *Public Health Nutr* 18 (4):596–609.
Cochet, B., A. Jung, M. Griessen, P. Bartholdi, P. Schaller, and A. Donath. 1983. Effects of lactose on intestinal calcium absorption in normal and lactase-deficient subjects. *Gastroenterology* 84 (5 Pt 1):935–40.
Crout, N. M., and G. Voigt. 1996. Modeling the dynamics of radioiodine in dairy cows. *J Dairy Sci* 79 (2):254–59.
Da Silva, M. S., and I. Rudkowska. 2014. Dairy products on metabolic health: Current research and clinical implications. *Maturitas* 77 (3):221–28.
Da Silva, M. S., and I. Rudkowska. 2015. Dairy nutrients and their effect on inflammatory profile in molecular studies. *Mol Nutr Food Res* 59 (7):1249–63.
Dangin, M., C. Guillet, C. Garcia-Rodenas, P. Gachon, C. Bouteloup-Demange, K. Reiffers-Magnani, J. Fauquant, O. Ballevre, and B. Beaufrere. 2003. The rate of protein digestion affects protein gain differently during aging in humans. *J Physiol* 549 (Pt 2):635–44.
Dupont, D., O. Ménard, S. Le Feunteun, and D. Rémond. 2014. Comment la structure des gels laitiers régule-t-elle la biodisponibilité des acides aminés? *Innovations Agronomiques* 36:57–68.
Ebringer, L., M. Ferencik, and J. Krajcovic. 2008. Beneficial health effects of milk and fermented dairy products: Review. *Folia Microbiol (Praha)* 53 (5):378–94.
Ejtahed, H. S., S. Shab-Bidar, F. Hosseinpanah, P. Mirmiran, and F. Azizi. 2016. Estimation of vitamin D intake based on a scenario for fortification of dairy products with vitamin D in a Tehranian population, Iran. *J Am Coll Nutr* 1–9 35 (5):383–91.
Emiliano Laino, J., M. Juarez del Valle, G. Savoy de Giori, and J. G. Joseph LeBlanc. 2013. Development of a high folate concentration yogurt naturally bio-enriched using selected lactic acid bacteria. *LWT-Food Sci Technol* 54 (1):1–5.
Ethgen, O., M. Hiligsmann, N. Burlet, and J. Y. Reginster. 2016. Cost-effectiveness of personalized supplementation with vitamin D-rich dairy products in the prevention of osteoporotic fractures. *Osteoporos Int* 27 (1):301–8.

Fisberg, M., and R. Machado. 2015. History of yogurt and current patterns of consumption. *Nutr Rev* 73 (Suppl 1):4–7.
Gaucheron, F. 2011. Milk and dairy products: A unique micronutrient combination. *J Am Coll Nutr* 30 (5 Suppl 1):400S–9S.
Gaudichon, C., S. Mahé, N. Roos, R. Benamouzig, C. Luengo, J. F. Huneau, H. Sick, C. Bouley, J. Rautureau, and D. Tome. 1995. Exogenous and endogenous nitrogen flow rates and level of protein hydrolysis in the human jejunum after [15N]milk and [15N] yoghurt ingestion. *Br J Nutr* 74 (2):251–60.
Gaudichon, C., N. Roos, S. Mahé, H. Sick, C. Bouley, and D. Tome. 1994. Gastric emptying regulates the kinetics of nitrogen absorption from 15N-labeled milk and 15N-labeled yogurt in miniature pigs. *J Nutr* 124 (10):1970–77.
Guarner, F., G. Perdigon, G. Corthier, S. Salminen, B. Koletzko, and L. Morelli. 2005. Should yoghurt cultures be considered probiotic? *Br J Nutr* 93 (6):783–86.
Gueguen, L., and A. Pointillart. 2000. The bioavailability of dietary calcium. *J Am Coll Nutr* 19 (2 Suppl):119S–36S.
Haug, A., A. T. Hostmark, and O. M. Harstad. 2007. Bovine milk in human nutrition: A review. *Lipids Health Dis* 6:25.
Heaney, R. P. 1998. Excess dietary protein may not adversely affect bone. *J Nutr* 128 (6):1054–57.
Heaney, R. P. 2000. Calcium, dairy products and osteoporosis. *J Am Coll Nutr* 19 (2 Suppl):83S–99S.
Hewitt, D., and H. J. Bancroft. 1985. Nutritional value of yogurt. *J Dairy Res* 52 (1):197–207.
Hill, C., F. Guarner, G. Reid, G. R. Gibson, D. J. Merenstein, B. Pot, L. Morelli, et al. 2014. Expert consensus document: The international scientific association for probiotics and prebiotics consensus statement on the scope and appropriate use of the term probiotic. *Nat Rev Gastroenterol Hepatol* 11 (8):506–14.
Ines Venica, C., M. C. Perotti, and C. V. Bergamini. 2014. Organic acids profiles in lactose-hydrolyzed yogurt with different matrix composition. *Dairy Sci Technol* 94 (6):561–80.
Kalač, P., and E. Samková. 2010 The effects of feeding various forages on fatty acid composition of bovine milk fat: A review. *Czech J. Anim. Sci.* 55 (12):521–37.
Kazmi, S. A., R. Viethb, and D. Rousseauc. 2007. Vitamin D3 fortification and quantification in processed dairy products. *Int Dairy J* 17:753–59.
Koopman, R., S. Walrand, M. Beelen, A. P. Gijsen, A. K. Kies, Y. Boirie, W. H. Saris, and L. J. van Loon. 2009. Dietary protein digestion and absorption rates and the subsequent postprandial muscle protein synthetic response do not differ between young and elderly men. *J Nutr* 139 (9):1707–13.
Korhonen, H., and A. Pihlanto. 2006. Bioactive peptides: Production and functionality. *Int Dairy J* 16:945–60.
Lamothe, S., N. Azimy, L. Bazinet, C. Couillard, and M. Britten. 2014. Interaction of green tea polyphenols with dairy matrices in a simulated gastrointestinal environment. *Food Funct* 5 (10):2621–31.
Lecerf, J-M., and P. Legrand. 2015. Les effets des nutriments dépendent-ilsdes aliments qui les portent? L'effet matrice. *Cahiers de nutrition et de diététique* 50 (3):158–64.
Legrand, P. 2008. Intérêt nutritionnel des principaux acides gras des lipides du lait. *Cerin* 105:1–6.
Marette, A., and E. Picard-Deland. 2014. Yogurt consumption and impact on health: Focus on children and cardiometabolic risk. *Am J Clin Nutr* 99 (5):1243S–47S.
Mekmene, O., Y. Le Graet, and F. Gaucheron. 2010. Theoretical model for calculating ionic equilibria in milk as a function of pH: Comparison to experiment. *J Agric Food Chem* 58 (7):4440–47.
Nagpal, R., P. Behare, R. Rana, A. Kumar, M. Kumar, S. Arora, F. Morotta, S. Jain, and H. Yadav. 2011. Bioactive peptides derived from milk proteins and their health beneficial potentials: An update. *Food Funct* 2 (1):18–27.

Nygren-Babol, L., and M. Jagerstad. 2012. Folate-binding protein in milk: A review of biochemistry, physiology, and analytical methods. *Crit Rev Food Sci Nutr* 52 (5):410–25.

Palmquist, D. L., A. D. Beaulieu, and D. M. Barbano. 1993. Feed and animal factors influencing milk fat composition. *J Dairy Sci* 76 (6):1753–71.

Park, Y. W., and G. F. W. Haenlein. 2013. *Milk and Dairy Products in Human Nutrition Production, Composition, and Health*. Chichester: Wiley.

Parra, M. D., B. E. Martinez de Morentin, J. M. Cobo, I. Lenoir-Wijnkoop, and J. A. Martinez. 2007. Acute calcium assimilation from fresh or pasteurized yoghurt depending on the lactose digestibility status. *J Am Coll Nutr* 26 (3):288–94.

Parvez, S., K. A. Malik, S. Ah Kang, and H. Y. Kim. 2006. Probiotics and their fermented food products are beneficial for health. *J Appl Microbiol* 100 (6):1171–85.

Peres, J. M., S. Bouhallab, F. Bureau, J. L. Maubois, P. Arhan, and D. Bougle. 1997. Absorption digestive du fer lié au caséinophosphopeptide 1–25 de la b-caséine. *Le Lait* 77:433–40.

Rai, A. K., S. Sanjukta, and K. Jeyaram. 2015. Production of angiotensin I converting enzyme inhibitory (ACE-I) peptides during milk fermentation and their role in reducing hypertension. *Crit Rev Food Sci Nutr*. In press. doi:10.1080/10408398.2015.1068736.

Rozenberg, S., J. J. Body, O. Bruyere, P. Bergmann, M. L. Brandi, C. Cooper, J. P. Devogelaer, et al. 2016. Effects of dairy products consumption on health: Benefits and beliefs-a commentary from the Belgian Bone Club and the European Society for Clinical and Economic Aspects of Osteoporosis, Osteoarthritis and Musculoskeletal Diseases. *Calcif Tissue Int* 98 (1):1–17.

Rychen, G., D. Mpassi, S. Jurjanz, M. Mertes, I. Lenoir-Wijnkoop, J. M. Antoine, and F. Laurent. 2002. 15N as a marker to assess portal absorption of nitrogen from milk, yogurt and heat-treated yogurt in the growing pig. *J Dairy Res* 69 (1):95–101.

Schaafsma, G. J., H. R. Dekker, and H. de Ward. 1988. Nutritional aspects of yogurt. 2. Bioavailability of essential minerals and trace elements. *Neth Milk Dairy J* 42:135–46.

Schanbacher, F. L, R. S. Talhouk, and F. A. Murray. 1997. Biology and origin of bioactive peptides in milk. *Liv Prod Sci* 50:105–23.

Schuette, S. A., N. J. Yasillo, and C. M. Thompson. 1991. The effect of carbohydrates in milk on the absorption of calcium by postmenopausal women. *J Am Coll Nutr* 10 (2):132–39.

Shahani, K. M., and R. C. Chandan. 1979. Nutritional and healthful aspects of cultured and culture-containing dairy foods. *J Dairy Sci* 62 (10):1685–94.

Shakur, Y. A., W. Lou, and M. R. L'Abbe. 2014. Examining the effects of increased vitamin D fortification on dietary inadequacy in Canada. *Can J Public Health* 105 (2):e127–32.

Shantha, N. C., L. N. Ram, J. O'Leary, C. L. Hicks, and E. A. Decker. 1995. Conjugated linoleic acid concentrations in dairy products as affected by processing and storage. *J Food Sci* 60:695–98.

Tamime, A. Y., and R. K. Robinson. 2007. *Yoghurt: Science and Technology* (3rd Edition). Boca Raton, FL: Woodhead Publishing.

Tamime, A. Y., A. Skriver, and L. M. Nilsson. 2006. Types of fermented milks. *Fermented Milks*. Edited by Tamime A. Y. Ames, IA: Blackwell Science.

Tessari, P., E. Kiwanuka, M. Cristini, M. Zaramella, M. Enslen, C. Zurlo, and C. Garcia-Rodenas. 2007. Slow versus fast proteins in the stimulation of beta-cell response and the activation of the entero-insular axis in type 2 diabetes. *Diabetes Metab Res Rev* 23 (5):378–85.

Teucher, B., G. Majsak-Newman, J. R. Dainty, D. McDonagh, R. J. FitzGerald, and S. J. Fairweather-Tait. 2006. Calcium absorption is not increased by caseinophosphopeptides. *Am J Clin Nutr* 84 (1):162–66.

Tome, D. 2012. Criteria and markers for protein quality assessment: A review. *Br J Nutr* 108 (Suppl 2):S222–29.

Trinidad, T. P., T. M. Wolever, and L. U. Thompson. 1996. Availability of calcium for absorption in the small intestine and colon from diets containing available and unavailable carbohydrates: An in vitro assessment. *Int J Food Sci Nutr* 47 (1):83–88.
Unal, G., S. N. El, and S. Kilic. 2005. In vitro determination of calcium bioavailability of milk, dairy products and infant formulas. *Int J Food Sci Nutr* 56 (1):13–22.
Vasbinder, A. J. 2002. *Casein Whey Protein Interactions in Heated Milk*. Utrecht: Universiteit Utrecht.
Vegarud, G. E., T. Langsrud, and C. Svenning. 2000. Mineral-binding milk proteins and peptides; occurrence, biochemical and technological characteristics. *Br J Nutr* 84 (Suppl 1):S91–S98.
Vignola, C. L. 2002. Science et technologie du lait, transformation du lait. *Fondation de technologie laitière du Québec*. Montreal, QC: Presses Internationales Polytechnique.
Visioli, F., and A. Strata. 2014. Milk, dairy products, and their functional effects in humans: A narrative review of recent evidence. *Adv Nutr* 5 (2):131–43.
Wang, Y. W., and P. J. Jones. 2004. Conjugated linoleic acid and obesity control: Efficacy and mechanisms. *Int J Obes Relat Metab Disord* 28 (8):941–55.
Williams, E. B., B. Hooper, A. Spiro, and S. Stanner. 2015. The contribution of yogurt to nutrient intakes across the life course. *Nutr Bull* 40 (1):9–32.
Yildiz, F. 2010. *Development and Manufacture of Yogurt and Other Functional Dairy Products*. Boca Raton, FL: Taylor & Francis.
Zemel, M., D. Teegarden, M. Van Loan, D. Schoeller, V. Matkovic, R. Lyle, and B. Craig. 2009. Dairy-rich diets augment fat loss on an energy-restricted diet: A multicenter trial. *Nutrients* 1 (1):83.

2 Yogurt Consumption

2.1 FOOD-BASED DIETARY GUIDELINES FOR DAIRY AND YOGURT

Dairy products are recognized by international health authorities and scientific institutions as part of a healthy diet at all life stages: children, teenagers, adults, pregnant women, and older persons. Recommendations for the consumption of dairy products are mostly based on meeting the recommended dietary allowance (RDA) for calcium (Dror and Allen 2014) and for their contribution to bone health (Public Health England et al. 2013). Many health authorities currently recommend two to four servings of dairy products each day. For example, two to three servings of low-fat dairy products per day in the United States, three servings of dairy products per day in France, two servings per day of nonfat and low-fat dairy in Mexico, four servings per day in Germany, and so on. Recommendations for the consumption of dairy products also vary between age groups; guidelines for children, adolescents, and adults vary between two to three, three to seven, and two to three servings per day, respectively (Dror and Allen 2014). Table 2.1 outlines examples of food-based dietary guidelines for dairy foods that are provided by authoritative national health organizations in different countries.

The recommended serving sizes vary between countries and one serving of yogurt does not always correspond to 1 unit (e.g., cup) of yogurt. For example, in France one serving of yogurt corresponds to 1 unit of yogurt (125 g per unit), but in the United States one serving of yogurt corresponds to 2 units of yogurts (100–125 g per unit). Moreover, because overweight and obesity are important health issues, dietary guidelines by many national authorities emphasize recommendations to select nonfat or low-fat dairy products: Argentina, Canada, France, Germany, India, Mexico, the United Kingdom, and the United States (Table 2.1). The Ministry of Health of Brazil and Public Health England have made specific recommendations about avoiding sweetened milks and yogurts (Table 2.1). Yogurt is often listed as a dairy option or an alternative to milk; however, not all national guidelines give specific recommendations for yogurt consumption. For example, the German Nutrition Society lists milk and cheese as the only examples for daily milk and milk product consumption. However, on the German Nutrition Society website, yogurt is illustrated in the German nutrition circle and detailed information about the milk and milk products group describes yogurt, kefir, or buttermilk as being daily dairy alternatives (German Nutrition Society 2013). The National Institute of Nutrition in India specifically recommends yogurt, curd, or soy as milk replacements for those who are intolerant to milk (National Institute of Nutrition 2011).

TABLE 2.1
Examples of Recommendations for Dairy and Yogurt Consumption Given by National Health Agencies

Country	Daily Dairy Recommendations	Source
Argentina	Three portions (milk, cheese, or yogurt, preferably skim milk) • 500 mL of milk • 500 mL of yogurt • 30 g of fresh cheese	Guías Alimentarias para la Población Argentina, 2016 (Dietary guidelines for the Argentinian population) Ministero de Salud (Ministry of Health) http://www.msal.gob.ar/images/stories/bes/graficos/0000000817cnt-2016-04_Guia_Alimentaria_completa_web.pdf
Brazil	No specific quantity of daily servings recommended for the milk and cheese group The milk and cheese group includes minimally processed foods (cow's milk, cheese curds, plain yogurt, and cheeses), whereas milk and yogurts that have been sweetened, colored, and flavored are considered as ultra-processed and it is recommended to avoid them	Guia Alimentar para a População Brasléira, 2014 (Dietary guidelines for the Brazilian population) Ministério da Saúde (Ministry of Health of Brazil) http://www.foodpolitics.com/wp-content/uploads/Brazilian-Dietary-Guidelines-2014.pdf
Canada	Two to four servings of milk and alternatives depending on age and sex Recommends 500 mL of milk every day and selecting low-fat alternatives • 250 mL of milk or fortified soy beverage • 125 mL canned milk • 175 g of yogurt or kefir • 50 g of cheese	Eating Well with Canada's Food Guide, 2007 Health Canada http://www.hc-sc.gc.ca/fn-an/alt_formats/hpfb-dgpsa/pdf/food-guide-aliment/print_eatwell_bienmang-eng.pdf
France	Three servings for adults and four for children, adolescents, and seniors > 55 years (milk, cheese, yogurt, fromage blanc, and fermented milks) Choose skimmed or reduced-fat dairy products; eat a variety of dairy each day • 125 g of yogurt • 100 g of fromage blanc • 30 g of cheese	La santé vient en mangeant: le guide nutrition pour tous, 2002 Ministère des Affaires sociales et de la Santé Santé publique France http://www.mangerbouger.fr/PNNS/Guides-et-documents/Guides-nutrition

(Continued)

TABLE 2.1 (CONTINUED)
Examples of Recommendations for Dairy and Yogurt Consumption Given by National Health Agencies

Country	Daily Dairy Recommendations	Source
Germany	Four servings of milk and milk products • 200–250 g of low-fat milk and milk products (yogurt, kefir, and buttermilk may be selected instead of milk) • 50–60 g of low-fat cheese	*Vollwertig essen und trinken nach den 10 Regeln der DGE*, 2013 (Ten guidelines for wholesome eating and drinking) Developed by the German Nutrition Society and endorsed by the Ministries of Health and Agriculture https://www.dge.de/ernaehrungspraxis/vollwertige-ernaehrung/ernaehrungskreis/
India	Three portions for adults and five portions for children Consume at least 250 mL boiled or pasteurized milk Milk can be replaced by an equal amount of curd, yogurt, or soy milk if it is not tolerated Skimmed milk should be used rather than whole milk	*Dietary Guidelines for Indians - A Manual*, 2011 National Institute of Nutrition http://ninindia.org/dietaryguidelinesforninwebsite.pdf
Mexico	Two portions of dairy (milk, cheese, or yogurt) Milk should be nonfat or low fat (1% milk fat) • 250 mL of milk or yogurt • 125 mL of evaporated milk • 45 mL of milk powder • 30 g of cheese	*Guías Alimentarias y de Actividad Física en contexto de sobrepeso y obesidad en la población mexicana*, 2015 (Dietary and physical activity guidelines in the context of overweight and obesity in the Mexican population), 2015 National Institute of Public Health, Ministry of Health, National Institute of Nutrition and Medical Sciences Salvador Zubirán, Universidad Iberoamericana, Ogali Nutrition Consultants, National Academy of Medicine http://guiasalimentacionyactividadfisica.org.mx/wp-content/uploads/2015/10/Guias-alimentarias-y-de-actividad-fisica.pdf
United Kingdom	No specific quantity of daily servings recommended for dairy (milk, cheese, and yogurt) and alternatives (soya drinks and soya yogurts) Choose lower fat and lower sugar options	The Eat Well Plate, 2007 Food Standards Agency and Public Health England http://www.nhs.uk/Livewell/Goodfood/Pages/milk-dairy-foods.aspx
United States	500 mL milk-equivalents for children 2–3 years, 625 mL milk-equivalents for children 4–8 years, and 750 mL milk-equivalents of dairy for adolescents and adults Should include nonfat and low-fat (1% milk fat) milk, yogurt, and cheese or fortified soy beverages	*Dietary Guidelines for Americans: 2015-2020* Department of Health and Human Services and Department of Agriculture http://health.gov/dietaryguidelines/2015/

2.2 DAIRY AND YOGURT CONSUMPTION

Dairy product consumption has been increasing worldwide; however, these increases have been driven mainly by developing countries (e.g., Brazil and China), going from 3.4% of energy in 1961 to 4.4% in 2007, whereas intake has remained relatively constant in developed countries at just over 14% of energy. A large percentage of daily dietary energy, protein, and fat comes from milk products in Europe, as well as Oceania and the Americas (Muehlhoff et al. 2013). Among European Union countries, dairy intake is relatively high, averaging 266 g/day, with some of the highest intakes in Denmark and Finland, whose calcium intakes are very close to 1000 mg/day (Fisberg and Machado 2015). The actual contribution of dairy products to the intake of calcium differs between countries. For example, in several occidental countries (e.g., Canada, Germany, and France), dairy products are the main source of dietary calcium (Johnson-Down et al. 2006, Hébel 2007). In fact, a cross-sectional study found that milk, cheese, yogurt, and lattes accounted for 49% of dietary intakes of calcium for American adults and milk, cheese, and yogurt represented 55% of calcium intakes for their children (Cluskey et al. 2015). However, in China and India, vegetables are the main sources of calcium at the national level (Li et al. 2005, National Institute of Nutrition 2011). A high percentage of Americans in different age groups do not meet the recommended intakes for dairy. For example, as few as 10% of females over 14 years consume adequate amounts of dairy foods (Webb et al. 2014).

In many countries, dietary intakes of dairy products fall short of recommendations for dairy, which is often accompanied by shortfalls in calcium. For example, >33% of children and >70% of seniors (≥ 71 years) do not consume the recommended two portions of milk per day in Canada (Garriguet 2004). Calcium is among the nutrients with the highest prevalence of inadequacies in Canada, which has proportions of its population with inadequate intakes ranging from 26.5% to as high as 86.9%, depending on the sex and age group (Health Canada 2012). Studies have demonstrated that the recommended intakes of dairy and the RDA for calcium are not being consumed by the majority of Americans or French (Institut de Veille Sanitaire 2007, Miller et al. 2001, USDA Agriculture 2010). Among American children, dairy products provide valuable nutrients; however, intakes have declined in many populations, with a trend toward even lower intakes with increasing age (Dror and Allen 2014). In the United States, dietary calcium and vitamin D recommendations have been increased by the U.S. Institute of Medicine (IOM) (Ross et al. 2011), which emphasizes the importance of consuming dairy products. The dietary reference intakes for calcium are based on evidence related to bone health, mainly from the results of calcium balance studies. The IOM report states that there is no additional health benefit associated with vitamin D or calcium intakes above the level of the new RDA. Yogurt and dairy product avoidance could have a negative impact on calcium and vitamin D intakes in infants, children, and adolescents. In the United States, removing milk and milk products from the diet requires careful replacement with other food sources of calcium, including fortified foods. It is unrealistic for most people to consume enough plant foods to achieve the RDA of calcium within the context of an American diet (USDA Agriculture 2010). In

Europe, the avoidance of conventional dairy products without supplementation or appropriate adaptation of dietary habits may result in low intakes of calcium, vitamin D, and riboflavin (Ross et al. 2011, EFSA Panel on Dietetic Products 2010). Furthermore, consuming a diverse range of dairy (including yogurt) products helps individuals optimize their nutrient intake, particularly for calcium and phosphorus (Moreno Aznar et al. 2013). Moreover, each type of dairy product contributes to essential nutrient intakes in different proportions in different populations. For example, in France, milk contributes more than yogurt and cheese to intakes of vitamin B2, vitamin B12, calcium, and phosphorus in children. However, in French adults, cheese contributes more than yogurt and milk to intakes of vitamin B12, calcium, and phosphorus (French are among the world's largest consumers of cheese). For example, "ultra-frais" yogurt and other fermented milks, fresh cheeses, and desserts contribute to 5% and 7% of total carbohydrate intake for adults and children, respectively, whereas the contribution of other dairy products is negligible (Hébel 2007).

The United States is the largest processor of milk in the world and over the last years it appears that its production of fluid milk has decreased, while production and consumption of refrigerated yogurt has increased (Chandan and Kilara 2013). There have been similar trends in Canada, with the per capita consumption of milk decreasing from 90.05 L to 70.64 L between 1996 and 2015 and the per capita yogurt consumption increasing from 3.17 L to 10.53 L over the same time period (Government of Canada 2016). It is believed that the increase in yogurt popularity has been fostered by the perception that it is a health food product (Chandan and Kilara 2013), whereas common barriers to milk consumption have been attributed to concerns over gastrointestinal side effects (Mobley et al. 2014).

Increasing yogurt consumption presents an opportunity to counter deficits in dairy consumption and shortfalls in nutrient intakes with a good source of calcium, protein, and live bacteria that provide health benefits to the host. In Europe, yogurt products make up almost one third of all dairy products consumed, whereas in the United States, it only accounts for 5% of dairy products (El-Abbadi et al. 2014). The average intake of yogurt in Brazil was estimated to be very low at approximately 0.1 portions per day and did not appear to contribute significantly to total nutrient intakes (Murphy et al. 2016). Similarly, due to the relatively low intakes of yogurt in the American diet, it generally does not contribute to significant intakes of dairy servings in any age group (Quann et al. 2015). However, among yogurt consumers, yogurt consumption was associated with higher intakes of three nutrients of concern: calcium, potassium, and fiber. Furthermore, adding low-fat or nonfat yogurt to the daily diet was thought to further increase intakes of nutrients of concern, helping Americans to reach adequate nutritional status and improve overall health (Webb et al. 2014).

Using 4-day food records from multiple years of the National Diet and Nutrition Survey in the United Kingdom, yogurt consumption across age groups was studied. The yogurt group also included fromage frais and dairy desserts. Overall, the report found that yogurt consumption was most frequent in young children (3 years and under) and least frequent in teenagers (11–18 years) and adults (19–49 years). In young children, however, yogurt only accounted for 42%–51% of products consumed in the yogurt group, which included fromage frais and dairy desserts. In contrast, yogurt made up over 90% of the yogurt group for adults (Williams et al. 2015). Another study in the United Kingdom corroborated that yogurt is frequently consumed by children in the United Kingdom, with as much as 56% of children (9–18 years) consuming yogurt (Green et al. 2015).

2.3 NUTRIENT DENSITY

The terms *nutrient dense* and *nutrient density* are often ambiguous, as no standard definition exists and there is no consensus over what constitutes a food that is nutrient dense (Nicklas et al. 2014). Many different tools appraising the nutrient profile of foods exist. Table 2.2 lists different nutrient density profiling systems that have been used. Generally, foods are positively scored when nutrients or criteria that promote health such as fruits, calcium, or iron are present, whereas foods are negatively scored when nutrients or criteria associated with negative health outcomes are present, such as high calories, sodium, saturated fats, and added sugars. Nutrient profiling systems may vary significantly in the number and types of nutrients and criteria included in the algorithm. For example, added sugar is an undesirable food component in the Office of Communications (Ofcom) (United Kingdom) and the Ratio of Recommended to Restricted Foods (RRR) (United States), but is absent from the Nutritious Food Index (Australia) or the Naturally Nutrient Rich Score (United States). Nutrient density scores may also vary depending on whether they are presented as a value based on weight (100 g) of a food or energy (100 kcal) in a food.

Based on the food components used to determine nutrient density that are outlined in Table 2.2, unsweetened, low-fat yogurt would be unanimously considered as a nutrient-dense food, because of its high vitamin, mineral, and calcium content and its low content in sugar, saturated fats, and energy. Although profiling systems have as an aim to easily identify the most healthful foods, limitations exist. For example, nutrient density profiling systems may label foods such as sweetened whole-fat yogurt as non-nutrient-dense foods despite the fact that it contributes valuable nutrients to the diet (Nicklas et al. 2014). A well-known method used in the United States, the Nutrient Rich Food score (NRF9.3), gives both sweetened and whole-fat yogurts poor nutrient density scores (Fulgoni et al. 2009), whereas the French system, SAIN (Nutrient Adequacy Score for Individual Foods), LIM (Nutrients to Limit) (Darmon et al. 2009), gives whole-fat yogurt a poor score, but sweetened yogurt still receives a good nutrient score. The Food Standards Agency in the United Kingdom has developed the Ofcom model for identifying less healthy foods to provide guidance on marketing foods on TV to children. Under the Ofcom model, less healthy foods would have a score of four points or more; therefore, whole-fat yogurt would be considered "less healthy" and would be subject to marketing restrictions. Under the NRF9.3 system, a sweetened low-fat yogurt only has a nutrient-rich food score of 2.4, whereas a nonfat plain yogurt has a high nutrient-rich food score of 70.4 (Table 2.3). Under the SAIN, LIM system, the plain, nonfat, and sweetened low-fat yogurts are considered as class 1 (SAIN > 5 and LIM ≤ 7.5) foods with the most favorable nutrient profiles, whereas sweetened whole-fat yogurt is a class 4 (SAIN < 5 and LIM > 7.5) food with the least favorable nutrient profile, containing

TABLE 2.2
Examples of Tools Used to Calculate the Nutrient Density/Quality of Foods

Tool	Description
Nutritional Quality Index (NQI) American index relating nutrients in a food to its energy content (Hansen et al. 1979)	Based on U.S. recommended dietary allowances (RDA), it is calculated separately for each nutrient
Calorie for nutrient (CFN) American ratio of calories to mean percentage daily value (Lachance and Fisher 1986)	Based on the adequacy of 11 key nutrients (protein, thiamin, riboflavin, niacin, vitamin C, vitamin A, calcium, magnesium, iron, zinc, and folic acid)
Nutritious Food Index (NFI) Australian index that ranks foods into different levels of nutrient desirability (Gazibarich and Ricci 1998)	Weighs 13 desirable food components (calcium, iron, zinc, fiber, folate, magnesium, potassium, niacin, riboflavin, thiamin, vitamin C, vitamin A, and phosphorus) against 4 undesirable food components (total fat, saturated fat, sodium, and cholesterol)
Ratio of Recommended to Restricted Foods (RRR) American index that ranks foods into different levels of nutrient desirability (Scheidt and Daniel 2004)	Weighs six desirable food components (protein, dietary fiber, calcium, iron, vitamin A, and vitamin D) against five nondesirable food components (calories, sugars, cholesterol, saturated fats, and sodium)
Naturally Nutrient Rich Score (NNR) American nutrients-to-calorie ratio (Drewnowski 2005)	Based on the average percentage daily values of 14 key nutrients (protein, vitamin A, vitamin C, calcium, iron, zinc, folate, thiamine, riboflavin, vitamin B-12, vitamin D, vitamin E, MUFA, and potassium)
Nutrient rich food index (NRF) American nutrient-to-calorie ratio (Drewnowski and Fulgoni 2008)	Based on a ratio of beneficial nutrients to nutrients to limit: 3–15 beneficial nutrients (e.g., protein, fiber, vitamin C, calcium, and iron) and 3 nutrients to limit (saturated fat, added sugar, and sodium)
Ofcom British system for identifying healthy foods from foods rich in fat, sodium, or sugar for the purposes of restricting the marketing of less healthy foods to children (Rayner et al. 2009)	Classifies foods based on four negative nutrients (energy, saturated fat, total sugar, and sodium) and three positive nutrients (nonstarch polysaccharide fiber, protein, and 'fruits, vegetables, and nuts')
SAIN, LIM System French diet modeling with linear programming tool to validate nutrient profiles and categorize foods into four classes (Darmon et al. 2009)	Based on two independent scores that include qualifying or positive nutrients (SAIN) and disqualifying or negative nutrients (LIM). SAIN is composed of five basic nutrients (protein, fiber, vitamin C, calcium, and iron) and four optional nutrients (vitamin D, vitamin E, alpha-linoleic acid, and monounsaturated fatty acids), whereas LIM is composed of three nutrients to limit (saturated fatty acids, added sugars, and sodium)
Nutrient Profiling Scoring Criterion (NPSC) Australian and New Zealand food standards for health-related claims (Food Standards Australia New Zealand 2016)	Points are allocated based on food components (calories, saturated fat, sodium, and total sugar) and then may be modified based on (fruit and vegetables, fiber, and protein)

TABLE 2.3
Examples of Nutrient Density Scores for Nonfat, Low-Fat, Whole-Fat, and Sweetened French Yogurts According to Common Nutrient Profiling Systems

Yogurt Type	NRF9.3 score	SAIN score	LIM score	Ofcom score
Plain, nonfat	70.4	11.4	0.8	−2
Plain, lowfat	55.3	9.7	1.6	−1
Sweetened, lowfat	2.4	7.8	7.5	2
Sweetened, wholefat, fruit	−2.8	3.9	10.4	6

Note: Higher nutrient scores for NRF9.3 denote higher nutrient density per 100 kcal; foods with the most favorable nutrient profiles have SAIN scores >5 and LIM scores ≤7.5; "less healthy" foods have Ofcom scores ≥4.

high amounts of nutrients that should be limited (Darmon et al. 2009). The NRF9.3, SAIN, LIM, and Ofcom nutrient profiling systems described in Table 2.3, are some of the most common methods used to profile the nutritional quality of foods.

Despite the limitations of potentially misclassifying nutritious foods, the use of the NRF system has been successful in improving the diet of consumers in a randomized controlled trial. Consumers who were given NRF education had higher Healthy Eating Index scores for fruit, whole grains, saturated fats, and added sugars compared with a control group that received standard nutrition education (Glanz et al. 2012). A study quantified the relative contributions of foods to encourage and foods to limit using individual diet optimization and nutrient profiling techniques based on the SAIN, LIM system. The relative proportions of four nutrient profiling classes were evaluated before and after the optimization process. The contribution of milk, fruits and vegetables, whole grains, and fish significantly increased, whereas the contribution of refined grains, meats, mixed dishes, sugars, and fats decreased. Nutrient profiling methods that adequately identify the nutrient density of foods can be important tools for nutrition education (Maillot et al. 2011).

2.4 NUTRIENT ADEQUACY

It is important to consider the duality between nutrient density reported by tools listed in Table 2.3 and the nutritional adequacy of a food. A food such as sweetened yogurt, which may have a lower nutrient density score, is still a source of key nutrients in the diet (Figure 2.1) and yogurts are considered by many as a nutrient-rich food (Erickson and Slavin 2015, Nicklas et al. 2014). Furthermore, yogurt consumption assists individuals in meeting recommended intakes of nutrients of concern in the American diet and elsewhere in the world, particularly calcium, protein, and potassium. For example, in France, dairy foods are the primary source of dietary calcium and can be provided by a wide variety of yogurt products (Drewnowski et al. 2015). A 6 oz serving of yogurt would help children 6–11 years old to achieve recommended intakes for calcium, as well as increase intakes of potassium and vitamin D for all children, especially when paired with fruits or vegetables (Hess and Slavin

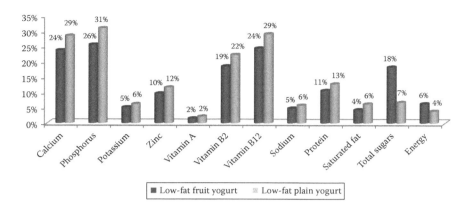

FIGURE 2.1 Contribution of 125 g servings of low-fat fruit flavored and plain yogurts to percentage daily values of nutrients and energy intakes in adults. (Data from the Institute of Medicine reference intakes for nutrients [The National Academies of Sciences, Dietary reference intakes tables and application, 2016. http://www.nationalacademies.org/hmd/Activities/Nutrition/SummaryDRIs/DRI-Tables.aspx.] and the USDA Food Composition Database [U.S. Department of Agriculture, Economic Research Service, Dairy data, 2016. http://www.ers.usda.gov/data-products/dairy-data.aspx]). Percentage daily values based on average values for men and women aged 31–55 and energy intake was based on a standard 2000 kcal diet.

2014). A diet study in the United Kingdom showed that the yogurt group (yogurt, fromage frais, and dairy desserts) contributed to significant intakes of vitamin B12, riboflavin, iodine, and phosphorus in children from 4 months to 10 years old. In very young children (4–18 months old), yogurt was also a significant source of non-milk extrinsic sugars, which may be attributed to the lack of variety of foods at this age. In women >65 years, yogurt made small contributions to phosphorus, iodine, calcium, vitamin B12, and riboflavin. In a modeling exercise, adding a 125 g portion per day of low-fat fruit yogurt to the diet of teenagers significantly reduced the proportion of teens who did not meet the recommended nutrient intakes for calcium, potassium, iodine, zinc, and magnesium; however, without food replacement, it also coincided with an increase in sugar and energy intake (Williams et al. 2015).

According to the nutrient-rich food score, a plain nonfat yogurt would have a higher nutrient-rich score than a vanilla-flavored nonfat yogurt (Drewnowski and Fulgoni 2014). For this reason, among Hispanic preschool children in western Illinois, yogurt was labeled under "unhealthy snacks" due to its energy density, but its nutrient density was not considered (Longley et al. 2014). Some varieties of yogurt in the United States are indeed energy dense, with the addition of large amounts of added sugar, but the added sugar content is highly variable (Erickson and Slavin 2015). Despite the energy density of some varieties of yogurt, overall, the yogurt group was associated with increased calcium, vitamin D, and protein intakes, as well as less fat and saturated fat intakes in U.S. children. It is suggested that yogurt consumption is a marker for healthy dietary patterns and that yogurt may replace more energy-dense snacks (Keast et al. 2015). There is some concern that restrictive guidelines on added sugars may lead to a reduction in intakes of nutrient-dense foods such as yogurt (Erickson and Slavin 2015), which is fairly consistently associated with healthier dietary patterns regardless of sugar or fat content.

Despite yogurt's perceived healthfulness, many brands contain excessive quantities of added sugar and do not meet the IOM's standard for competitive foods in schools (Hess and Slavin 2014). International health organizations such as the World Health Organization (WHO) are increasingly recommending stricter limitations on added sugars to the diet to <10% of total energy and have even suggested conditional recommendations to limit added sugar to <5% of total energy intake (WHO 2015). These trends for stricter guidance on added sugar recommendations by health agencies are problematic for commonly consumed foods that are considered nutrient rich, such as sweetened yogurts. This is particularly true given that plain yogurt is considered to be tart and sugars are added to make the product more palatable. Furthermore, the U.S. Department of Agriculture (USDA) does not recommend reliance upon artificial sweeteners because of lack of evidence on their long-term safety, but rather recommends selecting dairy foods with little added sugar or sugar substitutes (Hess et al. 2016). In France, 50% of plain yogurt consumers are known to add sweeteners before consumption. A recent study tested the practice of adding sweeteners (white sugar, honey, and jam) to plain yogurt and found that plain yogurt consumers added more sugar to their yogurt (13.6 g of sugar per 125 g) than contained in presweetened yogurts (10.2 g of sugar per 125 g). The study also indicated that plain yogurt consumers had a tendency to underestimate the amount of sugar that they added (Saint-Eve et al. 2016).

Similar to added sugars, whole-fat yogurts would receive lower nutrient density scores than nonfat yogurts despite their high contributions to other important nutrients such as calcium (Figure 2.1). Based on food intake studies, it would be difficult for Americans to meet recommended intakes of nutrients of concern (i.e., calcium, potassium, magnesium, riboflavin, and vitamin D) if they followed a dietary pattern that did not include dairy products. Both milk and yogurt have roles to play in the American diet in helping individuals to meet recommended intakes of key nutrients, regardless of their fat content (Weaver 2014). While international food-based dietary guidelines recommend that the public select nonfat and low-fat dairy products (Table 2.1), there is emerging evidence indicating that some dairy fats may have health benefits (Kratz et al. 2013). According to Hess and Slavin (2014), relaxing the fat restrictions for yogurts (nonfat and low fat) may add palatability, permitting manufacturers to commit to making a less discernible decrease of sugar in yogurt products (Hess and Slavin 2014). This is important, given that dairy products are an important contributor to children and adults' diet quality by providing substantial amounts of high-quality proteins, essential fatty acids, nonessential fatty acids, and micronutrients such as calcium, phosphorus, magnesium, zinc, vitamin A, vitamin B12, and riboflavin (Dror and Allen 2014), and, depending on the population, iodine and vitamin D. In countries where the food supply is not fortified with iodine, dairy products can be an important source of this nutrient for specific populations (Williams et al. 2015). Dairy foods such as yogurt provide key nutrients that are consistently consumed in inadequate quantities, such as calcium. While calcium can be obtained from other food sources, they would need to be consumed in excessive quantities to deliver the RDA. In the context of an American diet, dairy-free calcium products do not provide adequate levels of other nutrients such as magnesium and potassium that are of high concern in this population (Rozenberg et al. 2016). Besides calcium intake, an overall higher diet quality in terms of adequacy to nutrient recommendations has also been observed with increased dairy consumption in the United States (Weinberg et al. 2004, Foote et al. 2004). It has also been demonstrated in the United States that yogurt consumers have a better diet quality (measured by the Dietary Guidelines for Americans Adherence Index [DGAI] score) than nonconsumers; they have a higher potassium intake and are less likely to have an inadequate intake of vitamin B2, vitamin B12, calcium, magnesium, and zinc (Wang et al. 2013).

A diet modeling study in a French population aimed to estimate the number portions of different dairy products that would be suitable for a nutritionally adequate diet. In optimizing dairy product intake, portions per week of milk (nonfat, low fat, whole fat, plain, and flavored) and yogurt (nonfat, low fat, whole fat, plain, flavored, with fruits, and the yogurt-like product fromage blanc) were increased and cheese was decreased in comparison with intakes that are normally observed in the population. Increasing milk by 0.7 portions and yogurt by 2.4 portions, decreasing cheese by 4.8 portions, and keeping milk desserts constant at 1.2 portions per week resulted in a significant decrease in energy and a significant increase in calcium, indicating that yogurt and milk products are less energy-dense options with superior nutrient profiles (higher nutrient density and fewer LIM) in comparison with cheese. The study concluded that increasing intakes of both milk and yogurt (regardless of fat and sugar content) while decreasing cheese intake would help achieve nutrition adequacy in populations (Clerfeuille et al. 2013).

While the main source of calcium in the French diet is dairy, the French population does not meet the recommended three portions of dairy per day. Furthermore, the French cannot meet calcium intake guidelines without dairy products. While dairy products are generally all classified as nutrient-rich foods, there is considerable variability within the group with regard to saturated fatty acids, sugar, sodium, and energy content. Scores for nutrient costs based on a recent study modeled the energy, economic, and LIM costs of portions of different dairy products required to provide 15% of the daily value of calcium (800 g/day) in the French population. Per 100 g portion, the best energy, monetary, and LIM costs were supplied by the milk group (low-fat and skimmed milk). This was followed by plain and light yogurts, and then whole-fat milks, flavored milks, and sweetened yogurts. Light milk desserts also had a low-energy cost, but a greater monetary cost. Cheese varied greatly as a group; hard cheeses were excellent sources of calcium greater than or equal to milk, whereas soft, cream, and double-cream cheeses were poor in calcium. The cheese group had the poorest LIM scores. This type of modeling can help individuals select the most affordable, nutrient-rich dairy products in France (Drewnowski et al. 2015).

The consumption of take-away foods is increasing in different populations and these foods are often deficient in nutrients while being energy dense. Population groups at particular risk of nutritional deficiencies include children, teenagers, pregnant women, and older people, who often have higher nutrient requirements but lower energy needs. Moreover, it is important to note that obesity may also be associated with nutrient deficiencies (Markovic and Natoli 2009). The nutrient richness, taste, and smooth texture of yogurt and dairy products make them ideal foods that could be helpful in the diet of vulnerable populations such as frail elderly (van Staveren and de Groot 2011). Yogurt, in particular, given its condensed source of nutrients, may have an important role to play in healthy, active living for the elderly (El-Abbadi et al. 2014). Fermented products are also an interesting vehicle for fortification and can be an efficient tool to combat nutrient deficiencies (Shiby and Mishra 2013). For example, yogurt has been used in iron (Lysionek et al. 2002) and vitamin D fortification programs (Neyestani et al. 2015).

2.5 DIETARY PATTERNS, LIFESTYLE, AND SOCIODEMOGRAPHIC FACTORS

Yogurt consumption is not only associated with higher intakes of key nutrients and lower levels of inadequacy, but also healthier dietary patterns and lifestyle factors, making it a promising marker for healthy lifestyles. The following section will summarize the observational data from epidemiological studies that have presented associations between lifestyle factors, dietary patterns, and yogurt consumption in different parts of the world. Some of these associations appear to be fairly consistent across different regions and cultures in the world, indicating that yogurt consumption may be universally associated with certain dietary indicators for health.

2.5.1 DIETARY PATTERNS

In the United States, the diet of yogurt consumers can be characterized by a significantly higher percentage of energy contribution from the intake of fruits, vegetables, nuts and seeds, fish and seafood, and whole grains. It is further characterized by a lower percentage of energy contribution from intakes of processed meats, meat, and refined grains (Wang et al. 2013). Among children and adolescents, even at low levels of consumption (at least once per week), yogurt consumers were characterized by a higher diet quality score as defined by the healthy eating index (Zhu et al. 2015).

A study performed in elderly Spanish men ($n = 1,150$) and women ($n = 1,094$) characterized a dietary pattern associated with low energy density and evaluated its nutrient adequacy. Yogurt and low-fat milk, vegetables, fruits, legumes, and potatoes were fundamental to the diet low in energy density. Despite the lower energy content, the low energy-dense diet was better at achieving nutritional adequacy compared with higher energy-dense diets. Higher proportions of the elderly adults following the low energy-dense dietary pattern met dietary recommendations for fats, fiber, calcium, and other key micronutrients (vitamin C, vitamin E, thiamin, riboflavin, vitamin B6, folate, and magnesium) (Schroder et al. 2008).

In a French population, the Probability of Adequate Nutrient Intake (PANDiet) score and indicator of nutritional adequacy was positively associated with yogurt intake in both men and women (Camilleri et al. 2013). A healthy dietary pattern identified in a group of French adults was characterized by low sugar consumption and high fruit, yogurt, and soup intake. This pattern was associated with lower levels of inflammatory markers and higher microbial gene richness (Kong et al. 2014).

Among Italian adults, yogurt consumption was included among a group of healthy dietary habits, which coincided with lower intakes of processed meats, bread, rice, and sweet drinks, as well as higher intakes of fruits, vegetables, fish, olive oil, and tea (Ricceri et al. 2015). Among Spanish adults, more frequent yogurt consumption was significantly associated with greater adherence to the Mediterranean diet scores and fruit consumption (Martinez-Gonzalez et al. 2014).

Yogurt is consistently considered an important component of the prudent dietary pattern in many countries, suggesting better diet quality and overall health among yogurt consumers. In French Canadian adults, yogurt consumers, independent of fat content, had significantly higher prudent diet scores than nonconsumers (Cormier et al. 2015). Among pregnant Brazilian women, the prudent dietary pattern included milk, yogurt, cheese, fruit, crackers, and meat and fish (Coelho Nde et al. 2015). A prudent diet consisting of high fish, yogurt, pulses, rice, pasta, wine, fruits, and vegetables was associated with lower concentrations of biomarkers that correspond with low cardiovascular disease risk in Scotland (Wood et al. 2014).

In Japan, yogurt was associated with a Western breakfast pattern, which was inversely associated with circulating leptin and plasminogen activator inhibitor type-1 (Kashino et al. 2015). Among European adolescents, the intake of ready-to-eat cereals was associated with higher intakes of fruit, milk, and yogurt at breakfast (Michels et al. 2016). Adolescents with this dietary profile were also more likely to have better dietary habits and overall diet quality and were 57% less likely to be overweight. They had higher intakes of vitamins (B2, B5, B7, and D), minerals (calcium, phosphorus, and potassium), milk, yogurt, and fruit (Michels et al. 2015).

It is not yet clear whether the observational healthy dietary factors associated with yogurt consumption are independent of disease risk, or whether they contribute to mechanisms involved in disease prevention of diet-related diseases such as diabetes and obesity. It is therefore important to take dietary patterns and quality into account by controlling for dietary factors when examining the relationship between yogurt consumption and disease risk.

2.5.2 Lifestyle and Sociodemographic Factors

In a cross section of diabetic patients in Mauritius, yogurt intake was positively associated with family meal frequency, which is thought to be associated with an increased intake of fruits and vegetables (Ruhee and Mahomoodally 2015). In urban Pakistan, among a cross section of adults, a seafood and yogurt dietary pattern was identified; individuals who followed this pattern were less likely to have hypertension or use tobacco and were more likely to exercise, but were also more likely to have a higher body mass index (BMI) (Safdar et al. 2015, Safdar et al. 2013).

In two U.S. cohorts (Framingham Heart Study Offspring Cohort and Generation Three cohort), consuming yogurt was significantly associated with younger age and a lower proportion of regular smokers. Unexpectedly, the nonconsumers had a significantly higher physical activity score than consumers, although the difference was minimal (Wang et al. 2013). Another American study among children showed that there were significant differences in race and income-to-poverty ratio among children who frequently consumed yogurt. Frequent yogurt intake was also significantly greater in younger children (2–11 years) compared with adolescents (12–18 years) and among children who met physical activity recommendations (Zhu et al. 2015).

In a cohort of French Canadian adults, there was a significantly greater proportion of women categorized as yogurt consumers compared with men. There were, however, no significant differences between yogurt consumers and nonconsumers for other demographic variables: education, marital status, or personal income (Cormier et al. 2015).

Yogurt consumption among Italian adults was identified in a group of healthy dietary habits and was more common among individuals with greater education (Ricceri et al. 2015). Similarly, a subsequent study identifying 22.7% of Italians (18–97 years old) as yogurt consumers observed that higher yogurt intakes occurred among adults with more education. Yogurt consumers were also more physically active, had better knowledge of food and health, and read food labels more. This study indicated that Italian yogurt consumers had healthier lifestyle behaviors and were more educated than nonconsumers (D'Addezio et al. 2015).

In cohorts of Spanish adults from the Seguimiento University of Navarra (SUN) study, more frequent yogurt consumption was associated with greater time spent doing weekly physical activity, younger age, the female gender, and lower proportions of current and former smokers and married people. There were, however, no differences between frequencies of yogurt consumption and time spent sitting or watching TV. Contrary to what has been observed in other populations, more frequent yogurt consumption was associated with fewer years of education (Martinez-Gonzalez et al. 2014, Sayon-Orea et al. 2015).

In a cross-sectional study of Brazilian adults, yogurt consumption was more likely among individuals who were nonsmokers, had a higher per capita income, were of the female gender, and were between 20 and 39 years old (Possa et al. 2015). In another Brazilian cross-sectional study, adults over 45 years had higher intakes of light yogurt than younger adults. Among younger adults, there was more seasonal variation in their consumption patterns and less light yogurt was consumed in the winter (Rossato et al. 2015). Even though the average daily yogurt intake in Brazil is very low, it appears to be consumed significantly more by urban-dwelling than rural-dwelling Brazilians (Murphy et al. 2016).

Taken together, the studies summarized highlight commonalities between yogurt consumers, such as a higher income. However, some differences in lifestyle between yogurt consumers were also observed for physical activity and education. Nevertheless, knowing that there may be significant differences between yogurt consumers and nonconsumers, it is important to take lifestyle variables into account when investigating the relationship between yogurt consumption and disease risk in order to minimize the possibility of confounding these complex relationships.

2.6 CONCLUSIONS

- Health authorities generally unanimously recognize yogurt as an optional serving of daily recommended dairy products that play a role as part of a healthy diet; it contributes key nutrients such as calcium, phosphorus, thiamin, vitamin B12, and protein. However, the daily recommended

portions of dairy products and the portion size of yogurt varies between countries. Most health organizations emphasize consuming nonfat or low-fat dairy and an increasing number of organizations are also recommending unsweetened dairy.
- Dairy product consumption varies greatly across populations (e.g., 61.6 cups per person per year in the United States versus 280 cups per year per person in France) and in Occidental countries dairy foods (milk, yogurt, and cheese) are the primary sources of dietary calcium.
- Yogurt and dairy products contain substantial amounts of macronutrients, vitamins, and minerals and are generally nutrient-dense foods. Even if there is no standard definition of a nutrient-dense food, existing nutrient density systems classify plain yogurt as nutrient dense. Sweetened and whole-fat yogurts, however, may not always be considered nutrient-dense foods.
- In American (or Westernized) diets, it would be difficult to consume adequate intakes of nutrients of concern with a dairy-free diet. In this context, yogurt consumption helps consumers to achieve recommended intakes of calcium, potassium, magnesium, and riboflavin, as well as vitamin D (in fortified yogurts).
- An overall higher diet quality has been observed with increased dairy and yogurt consumption. However, several populations do not reach the recommended intake of dairy products. Dairy product avoidance could have a negative effect on health, since these products are a source of essential nutrients (especially calcium). Scientific institutions and regulatory authorities in Western countries increased the recommendations for calcium and vitamin D intake in 2011.
- Fermented products, such as yogurt, are a vehicle for fortification and can be an efficient tool to combat nutrient deficiencies, that is, vitamin D.
- Yogurt consumers across various distinct populations appear to have healthier dietary patterns, nutrient adequacy, and lifestyles compared with nonconsumers.

REFERENCES

Camilleri, G. M., E. O. Verger, J. F. Huneau, F. Carpentier, C. Dubuisson, and F. Mariotti. 2013. Plant and animal protein intakes are differently associated with nutrient adequacy of the diet of French adults. *J Nutr* 143 (9):1466–73.

Chandan, R. C., and A. Kilara. 2013. *Manufacturing Yogurt and Fermented Milks*. Hoboken, NJ: Wiley-Blackwell.

Clerfeuille, E., M. Maillot, E. O. Verger, A. Lluch, N. Darmon, and N. Rolf-Pedersen. 2013. Dairy products: How they fit in nutritionally adequate diets. *J Acad Nutr Diet* 113 (7):950–56.

Cluskey, M., S. S. Wong, R. Richards, M. Ballejos, M. Reicks, G. Auld, C. Boushey, C. Bruhn, S. Misner, B. Olson, and S. Zaghloul. 2015. Dietary sources of calcium among parents and their early adolescent children in the United States by parent race/ethnicity and place of birth. *J Immigr Minor Health* 17 (2):432–40.

Coelho Nde, L., D. B. Cunha, A. P. Esteves, E. M. Lacerda, and M. M. Theme Filha. 2015. Dietary patterns in pregnancy and birth weight. *Rev Saude Publica* 49:62.

Cormier, H., E. Thifault, V. Garneau, A. Tremblay, V. Drapeau, L. Perusse, and M. C. Vohl. 2016. Association between yogurt consumption, dietary patterns, and cardio-metabolic risk factors. *Eur J Nutr* 55 (2):577–87.

D'Addezio, L., L. Mistura, S. Sette, and A. Turrini. 2015. Sociodemographic and lifestyle characteristics of yogurt consumers in Italy: Results from the INRAN-SCAI 2005–06 survey. *Med J Nutrition Metab* 8 (2):119–29.

Darmon, N., F. Vieux, M. Maillot, J. L. Volatier, and A. Martin. 2009. Nutrient profiles discriminate between foods according to their contribution to nutritionally adequate diets: A validation study using linear programming and the SAIN, LIM system. *Am J Clin Nutr* 89 (4):1227–36.

Drewnowski, A. 2005. Concept of a nutritious food: Toward a nutrient density score. *Am J Clin Nutr* 82 (4):721–32.

Drewnowski, A., and V. L. Fulgoni, 3rd. 2008. Nutrient profiling of foods: Creating a nutrient-rich food index. *Nutr Rev* 66 (1):23–39.

Drewnowski, A., and V. L. Fulgoni, 3rd. 2014. Nutrient density: Principles and evaluation tools. *Am J Clin Nutr* 99 (5 Suppl):1223S–28S.

Drewnowski, A., W. Tang, and R. Brazeilles. 2015. Calcium requirements from dairy foods in France can be met at low energy and monetary cost. *Br J Nutr* 114 (11):1920–28.

Dror, D. K., and L. H. Allen. 2014. Dairy product intake in children and adolescents in developed countries: Trends, nutritional contribution, and a review of association with health outcomes. *Nutr Rev* 72 (2):68–81.

EFSA Panel on Dietetic Products, Nutrition and Allergies. 2010. Scientific opinion on lactose thresholds in lactose intolerance and galactosemia. *EFSA Journal* 8 (9):1777.

El-Abbadi, N. H., M. C. Dao, and S. N. Meydani. 2014. Yogurt: Role in healthy and active aging. *Am J Clin Nutr* 99 (5 Suppl):1263S–70S.

Erickson, J., and J. Slavin. 2015. Total, added, and free sugars: Are restrictive guidelines science-based or achievable? *Nutrients* 7 (4):2866–78.

Fisberg, M., and R. Machado. 2015. History of yogurt and current patterns of consumption. *Nutr Rev* 73 (Suppl 1):4–7.

Food Standards Australia New Zealand. 2016. Nutrient content claims and health claims. Accessed May 18. http://www.foodstandards.gov.au/consumer/labelling/nutrition/Pages/default.aspx.

Foote, J. A., S. P. Murphy, L. R. Wilkens, P. P. Basiotis, and A. Carlson. 2004. Dietary variety increases the probability of nutrient adequacy among adults. *J Nutr* 134 (7):1779–85.

Fulgoni, V. L., 3rd, D. R. Keast, and A. Drewnowski. 2009. Development and validation of the nutrient-rich foods index: A tool to measure nutritional quality of foods. *J Nutr* 139 (8):1549–54.

Garriguet, D. 2004. *Overview of Canadians' Eating Habits*. Edited by Statistics Canada. Ottawa: Governmemnt of Canada.

Gazibarich, B, and PF Ricci. 1998. Towards better food choices: The nutritious food index. *Aust J Nutr Diet* 55:10–20.

German Nutrition Society. 2013. *Nutrition Circle*. Bonn, Germany: Deutsche Gesellschaft für Ernährung.

Glanz, K., J. Hersey, S. Cates, M. Muth, D. Creel, J. Nicholls, V. L. Fulgoni, 3rd, and S. Zaripheh. 2012. Effect of a nutrient rich foods consumer education program: Results from the nutrition advice study. *J Acad Nutr Diet* 112 (1):56–63.

Goverment of Canada. 2016. Consumption of dairy products. Accessed May 15. http://www.dairyinfo.gc.ca/index_e.php?s1=dff-fcil&s2=cons&s3=conscdn.

Green, B. P., L. Turner, E. Stevenson, and P. L. S. Rumbold. 2015. Short communication: Patterns of dairy consumption in free-living children and adolescents. *J Dairy Sci* 98 (6):3701–5.

Hansen, R. G., B. W. Wyse, and A. W. Sorenson. 1979. *Nutrition Quality Index of Food*. Westport, CT: AVI Publishing.

Health Canada. 2012. *Do Canadian Adults Meet Their Nutrient Requirements Through Food Intake Alone*? Ottawa: Government of Canada.
Hébel, P. 2007. *Comportements et Consommations Alimentaires en France*. Paris: CRÉDOC.
Hess, J., and J. Slavin. 2014. Snacking for a cause: Nutritional insufficiencies and excesses of U.S. children, a critical review of food consumption patterns and macronutrient and micronutrient intake of U.S. children. *Nutrients* 6 (11):4750–59.
Hess, J. M., S. S. Jonnalagadda, and J. L. Slavin. 2016. Dairy foods: Current evidence of their effects on bone, cardiometabolic, cognitive, and digestive health. *Compr Rev Food Sci Food Saf* 15 (2):251–68.
Institut de Veille Sanitaire. 2007. Etude nationale nutrition santé, 2006: Situation nutritionnelle en France en 2006 selon les indicateurs d'objectif et les repères du programme national nutrition santé (pnns). Paris.
Johnson-Down, L., H. Ritter, L. J. Starkey, and K. Gray-Donald. 2006. Primary food sources of nutrients in the diet of Canadian adults. *Can J Diet Pract Res* 67 (1):7–13.
Kashino, I., A. Nanri, K. Kurotani, S. Akter, K. Yasuda, M. Sato, H. Hayabuchi, and T. Mizoue. 2015. Association of dietary patterns with serum adipokines among Japanese: A cross-sectional study. *Nutr J* 14:58.
Keast, D. R., K. M. Hill Gallant, A. M. Albertson, C. K. Gugger, and N. M. Holschuh. 2015. Associations between yogurt, dairy, calcium, and vitamin D intake and obesity among U.S. children aged 8–18 years: Nhanes, 2005–2008. *Nutrients* 7 (3):1577–93.
Kong, L. C., B. A. Holmes, A. Cotillard, F. Habi-Rachedi, R. Brazeilles, S. Gougis, N. Gausseres, et al. 2014. Dietary patterns differently associate with inflammation and gut microbiota in overweight and obese subjects. *PLoS One* 9 (10):e109434.
Kratz, M., T. Baars, and S. Guyenet. 2013. The relationship between high-fat dairy consumption and obesity, cardiovascular, and metabolic disease. *Eur J Nutr* 52 (1):1–24.
Lachance, P. A., and M. C. Fisher. 1986. Educational and technological innovations required to enhance the selection of desirable nutrients. *Clin Nutr* 5:257–64.
Li, L. M., K. Q. Rao, L. Z. Kong, C. H. Yao, H. D. Xiang, F. Y. Zhai, G. S. Ma, and X. G. Yang. 2005. A description on the Chinese national nutrition and health survey in 2002. *Zhonghua Liu Xing Bing Xue Za Zhi* 26 (7):478–84.
Longley, C. E., L. H. McArthur, and D. Holbert. 2014. Rural Latino parents offer preschool children few nutrient-dense snacks: A community-based study in western Illinois. *Hisp Health Care Int* 12 (4):189–97.
Lysionek, A. E., M. B. Zubillaga, M. J. Salgueiro, A. Pineiro, R. A. Caro, R. Weill, and J. R. Boccio. 2002. Bioavailability of microencapsulated ferrous sulfate in powdered milk produced from fortified fluid milk: A prophylactic study in rats. *Nutrition* 18 (3):279–81.
Maillot, M., A. Drewnowski, F. Vieux, and N. Darmon. 2011. Quantifying the contribution of foods with unfavourable nutrient profiles to nutritionally adequate diets. *Br J Nutr* 105 (8):1133–37.
Markovic, T. P., and S. J. Natoli. 2009. Paradoxical nutritional deficiency in overweight and obesity: The importance of nutrient density. *Med J Aust* 190 (3):149–51.
Martinez-Gonzalez, M. A., C. Sayon-Orea, M. Ruiz-Canela, C. de la Fuente, A. Gea, and M. Bes-Rastrollo. 2014. Yogurt consumption, weight change and risk of overweight/obesity: The SUN cohort study. *NMCD* 24 (11):1189–96.
Michels, N., S. De Henauw, L. Beghin, M. Cuenca-Garcǐa, M. Gonzalez-Gross, L. Hallstrom, A. Kafatos, et al. 2016. Ready-to-eat cereals improve nutrient, milk and fruit intake at breakfast in European adolescents. *Eur J Nutr* 55 (2):771–9.
Michels, N., S. De Henauw, C. Breidenassel, L. Censi, M. Cuenca-García, M. Gonzalez-Gross, F. Gottrand, et al. 2015. European adolescent ready-to-eat-cereal (RTEC) consumers have a healthier dietary intake and body composition compared with non-RTEC consumers. *Eur J Nutr* 54 (4):653–64.

Miller, G. D., J. K. Jarvis, and L. D. McBean. 2001. The importance of meeting calcium needs with foods. *J Am Coll Nutr* 20 (2 Suppl):168S–85S.

Mobley, A. R., J. D. Jensen, and M. K. Maulding. 2014. Attitudes, beliefs, and barriers related to milk consumption in older, low-income women. *J Nutr Educ Behav* 46 (6):554–59.

Moreno Aznar, L. A., P. C. Ral, R. M. Ortega Anta, J. J. Díaz Martín, E. Baladia, J. Basulto, S. Bel Serrat, et al. 2013. Scientific evidence about the role of yogurt and other fermented milks in the healthy diet for the Spanish population. *Nutr Hosp* 28 (6):2039–89.

Muehlhoff, E., A. Bennett, and D. McMahon, eds. 2013. *Milk and Dairy Products in Human Nutrition*. Rome: FAO.

Murphy, M. M., L. M. Barraj, L. D. Toth, L. S. Harkness, and D. R. Bolster. 2016. Daily intake of dairy products in Brazil and contributions to nutrient intakes: A cross-sectional study. *Public Health Nutr* 19 (3):393–400.

National Institute of Nutrition. 2011. *Dietary Guidelines for Indians: A Manual*. Hyderabad, Telangana: National Institute of Nutrition.

Neyestani, T. R., B. Nikooyeh, A. Kalayi, M. Zahedirad, and N. Shariatzadeh. 2015. A vitamin D-calcium-fortified yogurt drink decreased serum pth but did not affect osteocalcin in subjects with type 2 diabetes. *Int J Vitam Nutr Res* 85 (1–2):61–69.

Nicklas, T. A., A. Drewnowski, and C. E. O'Neil. 2014. The nutrient density approach to healthy eating: Challenges and opportunities. *Public Health Nutr* 17 (12):2626–36.

Possa, G., M. A. de Castro, D. M. Lobo Marchioni, R. M. Fisberg, and M. Fisberg. 2015. Probability and amounts of yogurt intake are differently affected by sociodemographic, economic, and lifestyle factors in adults and the elderly: Results from a population-based study. *Nutr Res* 35 (8):700–6.

Public Health England, Welsh Government, Scottish Government, and Food Standards Agency in Northern Ireland. 2013. *Your Guide to the Eatwell Plate: Helping You Eat a Healthier Diet*. Public Health England.

Quann, E. E., V. L. Fulgoni, 3rd, and N. Auestad. 2015. Consuming the daily recommended amounts of dairy products would reduce the prevalence of inadequate micronutrient intakes in the United States: Diet modeling study based on NHANES 2007–2010. *Nutr J* 14 (1):90.

Rayner, M., P. Scarborough, and P. Lobstein. 2009. The UK Ofcom nutrient profiling model: Defining "healthy" and "unhealthy" food and drinks for TV advertising to children. Accessed May 22, 2016. https://www.ndph.ox.ac.uk/bhfcpnp/about/publications-and-reports/group-reports/uk-ofcom-nutrient-profile-model.pdf.

Ricceri, F., M. T. Giraudo, S. Sieri, V. Pala, G. Masala, I. Ermini, M. C. Giurdanella, et al. 2015. Dietary habits and social differences: The experience of EPIC-italy. *Epidemiol Prev* 39 (5–6):315–21.

Ross, A. C., C. L. Taylor, and A. L. Yaktine,. 2011. *Dietary Reference Intakes for Vitamin D and Calcium*. Edited by Food and Nutrition Board. Institute of Medicine of the National Academies. Washington, DC: The National Academies Press.

Rossato, S. L., M. T. Olinto, R. L. Henn, L. B. Moreira, S. A. Camey, L. A. Anjos, V. Wahrlich, et al. Seasonal variation in food intake and the interaction effects of sex and age among adults in southern Brazil. *Eur J Clin Nutr* 69 (9):1015–22.

Rozenberg, S., J. J. Body, O. Bruyere, P. Bergmann, M. L. Brandi, C. Cooper, J. P. Devogelaer, et al. 2016. Effects of dairy products consumption on health: Benefits and beliefs-a commentary from the Belgian Bone Club and the European Society for Clinical and Economic Aspects of Osteoporosis, Osteoarthritis and Musculoskeletal Diseases. *Calcif Tissue Int* 98 (1):1–17.

Ruhee, D., and F. Mahomoodally. 2015. Relationship between family meal frequency and individual dietary intake among diabetic patients. *J Diabetes Metab Disord* 14:66.

Safdar, N. F., E. Bertone-Johnson, L. Cordeiro, T. H. Jafar, and N. L. Cohen. 2013. Dietary patterns of Pakistani adults and their associations with sociodemographic, anthropometric and life-style factors. *J Nutr Sci* 2:e42.

Safdar, N. F., E. R. Bertone-Johnson, L. Cordeiro, T. H. Jafar, and N. L. Cohen. 2015. Dietary patterns and their association with hypertension among Pakistani urban adults. *Asia Pac J Clin Nutr* 24 (4):710–19.

Saint-Eve, A., H. Leclercq, S. Berthelo, B. Saulnier, W. Oettgen, and J. Delarue. 2016. How much sugar do consumers add to plain yogurts? Insights from a study examining French consumer behavior and self-reported habits. *Appetite* 99:277–84.

Sayon-Orea, C., M. Bes-Rastrollo, A. Marti, A. M. Pimenta, N. Martin-Calvo, and M. A. Martinez-Gonzalez. 2015. Association between yogurt consumption and the risk of metabolic syndrome over 6 years in the SUN study. *BMC Public Health* 15:170.

Scheidt, D. M., and E. Daniel. 2004. Composite index for aggregating nutrient density using food labels: Ratio of recommended to restricted food components. *J Nutr Educ Behav* 36 (1):35–39.

Schroder, H., J. Vila, J. Marrugat, and M. I. Covas. 2008. Low energy density diets are associated with favorable nutrient intake profile and adequacy in free-living elderly men and women. *J Nutr* 138 (8):1476–81.

Shiby, V. K., and H. N. Mishra. 2013. Fermented milks and milk products as functional foods: A review. *Crit Rev Food Sci Nutr* 53 (5):482–96.

The National Academies of Sciences. 2016. Dietary reference intakes tables and application. Accessed April 15. http://www.nationalacademies.org/hmd/Activities/Nutrition/SummaryDRIs/DRI-Tables.aspx.

U.S. Department of Agriculture, Economic Research Service. 2016. Dairy data. USDA Accessed May 27. http://www.ers.usda.gov/data-products/dairy-data.aspx.

U.S. Department of Agriculture. 2010. *Dietary Guidelines for Americans*. Washington, DC: USDA.

Van Staveren, W. A., and L. C. de Groot. 2011. Evidence-based dietary guidance and the role of dairy products for appropriate nutrition in the elderly. *J Am Coll Nutr* 30 (5 Suppl 1):429S–37S.

Wang, H., K. A. Livingston, C. S. Fox, J. B. Meigs, and P. F. Jacques. 2013. Yogurt consumption is associated with better diet quality and metabolic profile in American men and women. *Nutr Res* 33 (1):18–26.

Weaver, C. M. 2014. How sound is the science behind the dietary recommendations for dairy? *Am J Clin Nutr* 99 (5 Suppl):1217S–22S.

Webb, D., S. M. Donovan, and S. N. Meydani. 2014. The role of yogurt in improving the quality of the American diet and meeting dietary guidelines. *Nutr Rev* 72 (3):180–89.

Weinberg, L. G., L. A. Berner, and J. E. Groves. 2004. Nutrient contributions of dairy foods in the United States, continuing survey of food intakes by individuals, 1994–1996, 1998. *J Am Diet Assoc* 104 (6):895–902.

WHO. 2015. *Information Note About Intake of Sugars Recommended in the WHO Guideline for Adults and Children*. Geneva: WHO Press.

Williams, E. B., B. Hooper, A. Spiro, and S. Stanner. 2015. The contribution of yogurt to nutrient intakes across the life course. *Nutr Bull* 40 (1):9–32.

Wood, A. D., A. A. Strachan, F. Thies, L. S. Aucott, D. M. Reid, A. C. Hardcastle, A. Mavroeidi, et al. 2014. Patterns of dietary intake and serum carotenoid and tocopherol status are associated with biomarkers of chronic low-grade systemic inflammation and cardiovascular risk. *Br J Nutr* 112 (8):1341–52.

Zhu, Y., H. Wang, J. H. Hollis, and P. F. Jacques. 2015. The associations between yogurt consumption, diet quality, and metabolic profiles in children in the USA. *Eur J Nutr* 54 (4):543–50.

Section II

Yogurt and Cardiometabolic Health

3 Weight Management and Obesity

The incidence of overweight and obesity is a major health concern worldwide. Even more worrisome is the fact that childhood obesity has increased dramatically since 1990 and is one of the most critical public health challenges of the twenty-first century (WHO 2012). Although genetic determinants can be involved in excessive weight gain, especially in some susceptible populations, it is clear that behavioral and environmental factors are keys to the rapid and epidemic rise of obesity in the world. Physical activity and a healthy diet are key factors in maintaining energy balance and preventing weight gain. Additionally, the substitution of nutrient-poor, energy-dense foods with nutrient-rich foods can have a positive impact on obesity prevention (Bowman and Vinyard 2004). Yogurt is a nutrient-dense food that can be incorporated into a healthy diet within a meal or as a snack and can help to manage appetite and body weight (Tremblay et al. 2015).

In the last few years, increasing attention has been paid to the impact of dairy product intake on weight maintenance and obesity. However, there is conflicting evidence regarding the relationship between dairy product consumption and body weight regulation. Some observational studies involving children and adolescents reported a significant inverse relationship between dairy consumption and measures of body composition (Barba et al. 2005, Novotny et al. 2003, Moore et al. 2008, Fiorito et al. 2006), while others have failed to detect such associations in the same populations (Berkey et al. 2005, Huh et al. 2010, Noel et al. 2011) or they have been confounded by energy intake (O'Sullivan et al. 2015). A systematic review of prospective cohort studies investigated the effects of dairy foods on overweight and obesity and identified 10 studies among children and adolescents. The authors concluded that while evidence demonstrated promising protective effects of dairy on overweight and obesity, it was not consistent enough to be entirely conclusive (Louie et al. 2011). Moreover, other reviews of the effects of milk and milk products on body weight in children and adolescents have shown contradictory results (Spence et al. 2011, Matthews et al. 2011). A meta-analysis conducted in 2014 has shown an inverse association between dairy food intake and adiposity in adolescents but no significant associations in preschool- and school-aged children (Dror 2014), which adds further ambiguity to the relationship between dairy foods and obesity in youth.

Two meta-analyses revealed that dairy products may have benefits in facilitating weight loss in adults in short-term or energy-restricted randomized controlled trials, but do not support the beneficial effect in long-term trials or studies without energy restriction (Chen et al. 2012, Abargouei et al. 2012). Similar findings were found in a subsequent meta-analysis of 41 randomized controlled trials examining the effects of increasing calcium (900 mg in supplements or 1,300 mg in three portions of dairy products) on weight. Increasing calcium intake through supplements or dairy products did not have an impact on short-term weight loss. The authors also concluded that fat loss was facilitated during energy-restricted diets by the consumption of three portions of dairy products per day (Booth et al. 2015). However, there is growing evidence from epidemiological data (five cross-sectional and seven prospective studies) showing a modest but significant inverse association between dairy product consumption and body weight gain in adults (Dougkas et al. 2011). This relationship has been supported, in part, by several reviews (Mozaffarian 2016, Moreno et al. 2015, Rozenberg et al. 2015).

Consuming more dairy products and fiber-rich foods and less refined grains, meat, and sugar-rich foods and drinks was associated with less weight gain in prospective cohort studies. The relationships between foods/dietary patterns and weight gain were stronger compared with those between macronutrients and weight gain (Fogelholm et al. 2012). Among dairy products, yogurt in particular has been associated with healthy dietary patterns and has shown to be beneficial for weight management (Rozenberg et al. 2015, Mozaffarian 2016). While few randomized controlled trials have evaluated the effect of yogurt on weight maintenance and obesity, prospective and cross-sectional studies evaluating food patterns provide interesting data on the relationship between yogurt and body weight. This chapter will report the existing studies that have investigated the relationship between weight, adiposity, and total yogurt consumption (fat free, low fat, full fat, unsweetened, sweetened, artificially sweetened, drinkable, high in protein, etc.). Summaries of observational adult studies for cross-sectional and prospective cohort studies that will be described are listed in Tables 3.1 and 3.2, respectively.

3.1 STUDIES IN CHILDREN AND ADOLESCENTS

Moreira et al. (2010) described the association between obesity, self-reported food consumption and gender, parental education, physical activity, and sleeping in 1976 Portuguese children. Food patterns that included fast food, sugar-sweetened beverages, and pastries were associated with TV viewing and male gender, while a higher level of maternal education and longer sleeping duration were positively associated with a dietary pattern that included fruits and vegetables. There were no associations between obesity and food patterns that included milk and milk puddings. Obesity was positively associated with the dietary pattern, including yogurt, cheese, and ice cream. These foods are commonly consumed by Portuguese children as savory snacks or desserts (Moreira et al. 2010).

A cross-sectional study performed on 1,000 Portuguese adolescents aimed to examine the independent associations between different dairy products and body mass index (BMI) and percentage body fat in adolescents. For boys and girls, respectively, total dairy product consumption was 2.6 ± 1.9 and 2.9 ± 2.5 servings per day, yogurt consumption was 0.5 ± 0.6 and 0.4 ± 0.7 servings per day, milk consumption was 1.7 ± 1.4 and 2.0 ± 1.7 servings per day, and cheese consumption was 0.4 ± 0.6 and 0.5 ± 0.8 servings per day. After adjusting for different factors, only milk intake was negatively associated with BMI and percentage of body fat in girls (Abreu et al. 2012a).

TABLE 3.1
Summary of Findings and Implications of Cross-Sectional Studies That Have Examined Weight and Adiposity in Relation to Yogurt Consumption

Cross Sectional Study	Population Age	Diet Assessment	Yogurt Intake	Findings	Implications	References
National Health and Nutrition Examination Survey (1999–2004)	Adults ≥ 18 years $n = 14,618$	One or two 24-hour recalls	100 g servings	For every serving of yogurt there was a 2–2.5-fold reduction in the prevalence odds of obesity and central obesity	Positive	(Beydoun et al. 2008)
Compilation of South Australia dietary intervention trials (2004–2007)	Adults $n = 720$	Food frequency questionnaire	Not reported	Yogurt consumption was inversely associated with percentage body fat, abdominal fat, waist circumference, and hip circumference	Positive	(Murphy et al. 2013)
Korean Health and Nutrition Examination Survey (2007–2009)	Adults 19–64 years $n = 7,173$	Food frequency questionnaire and 24-hour recalls	≥1 time/day vs. 0	Higher intakes of yogurt were associated with a lower prevalence of obesity	Positive	(Lee et al. 2014)
Observation of Cardiovascular Risk Factors in Luxembourg (ORISCAV-LUX) survey	Adults 18–69 years $n = 1,352$	Semiquantified 134-item 3-month food frequency questionnaire	125 g servings Yogurt tertiles	The highest tertile of whole-fat yogurt intake was associated with a lower odds ratio for abdominal and global obesity when compared with the lowest tertile. The highest tertile of low-fat yogurt intake was associated with a higher odds ratio for abdominal and global obesity when compared with the lowest tertile of yogurt intake	Positive for whole-fat yogurt Negative for low-fat yogurt	(Crichton and Alkerwi 2014)

(Continued)

TABLE 3.1 (CONTINUED)
Summary of Findings and Implications of Cross-Sectional Studies That Have Examined Weight and Adiposity in Relation to Yogurt Consumption

Cross Sectional Study	Population Age	Diet Assessment	Yogurt Intake	Findings	Implications	References
INFOGENE study	Adults 18–55 years $n = 664$	91-item 12-month food frequency questionnaire	175 g serving Yogurt consumers vs. nonconsumers (no yogurt over 12-month period)	Yogurt consumers had significantly lower weights, waist-to-hip ratios, and waist circumference than nonconsumers. Normal-weight individuals consumed significantly higher amounts of high-fat yogurt (≥2% MF) than overweight or obese individuals. There were no differences in the amounts of low-fat yogurt (<2% MF) consumption between normal-weight and overweight individuals. Overweight individuals consumed significantly higher amounts of fat-free yogurt (0% MF) than normal-weight individuals.	Positive for total yogurt consumption and high-fat yogurt Neutral for low fat yogurt Negative for fat-free yogurt	(Cormier et al. 2015)
Fenland study	Adults 30–55 years $n = 10,092$	Eating pattern snacking frequency questionnaire Food frequency questionnaire	Yogurt (g/10 MJ per day)	Overweight individuals had lower intakes of yogurt compared with normal-weight participants	Positive	(O'Connor et al. 2014)

TABLE 3.2
Summary of Findings and Implications of Prospective Cohort Studies That Have Examined Weight and Adiposity in Relation to Yogurt Consumption

Prospective Cohort Study and Follow-Up Period	Population Age[a]	Diet Assessment	Yogurt Intake	Findings	Implications	References
Quebec Family Study (6-year follow-up)	Adults 18–65 years $n = 248$	3-day diet records (baseline, 6 year)	Not reported	Each serving of low-fat yogurt (<2%) consumed was associated with a 0.54 cm increase in waist circumference	Negative for waist circumference	Drapeau et al. 2004
Supplementation en Vitamines et Mineraux Antioxidants (SU.VI.MAX) trial (6-year follow-up)	Adults 35–60 years $n = 13{,}017$	≥6 24-hour recalls	125 g serving	Inverse association between weight gain and increase in waist circumference and yogurt intake in men overweight at baseline Inverse association between weight gain and yogurt intake in women normal weight at baseline	Positive for weight in both sexes; positive for waist circumference in men; neutral for waist circumference in women	Vergnaud et al. 2008
Nurses' Health Study (NHS), Nurses' Health Study II (NHS-II), and Healthy Professionals Follow-Up Study (HPFS) (12–20-year follow-up)	Adults 18–65 years $n = 120{,}877$	Three to five food frequency questionnaires	Not reported	Weight increase over 4-year period inversely associated with each daily yogurt serving in all three cohorts	Positive for weight	Mozaffarian et al. 2011

(*Continued*)

TABLE 3.2 (CONTINUED)
Summary of Findings and Implications of Prospective Cohort Studies That Have Examined Weight and Adiposity in Relation to Yogurt Consumption

Prospective Cohort Study and Follow-Up Period	Population Age[a]	Diet Assessment	Yogurt Intake	Findings	Implications	References
Seguimiento Universidad de Navarra (Mean follow-up of 6.6 year)	Adults 37.1 years (SD 10.8) n = 8,516	Food frequency questionnaire	125 g servings categorised according to 0–2, >2–<5, 5–<7, 7 and >7 servings/week	No yearly differences in yearly weight change and yogurt consumption High consumption (>7 servings/week) of total- and whole-fat yogurt was associated with lower incidence of overweight and obesity compared with low consumption (0–2 servings/week)	Neutral for weight; positive for waist circumference overweight and obesity incidence	Martinez-Gonzalez et al. 2014
Framingham Heart Study Offspring Cohort (13 year follow-up)	Adults 26–64 years n = 3,440	Four semi-quantitative food frequency questionnaires	One cup (250 mL)	Lower weight (0.09 kg/year) and waist circumference increases (0.14 cm/year) associated with consuming ≥ 3 servings/week of yogurt vs. <1 serving/week	Positive for weight and waist circumference	Wang et al. 2014
Nurses' Health Study (NHS), Nurses' Health Study II (NHS II), and Healthy Professionals Follow-Up Study (HPFS) (16–24 year follow-up)	Adults n = 120,784	Validated food frequency questionnaire every 4 years	Yogurt (250 mL serving)	Increased intakes of total, sweetened, or plain/artificially sweetened yogurt were strongly linked to relative weight loss.	Positive for weight	Smith et al. 2015

[a] Where n equals sample size of the study.

A cross-sectional study was performed in 903 Azorean adolescents in order to assess the association between dairy products intake and abdominal obesity. Adolescent food intake was evaluated using a self-administered, semiquantitative food frequency questionnaire and dairy products consumption was categorized in <2 and ≥2 servings per day. A protective association was found between two or more servings of milk and yogurt and abdominal obesity in boys. This association was not confounded by other lifestyle factors or nutritional variables (e.g., calcium intake) (Abreu et al. 2012b).

The relationship between obesity indicators, nutrient intakes, and yogurt and dairy consumption was investigated in a representative sample of 3,786 U.S. children (8–18 years old). Almost 58% of children consumed less than two portions of dairy per day, falling below nutritional recommendations to consume three portions of dairy foods daily. The prevalence of yogurt consumption was very low, with 91.5% of the cohort not consuming any yogurt based on 2-day food recalls. High total dairy food consumption was associated with higher intakes of energy and saturated fat, but lower intakes of sugar and carbohydrates, whereas yogurt consumers had lower intakes of fat and saturated fat ($p = .05$). Yogurt consumption and high dairy consumption were both associated with higher intakes of calcium, vitamin D, protein, and potassium compared with nonconsumers ($p = .01$). In a model controlling for energy, gender, age, race-ethnicity, alcohol, and tobacco, yogurt consumers had significantly lower waist circumferences, subscapular skinfolds, BMI for age, and prevalence of overweight/obesity. When additional covariates (poverty income level, physical activity, and screen time) were included in the model, the prevalence of obesity was attenuated. For dairy consumption, only the subscapular skin folds were significantly lower in the high dairy consumption group (≥2 servings/day) compared with the group with the lowest intake (<1 serving/day) for both models. The same relationship was seen between subscapular skin folds and both calcium and vitamin D intake. Yogurt, dairy, calcium, and vitamin D were all independently associated with indices of obesity in children (Keast et al. 2015).

In a cohort of adolescents (12.5–17.5 years) from eight European cities, in the Healthy Lifestyle in Europe by Nutrition (HELENA) study, the relationship between dairy food consumption and cardiovascular disease (CVD) risk factors was investigated. A significant inverse association was found between dairy intake and waist circumference. Additionally, girls with the highest yogurt intakes had lower waist circumference z-score as well as greater cardiovascular fitness (Moreno et al. 2015).

3.2 STUDIES IN ADULTS

3.2.1 Cross-Sectional Studies

A cross-sectional study among U.S. adults was performed from National Health and Nutrition Examination Survey 1999–2004 data (sample sizes ranged from 4,519 for metabolic syndrome to 14,618 for obesity). This study evaluated the association between the consumption of a variety of dairy products and their related nutrients with obesity and central obesity. In a multivariate model adjusting for other dietary confounders, each 100 g serving of yogurt was associated with a decrease in the prevalence odds for obesity (OR=0.57; 95% CI 0.40, 0.82) and central obesity (OR=0.58; 95% CI 0.42, 0.81). In contrast, cheese was associated with a higher prevalence of these outcomes (Beydoun et al. 2008).

A cross-sectional study of 720 overweight and obese Australian adults found that dairy food consumption was inversely associated with BMI, waist circumference, and the percentage of body fat in a model adjusted for age, sex, and total energy intake. In a complete model that also controlled for other dairy products, yogurt was inversely associated with the percentage of body fat, waist circumference, and hip circumference. Additionally, low-fat milk was inversely associated with BMI and waist circumference (Murphy et al. 2013).

Data from the Korean National Health and Nutrition Examination Study (2007, 2008 and 2009) examined associations between dairy foods, calcium intake, and obesity in 7,173 adults aged 19–64 years. A reduced prevalence of obesity was found to be associated with the highest quintiles of total dairy, milk, yogurt, dairy calcium, and total calcium intakes compared with the lowest quintiles (Lee et al. 2014).

Similar findings were observed among 1,352 participants from the Observation of Cardiovascular Risk Factors in Luxembourg Study. The highest tertile of whole-fat yogurt, as well as total whole-fat dairy and whole-fat milk, was significantly associated with lower odds for global obesity, even following adjustment for age, sex, dietary, lifestyle, and metabolic covariates. Among low-fat dairy, only low-fat yogurt was inversely associated with global obesity. The same inverse relationship between whole-fat yogurt and abdominal obesity was also seen for low-fat yogurt (Crichton and Alkerwi 2014).

In a small cross-sectional study of 664 Canadian adults from the INFOGENE study, 85% of participants were yogurt consumers with intakes averaging approximately 82 g per day. This reflects a higher consumption than seen in other cohorts. Nevertheless, results are similar to other populations. Yogurt consumers had a significantly lower weight, waist-to-hip ratio, and waist circumference than nonconsumers (Cormier et al. 2015).

A cross-sectional study of 10,092 adults in the United Kingdom found that individuals with a BMI ≥ 25 had greater intakes of chips, sweets, chocolates, and ice cream, as well as lower intakes of yogurt and nuts. All associations, however, were completely attenuated following adjustment for snacking frequency (O'Connor et al. 2015).

3.2.2 Prospective Studies

Drapeau et al. (2004) evaluated in a prospective study whether changes in some dietary patterns over a 6-year follow-up period would be associated with weight changes. The age of the participants ranged from 18 to 65 years. Data from the Quebec Family study indicated that an increased consumption of whole fruit as well as skimmed milk and partly skimmed milk were the only two food patterns that were negatively correlated with the changes in body weight and adiposity indicators. Yogurt (<2% fat) was positively associated with changes in weight circumference, 0.42 cm for additional serving ($p = .003$) (Drapeau et al. 2004).

A prospective study aimed at investigating the relationships between different types of dairy products and calcium intake with body weight and waist circumference was performed on 1,245 men and 1,022 women for 6 years. Subjects were participants of the *Supplementation en Vitamines et Mineraux Antioxidants* (SU.VI.MAX) study. In overweight men, an inverse association was found, particularly with yogurt ($p = .01$ for weight and 0.03 for waist circumference changes) and milk consumption ($p = .02$ for both weight and waist circumference changes). However, positive relationships were found between milk consumption and waist circumference change in overweight women, and yogurt consumption and weight change in normal-weight women. The authors concluded that the relationship between dairy products and calcium intake with changes in weight and waist circumference may differ according to sex, initial body-weight status, and type of dairy products. Components in yogurt and dairy products other than calcium or specific dietary patterns associated with dairy consumption may have had an impact on the observed associations (Vergnaud et al. 2008).

A prospective study was conducted with three separate cohorts (Nurses' Health Study, Nurses' Health Study II, and Healthy Professionals Follow-Up Study) and included 120,877 U.S. healthy and nonobese women and men at baseline. The relationships between changes in lifestyle factors and weight were evaluated at 4-year intervals and multivariable adjustments were assessed. Within each 4-year period, subjects gained an average of 3.35 lb (5th to 95th percentile, −4.1 to 12.4). Weight change was inversely associated with yogurt (−0.82 lb), vegetables, whole grains, fruits, and nuts ($p \leq .005$ for each comparison). The relationship between 4-year weight change and selected commonly consumed foods is illustrated in Figure 3.1.

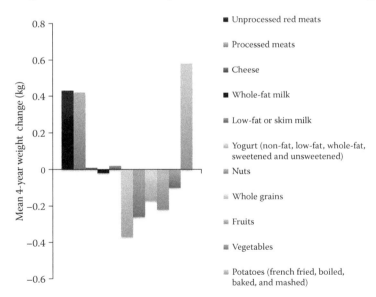

FIGURE 3.1 Mean 4-year changes in weight in relation to the consumption of common foods: multivariate adjusted pooled results from three American cohorts (Nurses' Health Study, Nurses' Health Study II, and Healthy Professionals Follow-Up Study). Four-year weight change adjusted for age, baseline BMI, sleep duration, changes in physical activity, alcohol use, television watching, smoking, and all other dietary variables. (Adapted from Mozaffarian et al. *N Engl J Med* 364 (25):2392–404, 2011.)

Significant associations with weight gain were not seen for other dairy foods. Moreover, no significant differences were seen for low-fat and skim milk versus whole-fat milk. However, the author pointed out the possibility that people who change their consumption of yogurt (or other foods) may have other behaviors that impact weight that were not measured (Mozaffarian et al. 2011).

The association between yogurt consumption and average weight gain was studied in a prospective cohort of 8,516 Spanish adults who were followed biennially in the Seguimiento Universidad de Navarra (SUN) project. In the study, dietary intake, measured with a 136-item food frequency questionnaire, was obtained at baseline and weights were recorded at baseline and then every 2 years. There were no statistically significant differences in the average yearly weight change and yogurt consumption frequency. However, over the follow-up period there was a marked decrease in risk for overweight and obesity for subjects consuming more than seven servings per week compared with zero to two servings per week of total yogurt (whole fat and low fat) or whole-fat yogurt (HR=0.8 [0.68–0.94] and HR=0.62 [0.47–0.82], respectively), but not low-fat yogurt (HR=0.84 [0.61–1.15]). Models were adjusted for sex, age, physical activity, TV viewing, sedentary activity, tobacco use, snacking, special diets, energy intake, adherence to the Mediterranean diet, marital status, education, and baseline BMI. Interestingly, this relationship was even stronger when subjects also reported high fruit consumption (Martinez-Gonzalez et al. 2014).

Dietary data, weight, and waist circumference were examined in 3,440 participants from the Framingham Heart Study Offspring Cohort from 1991 to 2008. Higher total dairy (≥ 3 servings/day) consumption was significantly associated with lower annual incremental weight gain ($p=.04$) after controlling for all covariates (age, sex, lifestyle factors, baseline weight, energy intake, and the Dietary Guidelines Adherence Index). Yogurt (≥ 3 servings/week) was the only dairy subgroup that remained significantly associated with a lower annual weight gain in the same model ($p=.03$). Waist circumference had similar relationships to total dairy and yogurt, with p-values of .05 and .03, respectively. Findings suggest that yogurt may play a role in the prevention of long-term weight gain and that its effects may be apparent at low doses (weekly vs. daily) (Wang et al. 2014).

A prospective study of three large U.S. cohorts (Nurse's Health Study, Nurse's Health Study II, and Health Professionals Follow-up Study) examined the relationship between 4-year changes of intakes of protein and carbohydrate foods and weight gain over a 16–24 year follow-up period. Over the follow-up, total yogurt, sweetened yogurt, and plain yogurt intakes did not change significantly in any of the cohorts. There was a weak positive association between changes in total yogurt and carbohydrate food intakes (Pearson correlation, $r=.12$). This correlation likely reflects the complex nutrient composition of yogurt containing both carbohydrates and protein. Total yogurt intake over the follow-up period was associated with a significant weight loss of 0.38–0.71 kg and remained significant even after adjusting for all covariates. The relative weight loss represents approximately 0.1–0.18 kg per year, which is likely to reflect weight management rather than clinically relevant weight loss. Regardless of whether carbohydrate intake increased, decreased, or stayed the same, yogurt was not associated with weight gain. This lack of association appeared to contradict relationships seen between other protein foods and carbohydrate foods. Furthermore, there was a trend toward greater weight loss when yogurt intakes coincided with an increase in carbohydrate intake (Smith et al. 2015).

3.2.3 Clinical Studies

In 2000, Zemel et al. observed that obese African-American adults who increased their calcium intake from 400 to 1,000 mg per day for 1 year with a yogurt-supplemented diet (two cups of yogurt per day) had a 4.9 kg reduction in body fat (Zemel et al. 2000). Another study from the group evaluated the impact of adding fat-free yogurt for 12 weeks to a reduced-calorie (−500 kcal/day) diet in obese adults with a low calcium intake (500–600 mg/day). The group who consumed yogurt (1,100 mg Ca/day) lost 22% more weight than the control group (400–500 mg Ca/day) (6.63 kg for yogurt group vs. 4.99 kg for control). In this study, the isocaloric substitution of yogurt for other foods significantly augmented fat loss and reduced central adiposity during energy restriction. This effect appears to be mediated by calcium supplementation in a population with a low calcium diet (Zemel et al. 2005).

A randomized controlled clinical trial was performed to compare the effects on anthropometric measurements and CVD risk factors of consuming a mix of low-glycemic index foods (such as yogurt, salad, and water) before (preload) or with a meal (control group). Subjects consumed similar amounts of macronutrients within a hypocaloric diet for 3 months. The body weight, waist circumference, and other CVD risk factors (triglyceride, total cholesterol, and systolic blood pressure) decreased more in the preload group ($p < .05$ for all). Moreover, fasting blood sugar and low-density lipoprotein cholesterol decreased significantly only in the preload group (Azadbakht et al. 2012).

A randomized comparative trial tested the differences in weight loss between two groups given energy-restricted diets. One group was asked to consume four to five portions of nonfat dairy per day, including two 6 oz portions of yogurt, and the other group was asked to consume three portions of nonfat dairy products per day. Both groups experienced significant weight loss following the 24-week weight-loss program; however, no differences in anthropometric outcomes were observed between intervention groups. An energy-restricted diet high in nonfat dairy, which included yogurt, was as effective as an energy-restricted diet with moderate nonfat dairy intake (Shlisky et al. 2015).

3.2.4 Reviews

A review by Jacques and Wang (2014) examined two randomized clinical trials (energy-restricted diets) and five prospective cohort studies that investigated the relationship between yogurt intake and weight. Results from the randomized clinical trials were similar, finding greater weight loss with yogurt interventions; however, the results were based on two short-term interventions involving weight loss under energy-restricted diets. Cohort studies had inconsistent outcomes and the authors concluded that the relationship between yogurt and weight remains ambiguous (Jacques and Wang 2014).

The latest systematic review of yogurt and weight management conducted in 2015 identified 14 eligible studies; 6 cohort studies, 7 cross-sectional studies, 6 randomized controlled trials, and 1 controlled trial. In epidemiological studies, yogurt intake was linked to lower BMI, body weight, weight gain, smaller waist circumference, and lower body fat. Findings from the randomized clinical trials remain inconclusive and do not permit a causal relationship between yogurt intake and weight loss; they included five nonsignificant weight losses, one nonsignificant weight gain, and one significant weight loss confounded by calcium intake (Eales et al. 2015). To date, no meta-analyses have been conducted of yogurt consumption and weight, obesity, or adiposity.

3.3 MECHANISMS OF ACTION

3.3.1 Studies on Satiety

Yogurt may influence energy balance by suppressing appetite, resulting in a reduced energy intake (Pei et al. 2015). Some studies have shown that yogurt may induce greater satiety than other foods, beverages, and snacks (Tsuchiya et al. 2006, Chapelot and Payen 2010, Almiron-Roig et al. 2009). A study with healthy women showed that yogurt had a greater effect on suppressing appetite compared with milk or cheese, but did not affect subsequent food intake compared with other dairy products. Moreover, yogurt led to reduced hunger, increased fullness, and delayed subsequent eating compared with snacks with a lower protein content (Douglas et al. 2012). However, in another study, a high-protein Greek yogurt (9 g) was insufficient to elicit protein-related improvements in markers of energy intake regulation compared with an isocaloric normal-protein regular yogurt (Ortinau et al. 2013). In a randomized crossover study, three 160 Kcal snacks (high-protein yogurt, high-fat crackers, and high-fat chocolate snacks) were tested for their satiating and hunger-reducing efficacy. No differences in feelings of fullness were noted. Yogurt was more effective in reducing feelings of afternoon hunger and in postponing dinner initiation by 30 minutes compared with the chocolate group. While yogurt appeared to be effective in enhancing satiety, the improved efficacy of yogurt over chocolate was likely related to its high protein content (Ortinau et al. 2014).

3.3.2 Micro- and Macronutrients and Their Physiological Effects

There is accumulating evidence suggesting that specific dairy product components affect physiological functions and food intake regulation. Epidemiological studies have shown that low calcium intake is a risk factor for overweight and obesity (Tremblay and Gilbert 2011). Moreover, evidence from intervention trials supports that calcium intake promotes weight loss (Dougkas et al. 2011, Heaney 2011). This effect might be explained by an increase in fat oxidation (Zemel et al. 2008), fecal loss, and the facilitation of appetite control (Tremblay and Gilbert 2011). Interestingly, a randomized placebo-controlled trial has shown that, during an energy-restricted diet program, milk supplementation, provided to female low-calcium consumers, attenuated weight loss-related increases in appetite (Gilbert et al. 2011). Moreover, a higher Ca:P ratio has been shown to contribute to a lower prevalence of central obesity (Pereira et al. 2013).

Other factors such as total energy intake (yogurt is low in energy), protein amount and source, and vitamin D status may act synergistically to regulate energy balance, promoting reduction or prevention of body fat accumulation (Teegarden 2005). Among dairy components, proteins have the greatest putative role in satiety. Indeed, proteins have been shown to be more satiating than other macronutrients in the short term, over 24 hours, and in the long term and thermogenesis plays a role in this effect (Westerterp-Plantenga 2003). The satiety effect depends not only on the dose and physical characteristics of protein (e.g., viscosity and gel strength), but could also depend on the source of protein (Solah et al. 2010, Ricci-Cabello et al. 2012). Whey proteins deliver a concentrated source of branched-chain amino acids, particularly L-leucine, and have the potential to impact both short- and long-term satiety (Marette and Picard-Deland 2014). Whey proteins have been shown to be more insulinotropic compared with casein or other animal and plant proteins, which could impact appetite and food intake (Nilsson et al. 2004). However, other studies have found similar effects between whey protein and casein on food intake and satiety (Veldhorst et al. 2009, Bowen et al. 2006). Thus, inconsistent data exists from human studies regarding the role of protein sources on satiety (Westerterp-Plantenga et al. 2012).

Mechanisms by which milk peptides could exert their effect on food intake via the gastrointestinal tract include the stimulation of gut hormone receptors (e.g., cholecystokinin [CCK; Pupovac and Anderson 2002] and glucagon-like peptide-1 [Aziz and Anderson 2003]). These hormones may affect organs and tissues after absorption into the bloodstream, slowing stomach emptying, perhaps via opioid receptors (Pupovac and Anderson 2002). Bioactive peptides could also act on adipocyte lipogenesis via the renin angiotensin system (Huth et al. 2006). Interestingly, glycomacropeptide (GMP) from whey protein has been shown to lead to appetite suppression in animal models (Ricci-Cabello et al. 2012). Moreover, alpha-lactalbumin could also play a role in appetite regulation. Indeed, a study reported that an alpha-lactalbumin-enriched yogurt drink suppressed hunger and the desire to eat more than a whey-enriched yogurt drink (Hursel et al. 2010). Furthermore, the branched-chain amino acids leucine, isoleucine, and valine, which are present in high proportions in dairy protein (about 21%–26%), could stimulate protein synthesis and preserve lean body mass during weight-loss regimens (Layman and Walker 2006).

Interestingly, it has been reported in a large European study that a modest increase in protein content and a modest reduction in the glycemic index in the diet led to an improved weight-loss maintenance and completion rate of the intervention (Larsen et al. 2010). Lactose, the main carbohydrate in yogurt, is classified as a low-glycemic index carbohydrate (glycemic index of lactose=46). Low-glycemic index foods may contribute to increased satiety and reduced energy intake by affecting blood glucose concentrations and insulin responses and by stimulating gut peptides (Dougkas et al. 2011).

Yogurt lipids could also play a role in protecting against obesity and weight gain. Diets rich in medium-chain fatty acids have been associated with a reduction in body fat in human subjects (Nagao and Yanagita 2008, Tsuji et al. 2001, St-Onge et al. 2000). A significant borderline inverse relationship between frequent whole-fat yogurt consumption (≥875 g/week) and adiposity compared with less frequent whole-fat yogurt intake (≤250 g/week) was observed in a Mediterranean population from a prospective cohort followed for 6 years; OR=0.85 (95% CI: 0.73–0.99) (Sayon-Orea et al. 2015). Dairy fat contains bioactive lipids that may play an important role in energy regulation and weight maintenance. For example, the antiobesogenic effects of conjugated linoleic acid (CLA) have been widely studied; consumption has been shown to reduce body fat in animals. However, results in humans are less conclusive (Plourde et al. 2008). CLA is thought to optimize energy balance through pathways that increase energy expenditure, prevent adipocyte differentiation, promote lipolysis, and enhance fat oxidation (Wang and Jones 2004). It has also been hypothesized that bioactive dairy fats could activate peroxisome proliferator-activated receptor (PPAR) pathways to promote energy balance (Parodi 2016).

3.3.3 Viscosity

Some researchers have been investigating the influence of food viscosity on the regulation of energy intake. The energy content of a food could depend on the food's characteristics, such as texture, which could influence subsequent food intake (Mars et al. 2009). Texture might affect the duration of sensory exposure and eating rate. However, it has been suggested that the eating rate is a more important determinant of short-term intake than the texture per se, especially when differences in textures are relatively small (Hogenkamp et al. 2010). More studies in this area are clearly needed before drawing any conclusions.

3.3.4 Gut Microbiota

Yogurt consumption could have an impact on the balance of indigenous microbiota (Alvaro et al. 2007, Garcia-Albiach et al. 2008), which might influence weight gain (Kinross et al. 2011). There is increasing evidence showing that the modulation of gut microbiota affects metabolism and has an impact on energy storage and obesity (Cani and Delzenne 2007, Tremaroli and Backhed 2012). It has been shown that metabolic syndrome phenotypes can be induced through fecal transplants, demonstrating the important role of the gut microbiota on obesity-related diseases (Cani and Delzenne 2007, Backhed et al. 2004, Turnbaugh et al. 2006). Different components in yogurt, particularly living ferments and probiotics, may act to balance the microbiota, contributing to energy balance (Marette and Picard-Deland 2014). Yogurt consumption may also limit the proliferation and adhesion of pathogenic bacteria, helping to restore a healthy gut microbiota and suppress inflammation (Pei et al. 2015).

3.4 CONCLUSIONS

- There is a growing interest in the relationship between yogurt and obesity, as evidenced by the number of publications on the topic over the last few years. To date, few systematic reviews have been conducted. Based on current evidence (observational studies and randomized clinical trials), it

appears that a large majority of published studies demonstrate a protective relationship between yogurt and weight gain; however, the level of evidence remains low. A meta-analysis would provide a stronger level of evidence from which more definite conclusions can be drawn.
- There appear to be few studies investigating the association between yogurt consumption and its impact on adiposity or weight gain in children and adolescents. Existing studies are cross-sectional in nature and do not always isolate yogurt from other dairy foods or specific eating patterns, making the relationship difficult to understand.
- There is potential for foods such as yogurt to contribute to both the nutritional quality of the diet as well as weight management. To gain a better comprehension of this relationship between yogurt and weight management, more clinical trials are needed.
- Yogurt components such as calcium, protein/bioactive peptides, and living ferments/bacteria could have an impact on body weight maintenance and obesity. Calcium has an established role in weight management and is a potentially important confounder to the yogurt–weight relationship. Future clinical trials and epidemiological studies should systematically control for this covariate.
- Yogurt may have a superior effect than other food, beverages, and snacks on inducing satiety due to its high protein content. Moreover, the substitution of nutrient-poor, energy-dense items with nutrient-rich foods such as yogurt can have a beneficial impact on weight maintenance and obesity.

REFERENCES

Abargouei, A. S., M. Janghorbani, M. Salehi-Marzijarani, and A. Esmaillzadeh. 2012. Effect of dairy consumption on weight and body composition in adults: A systematic review and meta-analysis of randomized controlled clinical trials. *Int J Obes (Lond)* 36 (12):1485–93.

Abreu, S., R. Santos, C. Moreira, P. C. Santos, S. Vale, L. Soares-Miranda, J. Mota, et al. 2012a. Milk intake is inversely related to body mass index and body fat in girls. *Eur J Pediatr* 171 (10):1467–74.

Abreu, S., R. Santos, C. Moreira, S. Vale, P. C. Santos, L. Soares-Miranda, A. I. Marques, et al. 2012b. Association between dairy product intake and abdominal obesity in Azorean adolescents. *Eur J Clin Nutr* 66 (7):830–35.

Almiron-Roig, E., D. Grathwohl, H. Green, and A. Erkner. 2009. Impact of some isoenergetic snacks on satiety and next meal intake in healthy adults. *J Hum Nutr Diet* 22 (5):469–74.

Alvaro, E., C. Andrieux, V. Rochet, L. Rigottier-Gois, P. Lepercq, M. Sutren, P. Galan, et al. 2007. Composition and metabolism of the intestinal microbiota in consumers and nonconsumers of yogurt. *Br J Nutr* 97 (1):126–33.

Azadbakht, L., F. Haghighatdoost, G. Karimi, and A. Esmaillzadeh. 2012. Effect of consuming salad and yogurt as preload on body weight management and cardiovascular risk factors: A randomized clinical trial. *Int J Food Sci Nutr* 64 (4):392–99.

Aziz, A., and G. H. Anderson. 2003. Exendin-4, a GLP-1 receptor agonist, interacts with proteins and their products of digestion to suppress food intake in rats. *J Nutr* 133 (7):2326–30.

Backhed, F., H. Ding, T. Wang, L. V. Hooper, G. Y. Koh, A. Nagy, C. F. Semenkovich, et al. 2004. The gut microbiota as an environmental factor that regulates fat storage. *Proc Natl Acad Sci USA* 101 (44):15718–23.

Barba, G., E. Troiano, P. Russo, A. Venezia, and A. Siani. 2005. Inverse association between body mass and frequency of milk consumption in children. *Br J Nutr* 93 (1):15–19.

Berkey, C. S., H. R. Rockett, W. C. Willett, and G. A. Colditz. 2005. Milk, dairy fat, dietary calcium, and weight gain: A longitudinal study of adolescents. *Arch Pediatr Adolesc Med* 159 (6):543–50.

Beydoun, M. A., T. L. Gary, B. H. Caballero, R. S. Lawrence, L. J. Cheskin, and Y. Wang. 2008. Ethnic differences in dairy and related nutrient consumption among U.S. adults and their association with obesity, central obesity, and the metabolic syndrome. *Am J Clin Nutr* 87 (6):1914–25.

Booth, A. O., C. E. Huggins, N. Wattanapenpaiboon, and C. A. Nowson. 2015. Effect of increasing dietary calcium through supplements and dairy food on body weight and body composition: A meta-analysis of randomised controlled trials. *Br J Nutr* 114 (7):1013–25.

Bowen, J., M. Noakes, C. Trenerry, and P. M. Clifton. 2006. Energy intake, ghrelin, and cholecystokinin after different carbohydrate and protein preloads in overweight men. *J Clin Endocrinol Metab* 91 (4):1477–83.

Bowman, S. A., and B. T. Vinyard. 2004. Fast food consumption of U.S. adults: Impact on energy and nutrient intakes and overweight status. *J Am Coll Nutr* 23 (2):163–68.

Cani, P. D., and N. M. Delzenne. 2007. Gut microflora as a target for energy and metabolic homeostasis. *Curr Opin Clin Nutr Metab Care* 10 (6):729–34.

Chapelot, D., and F. Payen. 2010. Comparison of the effects of a liquid yogurt and chocolate bars on satiety: A multidimensional approach. *Br J Nutr* 103 (5):760–67.

Chen, M., A. Pan, V. S. Malik, and F. B. Hu. 2012. Effects of dairy intake on body weight and fat: A meta-analysis of randomized controlled trials. *Am J Clin Nutr* 96 (4):735–47.

Cormier, H., E. Thifault, V. Garneau, A. Tremblay, V. Drapeau, L. Perusse, and M. C. Vohl. 2015. Association between yogurt consumption, dietary patterns, and cardio-metabolic risk factors. *Eur J Nutr* 55 (2):577–87.

Crichton, G. E., and A. Alkerwi. 2014. Whole-fat dairy food intake is inversely associated with obesity prevalence: Findings from the observation of cardiovascular risk factors in Luxembourg study. *Nutr Res* 34 (11):936–43.

Dougkas, A., C. K. Reynolds, I. D. Givens, P. C. Elwood, and A. M. Minihane. 2011. Associations between dairy consumption and body weight: A review of the evidence and underlying mechanisms. *Nutr Res Rev* 15:1–24.

Douglas, S. M., L. C. Ortinau, H. A. Hoertel, and H. J. Leidy. 2012. Low, moderate, or high protein yogurt snacks on appetite control and subsequent eating in healthy women. *Appetite* 60 (24):72–95.

Drapeau, V., J. P. Despres, C. Bouchard, L. Allard, G. Fournier, C. Leblanc, and A. Tremblay. 2004. Modifications in food-group consumption are related to long-term body-weight changes. *Am J Clin Nutr* 80 (1):29–37.

Dror, D. K. 2014. Dairy consumption and pre-school, school-age and adolescent obesity in developed countries: A systematic review and meta-analysis. *Obesity Rev* 15 (6):516–27.

Eales, J., I. Lenoir-Wijnkoop, S. King, H. Wood, F. J. Kok, R. Shamir, A. Prentice, M. Edwards, J. Glanville, and R. L. Atkinson. 2015. Is consuming yoghurt associated with weight management outcomes? Results from a systematic review. *Int J Obes (Lond)* 40 (5):731–46.

Fiorito, L. M., D. C. Mitchell, H. Smiciklas-Wright, and L. L. Birch. 2006. Girls' calcium intake is associated with bone mineral content during middle childhood. *J Nutr* 136 (5):1281–86.

Fogelholm, M., S. Anderssen, I. Gunnarsdottir, and M. Lahti-Koski. 2012. Dietary macronutrients and food consumption as determinants of long-term weight change in adult populations: A systematic literature review. *Food Nutr Res* 56: Online only. doi:10.3402/fnr.v56i0.19103.

Garcia-Albiach, R., M. J. Pozuelo de Felipe, S. Angulo, M. I. Morosini, D. Bravo, F. Baquero, and R. del Campo. 2008. Molecular analysis of yogurt containing *Lactobacillus delbrueckii* subsp. *bulgaricus* and *Streptococcus thermophilus* in human intestinal microbiota. *Am J Clin Nutr* 87 (1):91–96.

Gilbert, J. A., D. R. Joanisse, J. P. Chaput, P. Miegueu, K. Cianflone, N. Almeras, and A. Tremblay. 2011. Milk supplementation facilitates appetite control in obese women during weight loss: A randomised, single-blind, placebo-controlled trial. *Br J Nutr* 105 (1):133–43.

Heaney, R. P. 2011. Calcium and obesity: Effect size and clinical relevance. *Nutr Rev* 69 (6):333–34.

Hogenkamp, P. S., M. Mars, A. Stafleu, and C. de Graaf. 2010. Intake during repeated exposure to low- and high-energy-dense yogurts by different means of consumption. *Am J Clin Nut* 91 (4):841–47.

Huh, S. Y., S. L. Rifas-Shiman, J. W. Rich-Edwards, E. M. Taveras, and M. W. Gillman. 2010. Prospective association between milk intake and adiposity in preschool-aged children. *J Am Diet Assoc* 110 (4):563–70.

Hursel, R., L. van der Zee, and M. S. Westerterp-Plantenga. 2010. Effects of a breakfast yoghurt, with additional total whey protein or caseinomacropeptide-depleted alpha-lactalbumin-enriched whey protein, on diet-induced thermogenesis and appetite suppression. *Br J Nutr* 103:775–80.

Huth, P. J., D. B. DiRienzo, and G. D. Miller. 2006. Major scientific advances with dairy foods in nutrition and health. *J Dairy Sci* 89:1207–21.

Jacques, P. F., and H. Wang. 2014. Yogurt and weight management. *Am J Clin Nutr* 99 (5):1229S–34S.

Keast, D. R., K. M. Hill Gallant, A. M. Albertson, C. K. Gugger, and N. M. Holschuh. 2015. Associations between yogurt, dairy, calcium, and vitamin D intake and obesity among U.S. children aged 8–18 years: Nhanes, 2005–2008. *Nutrients* 7 (3):1577–93.

Kinross, J. M., A. W. Darzi, and J. K. Nicholson. 2011. Gut microbiome-host interactions in health and disease. *Genome Med* 3 (3):14.

Larsen, T. M., S. M. Dalskov, M. van Baak, S. A. Jebb, A. Papadaki, A. F. Pfeiffer, J. A. Martinez, T. Handjieva-Darlenska, M. Kunesova, M. Pihlsgard, S. Stender, C. Holst, W. H. Saris, and A. Astrup. 2010. Diets with high or low protein content and glycemic index for weight-loss maintenance. *N Engl J Med* 363 (22):2102–13.

Layman, D. K., and D. A. Walker. 2006. Potential importance of leucine in treatment of obesity and the metabolic syndrome. *J Nutr* 136 (1 Suppl):319S–23S.

Lee, H. J., J. I. Cho, H. S. Lee, C. I. Kim, and E. Cho. 2014. Intakes of dairy products and calcium and obesity in Korean adults: Korean National Health and Nutrition Examination Surveys (KNHANES) 2007–2009. *PLoS One* 9 (6):e99085.

Louie, J. C. Y., V. M. Flood, D. J. Hector, A. M. Rangan, and T. P. Gill. 2011. Dairy consumption and overweight and obesity: A systematic review of prospective cohort studies. *Obesity Rev* 12 (7):E582–E92.

Marette, A., and E. Picard-Deland. 2014. Yogurt consumption and impact on health: Focus on children and cardiometabolic risk. *Am J Clin Nutr* 99 (5):1243S–47S.

Mars, M., P. S. Hogenkamp, A. M. Gosses, A. Stafleu, and C. De Graaf. 2009. Effect of viscosity on learned satiation. *Physiol Behav* 98 (1–2):60–66.

Martinez-Gonzalez, M. A., C. Sayon-Orea, M. Ruiz-Canela, C. de la Fuente, A. Gea, and M. Bes-Rastrollo. 2014. Yogurt consumption, weight change and risk of overweight/obesity: The SUN cohort study. *NMCD* 24 (11):1189–96.

Matthews, V. L., M. Wien, and J. Sabate. 2011. The risk of child and adolescent overweight is related to types of food consumed. *Nutr J* 10:71.

Moore, L. L., M. R. Singer, M. M. Qureshi, and M. L. Bradlee. 2008. Dairy intake and anthropometric measures of body fat among children and adolescents in NHANES. *J Am Coll Nutr* 27 (6):702–10.

Moreira, P., S. Santos, P. Padrao, T. Cordeiro, M. Bessa, H. Valente, R. Barros, et al. 2010. Food patterns according to sociodemographics, physical activity, sleeping and obesity in Portuguese children. *Int J Environ Res Public Health* 7 (3):1121–38.

Moreno, L., S. Bel-Serrat, A. Santaliestra-Pasías, and Gloria Bueno. 2015. Dairy products, yogurt consumption, and cardiometabolic risk in children and adolescents. *Nutrition Rev* 73 (Suppl 1):8–14.

Mozaffarian, D. 2016. Dietary and policy priorities for cardiovascular disease, diabetes, and obesity: A comprehensive review. *Circulation* 133 (2):187–225.

Mozaffarian, D., T. Hao, E. B. Rimm, W. C. Willett, and F. B. Hu. 2011. Changes in diet and lifestyle and long-term weight gain in women and men. *N Engl J Med* 364 (25):2392–404.

Murphy, K. J., G. E. Crichton, K. A. Dyer, A. M. Coates, T. L. Pettman, C. Milte, A. A. Thorp, N. M. Berry, J. D. Buckley, M. Noakes, and P. R. Howe. 2013. Dairy foods and dairy protein consumption is inversely related to markers of adiposity in obese men and women. *Nutrients* 5 (11):4665–84.

Nagao, K., and T. Yanagita. 2008. Bioactive lipids in metabolic syndrome. *Prog Lipid Res* 47 (2):127–46.

Nilsson, M., M. Stenberg, A. H. Frid, J. J. Holst, and I. M. Bjork. 2004. Glycemia and insulinemia in healthy subjects after lactose-equivalent meals of milk and other food proteins: The role of plasma amino acids and incretins. *Am J Clin Nutr* 80 (5):1246–53.

Noel, S. E., A. R. Ness, K. Northstone, P. Emmett, and P. K. Newby. 2011. Milk intakes are not associated with percent body fat in children from ages 10 to 13 years. *J Nutr* 141 (11):2035–41.

Novotny R., S. Acharya, and J.S. Grove. 2003. Higher dairy intake is associated with lower body fat during adolescence. *FASEB J* 18:A2277.

O'Connor, L., S. Brage, S. J. Griffin, N. J. Wareham, and N. G. Forouhi. 2015. The cross-sectional association between snacking behaviour and measures of adiposity: The Fenland Study, UK. *Br J Nutr*:1–8.

Ortinau, L. C., J. M. Culp, H. A. Hoertel, S. M. Douglas, and H. J. Leidy. 2013. The effects of increased dietary protein yogurt snack in the afternoon on appetite control and eating initiation in healthy women. *Nutr J* 12 (1):71.

Ortinau, L. C., H. A. Hoertel, S. M. Douglas, and H. J. Leidy. 2014. Effects of high-protein vs. high-fat snacks on appetite control, satiety, and eating initiation in healthy women. *Nutr J* 13:97.

O'Sullivan, T. A., A. P. Bremner, H. K. Bremer, M. E. Seares, L. J. Beilin, T. A. Mori, P. Lyons-Wall, et al. 2015. Dairy product consumption, dietary nutrient and energy density and associations with obesity in Australian adolescents. *J Hum Nutr Diet* 28 (5):452–64.

Parodi, P. W. 2016. Cooperative action of bioactive components in milk fat with PPARs may explain its anti-diabetogenic properties. *Medical Hypotheses* 89:1–7.

Pei, R., D. A. Martin, D. M. DiMarco, and B. W. Bolling. 2015. Evidence for the effects of yogurt on gut health and obesity. *Crit Rev Food Sci Nutr*. In press. doi:10.1080/10408 398.2014.883356.

Pereira, D. D., R. P. Lima, R. T. de Lima, M. D. Goncalves, L. C. de Morais, S. D. Franceschini, R. G. Filizola, et al. 2013. Association between obesity and calcium:phosphorus ratio in the habitual diets of adults in a city of northeastern Brazil: An epidemiological study. *Nutr J* 12 (1):90.

Plourde, M., S. Jew, S. C. Cunnane, and P. J. H. Jones. 2008. Conjugated linoleic acids: Why the discrepancy between animal and human studies? *Nutrition Rev* 66 (7):415–21.

Pupovac, J., and G. H. Anderson. 2002. Dietary peptides induce satiety via cholecystokinin-A and peripheral opioid receptors in rats. *J Nutr* 132 (9):2775–80.

Ricci-Cabello, I., M. O. Herrera, and R. Artacho. 2012. Possible role of milk-derived bioactive peptides in the treatment and prevention of metabolic syndrome. *Nutr Rev* 70 (4):241–55.

Rozenberg, S., J. J. Body, O. Bruyere, P. Beergmann, M. L. Brandi, C. Cooper, J. P. Devogelaer, et al. 2015. Effects of dairy products consumption on health: Benefits and beliefs-a commentary from the Belgian Bone Club and the European Society for Clinical and Economic Aspects of Osteoporosis, Osteoarthritis and Musculoskeletal Diseases. *Calcif Tissue Int* 98 (1):1–17.

Sayon-Orea, C., M. Bes-Rastrollo, A. Marti, A. M. Pimenta, N. Martin-Calvo, and M. A. Martinez-Gonzalez. 2015. Association between yogurt consumption and the risk of metabolic syndrome over 6 years in the SUN study. *BMC Public Health* 15:170.

Shlisky, J. D., C. M. Durward, M. K. Zack, C. K. Gugger, J. K. Campbell, and S. M. Nickols-Richardson. 2015. An energy-reduced dietary pattern, including moderate protein and increased nonfat dairy intake combined with walking promotes beneficial body composition and metabolic changes in women with excess adiposity: A randomized comparative trial. *Food Sci Nutr* 3 (5):376–93.

Smith, J. D., T. Hou, D. S. Ludwig, E. B. Rimm, W. Willett, F. B. Hu, and D. Mozaffarian. 2015. Changes in intake of protein foods, carbohydrate amount and quality, and long-term weight change: Results from 3 prospective cohorts. *Am J Clin Nutr* 101 (6):1216–24.

Solah, V. A., D. A. Kerr, C. D. Adikara, X. Meng, C. W. Binns, K. Zhu, A. Devine, et al. 2010. Differences in satiety effects of alginate- and whey protein-based foods. *Appetite* 54 (3):485–91.

Spence, L. A., C. J. Cifelli, and G. D. Miller. 2011. The role of dairy products in healthy weight and body composition in children and adolescents. *Curr Nutr Food Sci* 7 (1):40–49.

St-Onge, M. P., E. R. Farnworth, and P. J. Jones. 2000. Consumption of fermented and non-fermented dairy products: Effects on cholesterol concentrations and metabolism. *Am J Clin Nutr* 71 (3):674–81.

Teegarden, D. 2005. The influence of dairy product consumption on body composition. *J Nut* 135 (12):2749–52.

Tremaroli, V., and F. Backhed. 2012. Functional interactions between the gut microbiota and host metabolism. *Nature* 489 (7415):242–49.

Tremblay, A., C. Doyon, and M. Sanchez. 2015. Impact of yogurt on appetite control, energy balance, and body composition. *Nutr Rev* 73 (Suppl 1):23–27.

Tremblay, A., and J. A. Gilbert. 2011. Human obesity: Is insufficient calcium/dairy intake part of the problem? *J Am Coll Nutr* 30 (5 Suppl 1):449S–53S.

Tsuchiya, A., E. Almiron-Roig, A. Lluch, D. Guyonnet, and A. Drewnowski. 2006. Higher satiety ratings following yogurt consumption relative to fruit drink or dairy fruit drink. *J Am Diet Assoc* 106 (4):550–57.

Tsuji, H., M. Kasai, H. Takeuchi, M. Nakamura, M. Okazaki, and K. Kondo. 2001. Dietary medium-chain triacylglycerols suppress accumulation of body fat in a double-blind, controlled trial in healthy men and women. *J Nutr* 131 (11):2853–59.

Turnbaugh, P. J., R. E. Ley, M. A. Mahowald, V. Magrini, E. R. Mardis, and J. I. Gordon. 2006. An obesity-associated gut microbiome with increased capacity for energy harvest. *Nature* 444 (7122):1027–31.

Veldhorst, M. A., A. G. Nieuwenhuizen, A. Hochstenbach-Waelen, K. R. Westerterp, M. P. Engelen, R. J. Brummer, N. E. Deutz, et al. 2009. A breakfast with alpha-lactalbumin, gelatin, or gelatin+trp lowers energy intake at lunch compared with a breakfast with casein, soy, whey, or whey-gmp. *Clin Nutr* 28 (2):147–55.

Vergnaud, A. C., S. Peneau, S. Chat-Yung, E. Kesse, S. Czernichow, P. Galan, S. Hercberg, et al. 2008. Dairy consumption and 6-y changes in body weight and waist circumference in middle-aged French adults. *Am J Clin Nutr* 88 (5):1248–55.

Wang, H., L. M. Troy, G. T. Rogers, C. S. Fox, N. M. McKeown, J. B. Meigs, and P. F. Jacques. 2014. Longitudinal association between dairy consumption and changes of body weight and waist circumference: The Framingham Heart Study. *International J Obes* 28 (2):299–305.

Wang, Y. W., and P. J. Jones. 2004. Conjugated linoleic acid and obesity control: Efficacy and mechanisms. *Int J Obes Relat Metab Disord* 28 (8):941–55.

Westerterp-Plantenga, M. S. 2003. The significance of protein in food intake and body weight regulation. *Curr Opin Clin Nutr Metab Care* 6 (6):635–38.

Westerterp-Plantenga, M. S., S. G. Lemmens, and K. R. Westerterp. 2012. Dietary protein: Its role in satiety, energetics, weight loss and health. *Br J Nutr* 108 (Suppl 2):S105–12.

WHO. 2012. Global strategy on diet, physical activity & health, childhood overweight and obesity. http://www.who.int/dietphysicalactivity/childhood/en/.

Zemel, M. B., J. Richards, S. Mathis, A. Milstead, L. Gebhardt, and E. Silva. 2005. Dairy augmentation of total and central fat loss in obese subjects. *Int J Obes (Lond)* 29 (4):391–97.

4 Type 2 Diabetes

Type 2 diabetes (T2D) is a chronic disease associated with dysfunctional glucose–insulin homeostasis. This disease occurs when the body does not efficiently use the insulin it makes (also known as insulin resistance) and when the pancreas fails to produce enough insulin to compensate for this insulin resistance. T2D is characterized by dyslipidemic and pro-inflammatory/pro-thrombotic states that contribute to the increased risk of cardiovascular disease (CVD) (Montecucco et al. 2008). Uncontrolled diabetes leads to hyperglycemia, which over time causes serious complications, including microvascular and macrovascular damage (e.g., retinopathy, nephropathy, ischemic heart disease, and stroke). T2D ranks high among diseases that cause individuals to become bedridden with serious complications and is a leading cause of death. The International Diabetes Federation (IDF) estimated that in 2015, 415 million adults (20–79 years) were living with diabetes and it accounted for at least USD 673 billion in health-care expenditures, which represents 12% of global health expenditures (IDF 2015). Until recently, T2D was only seen in adults, but it is now also occurring in children (WHO 2012). Thus, there is an urgent need for effective preventive strategies, which include dietary and lifestyle changes.

Dietary modifications are proposed as a primary target for the prevention and treatment of T2D. In the Framingham Heart Study Offspring Cohort, it was suggested that a diet that is rich in reduced-fat dairy, fruits, vegetables, and whole grains protects against insulin-resistant phenotypes among adults without diabetes (Liu et al. 2009). A systematic review and meta-analysis of seven prospective studies found that increasing dairy intake by one serving per day was associated with a 5% reduced risk for T2D. The risk reduction was higher for low-fat dairy products (Tong et al. 2011). However, the reduction in the risk of T2D following dairy consumption has not been consistently shown. A systematic review of randomized controlled trials examining dairy interventions on glucose metabolism identified 10 trials, of which 5 had no effects, 4 were positive for insulin sensitivity, and 1 was negative. Authors concluded that large longer-term trials are needed to establish any links between dairy intake and insulin sensitivity (Turner et al. 2015a). Despite sparse evidence for different types of dairy products, results seem to be promising and more consistent for fermented dairy foods (Nestel 2012, Sluijs et al. 2012). Details of selected observational studies evaluating the relationship between T2D risk and the consumption of yogurt (fat free, low fat, full fat, unsweetened, sweetened, artificially sweetened, drinkable, high in protein, etc.) will be discussed in the following sections. A large number of prospective cohort studies describing the relationship between yogurt consumption and incident T2D have been published and the studies described are summarized in Table 4.1 and Section 4.2.2.

TABLE 4.1
Summary of Findings and Implications from Prospective Cohort Studies in Adults That Have Examined Type 2 Diabetes Risk in Relation to Yogurt Consumption

Study and Follow-Up Period	Population Age[a] n	Diet Assessment	Yogurt Intake	Findings	Implications	References
The Coronary Artery Risk Development in Young Adults Study 10-year follow-up	Adults 18–30 years 3,157	700 item 28-day quantitative food frequency questionnaire	Eating occasion (amount not specified)	Yogurt consumption was not associated with abnormal glucose homeostasis or insulin resistance syndrome	Neutral	(Pereira et al. 2002)
The Health Professionals Follow-up Study 12-year follow-up	Men 40–75 years 41,254	130-item semiquantitative food frequency questionnaire over 1 year	Standard portion size (amount not specified)	Yogurt consumption was not associated with incident T2D	Neutral	(Choi et al. 2005)
The Women's Health Study 10-year follow-up	Women Middle-aged 37,183	131-item semiquantitative food frequency questionnaire	Daily servings (amount not specified)	There was a significantly lower risk for incident type 2 diabetes among women consuming ≥2 per week compared with those consuming <1 serving per month. The relationship had a significant linear trend	Positive	(Liu et al. 2006)
The Japanese Public Health Center-based Prospective Study 5-year follow-up	Adults Middle-aged and older 59,796	147-item food frequency questionnaire	gram/day	Yogurt was not associated with incident T2D in men, women, or both sexes	Neutral	(Kirii et al. 2009)
The Women's Health Initiative Observational Study 8-year follow-up	Women 50–79 years 80,076	122-item food frequency questionnaire over last 3 months	1 serving per day of medium portion size	There was a significantly lower risk for incident type 2 diabetes among women consuming yogurt 1/month to ≤3/months, >3/months to <2/weeks, and ≥2/weeks compared with those consuming <1 month. The relationship had a significant linear trend	Positive	(Margolis et al. 2011)
The European Prospective Investigation into Cancer and Nutrition Study Median 12.3-year follow-up	Adults 340,324	Quantitative dietary questionnaire or semiquantitative food frequency questionnaires	gram/day	Yogurt consumption was not associated with incident T2D	Neutral	(Slujis et al. 2012)

(Continued)

TABLE 4.1 (CONTINUED)
Summary of Findings and Implications from Prospective Cohort Studies in Adults That Have Examined Type 2 Diabetes Risk in Relation to Yogurt Consumption

Study and Follow-Up Period	Population Age[a]	n	Diet Assessment	Yogurt Intake	Findings	Implications	References
Whitehall II Prospective Cohort Study 10-year follow-up	Adults Mean age = 56 years (SD 6)	4,526	Food frequency questionnaire	gram/day	Yogurt consumption was not associated with incident T2D	Neutral	(Soedamah-Muthu et al. 2012)
The Australian Diabetes, Obesity and Lifestyle Study 5-year follow-up	Adults ≥ 25 years	5,582	121-item food frequency questionnaire	200 g serving	Yogurt consumption was not associated with incident T2D	Neutral	(Grantham et al. 2013)
The European Prospective Investigation into Cancer—Norfolk Study 11-year follow-up	Adults	4,000	Prospective 7-day food diary	gram/day	Yogurt consumption was significantly and inversely associated to incident T2D	Positive	(O'Connor et al. 2014)
PREDIMED Median 4.1-year follow-up	55–80 years	3,454	137-item semiquantitative food frequency questionnaire	125 g serving/day	Total yogurt, low-fat yogurt, and whole-fat yogurt were significantly associated with lower incidence of T2D	Positive	(Diaz-Lopez et al. 2015)
Nurses' Health Study (NHS), Nurses' Health Study II (NHS II), and Health Professionals Follow-Up Study (HPFS) 20 years, 18 years, and 22 years follow-up for NHS, NHS II, and HPFS, respectively	Adults Age: NHS, 30–55 years; NHS II 25–42 years; HPFS, 40–75 years n: NHS, 67,138 women; NHS II, 85,884 women; HPFS, 41,436 men		61-item food frequency questionnaire and 131-item expanded food frequency questionnaire	125 mL standard serving	NHS, significant inverse relationship between each serving of yogurt consumed and T2D incidence and significant linear trend; NHS II, nonsignificant inverse relationship and significant linear trend; HPFS, nonsignificant inverse relationship and nonsignificant linear trend; pooled cohorts, significant inverse relationship between each serving of yogurt consumed and T2D incidence and significant linear trend	Positive for NHS and pooled cohorts; neutral for NHS II and HPFS	(Chen et al. 2014)

[a] Where n equals sample size of the study.

4.1 STUDIES IN CHILDREN AND ADOLESCENTS

Metabolic parameters of pediatric populations in relation to yogurt consumption have rarely been examined. The relationship between yogurt consumption and metabolic data was examined in a cross section of 5,124 American children (2–18 years old) participating in the National Health and Nutrition Exam Survey (NHANES) (2003–2006). Yogurt consumption was assessed with a 12-month food frequency questionnaire and diet quality was based on a single 24-hour recall. Only 33.1% of children consumed yogurt at least once a week; this group was considered as frequent yogurt consumers. The group of frequent yogurt consumers was associated with improved indices of glucose metabolism compared with infrequent consumers; lower fasting glucose ($p < .001$), lower HOMA-IR ($p < .001$), and a higher insulin sensitivity check index ($p = .03$). None of the other metabolic parameters measured (weight, serum lipid profiles, C-reactive protein, and blood pressure) were associated with yogurt consumption (Zhu et al. 2015).

4.2 STUDIES IN ADULTS

4.2.1 Cross-Sectional Studies

The ATTICA cross-sectional study investigated the association between food groups and indices of glycemic control in around 3,000 men and women (18–90 years) without T2D and CVD. The intakes of yogurt, fruits, vegetables, legumes, milk, and cheese were not associated with levels of glycemic control indices. Low-fat dairy product consumption was not examined in this study. Red meat consumption was positively associated with hyperglycemia, hyperinsulinemia, and homeostatic model assessment (HOMA) levels (after adjusting for potential confounders). The authors suggested that the substitution of meat for yogurt, cheese, and vegetable sources of proteins could have beneficial effects on hyperinsulinemia and insulin resistance in nondiabetic subjects (Panagiotakos et al. 2005).

The Hoorn Study investigated the relationship between dairy consumption, body weight, and components of the metabolic syndrome, including body weight, among Dutch men and women (50–75 years). Yogurt consumption accounted for approximately 15% of total dairy product servings per day. There was no association between the consumption of yogurt and fasting glucose or 2-hour glucose tests (Snijder et al. 2007).

A cross-sectional study investigated dairy consumption and its relationship to glycemia, insulinemia, and newly diagnosed diabetes in a Brazilian cohort of 10,010 adults. Total dairy intake was inversely associated with fasting glucose, 2-hour post-load glucose, Hb A_{1c}, 2-hour post-load insulin, and HOMA-IR (insulin resistance) following adjustment for all major covariates. In subgroup analyses, significant inverse associations were seen between total fermented dairy, fasting glucose, and 2-hour post-load glucose; cheese and 2-hour post-load glucose; and yogurt and Hb A_{1c} (Drehmer et al. 2015).

4.2.2 Prospective Cohort Studies

The effects of yogurt and dairy products were assessed on various criteria of the metabolic syndrome in a cohort with 3,157 black and white adults (18–30 years) who were followed for 10 years in the Coronary Artery Risk Development in Young Adults (CARDIA) study. No significant relationships were observed between yogurt, glucose, and insulin parameters. However, yogurt consumption was low in comparison with other dairy products (around 1.8% of total dairy products) (Pereira et al. 2002).

After a 12-year follow-up in middle-aged and elderly men, Choi et al. (2005) showed that an increase of each additional serving of dairy per day was associated with a 9% lower risk for T2D, with the effect confined to low-fat dairy (corresponding relative risk was 0.88 [95% CI, 0.81–0.94]). In this study, no significant association was observed between yogurt consumption and T2D risk (Choi et al. 2005).

In women (≤45 years), an increase of each additional serving of dairy per day was associated with a 4% decrease in risk for T2D; however, it was not significant. A decrease of 18% of T2D risk was observed for consumption of more than two portions of yogurt per week compared with less than one portion per month (0.82; 95% CI, 0.70–0.97). This association remained significant following adjustments for confounding factors (Liu et al. 2006).

Calcium, vitamin D, and dairy intake in relation to T2D risk was evaluated in a Japanese cohort of 59,796 middle-aged and older men and women from the Japan Public Health Center-based Prospective Study, who were followed for 5 years, during which 1114 cases of T2D were documented. In women, the intake of dairy foods was significantly and inversely associated with the risk of T2D. In models adjusted for age and area, the odds ratio for the highest versus lowest intake category of yogurt was 0.72 (95% CI 0.55–0.93). However, in multivariable analyses adjusting for additional covariates, the association was attenuated. Among participants with a higher vitamin D intake, calcium intake was inversely associated with T2D risk (Kirii et al. 2009).

Margolis et al. (2011) performed a prospective study on an ethnically diverse group of 82,076 postmenopausal women. Yogurt intake and total, low-, and high-fat dairy product intakes were estimated with food frequency questionnaires at baseline and after 3 years of follow-up. Yogurt consumption was associated with a significant decrease in T2D risk. Indeed, consumption of more than one yogurt per month was associated with a lower risk of developing T2D (RR=0.61 [95% CI=0.41–0.92]; once per week, RR=0.55 [95% CI=0.37–0.82]; more than twice per week, RR=0.46 [95% CI=0.31–0.68]). Low-fat dairy product consumption was also inversely associated with an increased risk of T2D in those women, particularly those who were obese (Margolis et al. 2011).

The EPIC-Inter Act study, involving eight European countries of the European Prospective Investigation into Cancer and Nutrition ($n=340,234$), recently investigated the association between dairy products and the incidence of T2D in populations whose consumption varied considerably. Authors found no association between total dairy product intake or yogurt intake and T2D. However, in adjusted analyses that compared extreme quintiles, an inverse association between T2D was found for cheese intake and combined fermented dairy product intake (cheese, yogurt, and thick fermented milk; HR: 0.88; 95% CI: 0.78, 0.99; $p=.02$) (Sluijs et al. 2012, Forouhi 2015).

Another prospective study was performed involving the Whitehall II cohort (London-based office staff; $n=4,526$, mean age of 56 years, 72% men, 10-year follow-up) to evaluate the effect of different types of dairy product on the risk of T2D, cardiovascular heart diseases, and mortality. Dairy product intake was assessed using food frequency questionnaires. Incident T2D was diagnosed with oral glucose tolerance tests or based on self-reporting. No significant associations were found between intakes of total dairy, types of dairy products, and incident T2D. Fermented dairy products were inversely associated with overall mortality but not with diabetes risk (Soedamah-Muthu et al. 2012).

The effects of dairy foods on T2D risk were evaluated in The Australian Diabetes, Obesity and Lifestyle Study (AusDiab) over 5 years (baseline measurements: food frequency questionnaire, anthropometrics, and an oral glucose tolerance test). They found that high intakes of dairy food (milk, cheese, and yogurt) could significantly reduce the risk of diabetes incidence among men, but not women. High intakes of low-fat milk were associated with a lower risk of T2D in combined sexes and there was no association between yogurt consumption and 5-year incidence of T2D (Grantham et al. 2013).

The relationship between dairy product intake and T2D was investigated in a nested case-cohort of adults from the EPIC-Norfolk study. Dietary data was assessed with 7-day food diaries and cases of incident diabetes were recorded over an 11-year follow-up. Among dairy products, only low-fat dairy was inversely associated with T2D risk. Furthermore, low-fat fermented dairy products, especially yogurt, were significantly and inversely associated with T2D in adjusted models (O'Connor et al. 2014).

In a cohort of 3,454 elderly Spanish adults (55–80 years) at high risk of cardiovascular events from the prospective Prevención con Dieta Mediterránea (Prevention with a Mediterranean Diet [PREDIMED]) study, the association between dairy intake and T2D risk was studied. Over a median follow-up of 4.1 years, 270 cases of T2D were recorded. Total dairy and low-fat dairy, but not whole-fat dairy, were significantly and inversely associated with a lower risk for T2D. Low-fat milk was also inversely associated with T2D risk. Total yogurt, low-fat yogurt, and whole-fat yogurt intakes were all found to be inversely related to T2D risk (Díaz-López et al. 2015).

The relationship between dairy product consumption and T2D in adults was investigated by conducting a prospective study of three large American cohorts. A total of 15,156 incident cases over a maximum of 16–30 years (depending on the cohort) were recorded in the three pooled American cohorts (Nurses' Health Study, Nurses' Health Study II, and Health Professionals Follow-Up Study; $n = 194,458$ adults). Total dairy, low-fat dairy, and whole-fat dairy were not associated with T2D incidence. Yogurt, however, was consistently and strongly associated with a reduction of incident diabetes in the pooled cohorts by 17% for every serving per day of yogurt consumed in a multivariate model that controlled for lifestyle and dietary covariates as well as comorbidities (Chen et al. 2014).

4.2.3 Meta-Analyses and Systematic Reviews

The result from a meta-analysis of seven cohort studies indicated that there was an inverse association of daily intake of dairy products, especially low-fat dairy, with

T2D risk. Dose–response analysis showed that T2D risk could be reduced by 10% for low-fat dairy products and 5% for total dairy products. Moreover, a 17% decrease in T2D risk was observed for yogurt intake. However, the efficiency of this meta-analysis is limited because of the small number of yogurt studies included ($n = 3$) (Tong et al. 2011).

A systematic review and dose–response meta-analysis of 17 cohort studies evaluated the associations between different types of dairy products and T2D risk. This meta-analysis showed that a high intake of dairy was associated with a decreased risk of T2D. A significant inverse association was observed between high intakes of low-fat dairy, low-fat or skim milk and cheese, and yogurt compared with low intakes. However, the dose–response between the consumption of each 200 g of yogurt and the relative risk of T2D was not linear and not significant (RR = 0.78, 95% CI 0.60, 1.02). Yogurt analyses were based on 7 cohort studies totaling 19,082 cases among 254,892 participants (Aune et al. 2013). Another systematic review and meta-analysis published 1 month later investigated the same research question among 16 cohort studies and concluded that there was a modest protective effect of total dairy intake on T2D prevention. Low-fat dairy appeared to have a stronger inverse relationship to T2D. Yogurt subgroup analyses were also based on 7 studies, including 18,532 cases and 254,552 participants. An inverse relationship between high yogurt intake and T2D risk as well a dose–response indicated reduced risk for every 50 g of yogurt consumed (Gao et al. 2013). Both meta-analyses had similar findings in terms of an inverse relationship between yogurt intake and T2D risk, but the differences in dose response may be due to the inclusion of slightly different studies and the use of different reference doses: 200 g versus 50 g.

An updated meta-analysis of Aune et al.'s (2013) study was conducted to reflect longer new analyses, including longer follow-up periods and additional examination into specific dairy subtypes. The meta-analyses included a total of 14 prospective cohort studies with 459,790 adults and found that total dairy was not significantly associated with T2D. A total of nine prospective cohorts involving yogurt were analyzed and found that that for every serving per day of yogurt consumed there was a significant reduced risk of incident diabetes by 18% (Chen et al. 2014). The most recent meta-analysis to study the relationship between dairy foods and T2D incidence examined 22 cohort studies, of which 12 were yogurt cohorts ($n = 438{,}140$). Similar to findings in Chen et al. (2014), there was a 14% reduced risk of T2D associated with an intake of 80 g per day compared with 0 g per day. However, there were no further reductions in risk associated with intakes greater than 80 g per day (Gijsbers et al. 2016).

4.3 MECHANISMS OF ACTION

According to the Dietary Guidelines Advisory Committee, not consuming adequate quantities of dairy products could lead to an increased risk of T2D and moderate evidence supports that lower incidence of T2D is associated with dairy product intake (Committee DGA 2010). Several mechanisms explaining this relationship have been hypothesized, but remain poorly understood. It is plausible that numerous mechanisms may act together to confer protective properties, including lifestyle factors, dietary patterns, and nutrient components of dairy products. Lacroix and Li-Chan (2014) suggested that dietary patterns that are inversely associated with T2D generally include low-fat dairy and may contribute to the protective properties of dairy on T2D. Obesity in particular is an important risk factor for T2D and specific yogurt components such as lactic acid bacteria (LAB) may enhance the nutritional properties of dairy. For example, LAB have been shown to act on the gastrointestinal tract and obesity-related mechanisms. Various mechanisms with potential to impact T2D development are briefly described in the following sections.

4.3.1 Vitamins and Minerals

Vitamin D, calcium, and magnesium have an important role in glucose regulation (Lacroix and Li-Chan 2014) and have been shown to have positive effects on T2D. Increased intakes of calcium and vitamin D, from low-fat dairy products in particular, may be beneficial for enhancing insulin sensitivity and preventing T2D (Candido et al. 2013). Data from the Nurses' Health Study has shown that a combined daily intake of >1200 mg calcium and >800 IU vitamin D was associated with a 33% lower risk of T2D compared with an intake of <600 mg and 400 IU calcium and vitamin D, respectively (Pittas et al. 2006). In a nationally representative sample of more than 4000 Australians, a low-serum vitamin D concentration was associated with an increased risk of developing T2D and metabolic syndrome irrespective of potential confounders, including body mass index (BMI) (Gagnon et al. 2012). Moreover, other studies investigating the effect of yogurt enriched with vitamin D in T2D subjects have observed an improvement of glycemic status (Nikooyeh et al. 2011), lipid profile, and endothelial biomarkers (Shab-Bidar et al. 2011).

The mechanisms by which vitamin D may affect the risk of T2D are not clear, but could imply, among other mechanisms, insulin secretion (Zeitz et al. 2003, Scragg et al. 2004) and a reduction of pro-inflammatory mediators (Pittas et al. 2007). Vitamin D could also facilitate intestinal calcium absorption and regulate extracellular calcium. Calcium is essential for insulin-mediated intracellular processes in tissues that are responsive to insulin, such as adipose tissue and skeletal muscle (Ojuka 2004). Moreover, recent studies suggest that vitamin D can increase glucose uptake in insulin target cells through activation of insulin receptor signaling (Calle et al. 2008, Wright et al. 2004).

It has been shown that a diet high in magnesium-rich foods is associated with a lower risk of T2D in humans (van Dam et al. 2006, Villegas et al. 2009). Magnesium may reduce the risk of T2D by improving insulin sensitivity (Yokota 2005). An intervention trial involving nondiabetic volunteers demonstrated a significant association between low serum magnesium and relative insulin resistance, glucose intolerance, and hyperinsulinemia (Rosolova et al. 1997).

4.3.2 Glycemic Load

Low glycemic load and glycemic index diets have been suggested to have a beneficial impact on weight-loss maintenance (Larsen et al. 2010), insulin sensitivity, and lipid metabolism (Du et al. 2008), as well as low-grade inflammation in humans

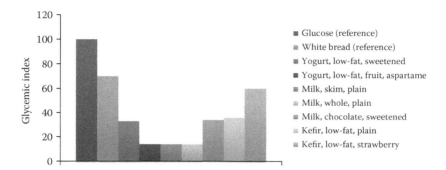

FIGURE 4.1 Mean glycemic index of sweetened, artificially sweetened and plain dairy products in reference to white bread and a glucose load. (From Miller et al., *Br J Nutr* 73 (4):613–23, 1995; Hoyt et al., *Br J Nutr* 93 (2):175–77, 2005, Ostman et al., *Am J Clin Nutr* 74 (1):96–100, 2001)

(Gogebakan et al. 2011). The mean glycemic index of yogurt and other dairy products is shown in Figure 4.1. Furthermore, it has been shown that a high-protein, low-carbohydrate pre-breakfast snack (30 g soya beans; 75 g yogurt) reduces the postprandial plasma glucose increment in people with T2D by 40% (Chen et al. 2010).

Interestingly, lactic acid present in yogurt may potentiate the beneficial effect of the low glycemic load on postprandial glycemia by reducing the gastric emptying rate (Liljeberg and Bjorck 1998, Ostman et al. 2001). The postprandial response of a yogurt meal compared with a reference meal resulted in a lower glucose peak and lower area under the curve (0–180 minutes post meal) (Lindstrom et al. 2015).

4.3.3 Proteins

Yogurt and milk bioactive peptides could improve defective insulin secretion in T2D, leading to better glucose control and food intake regulation. Yogurt peptides could release hormones such as glucose-dependent insulinotropic polypeptide and glucagon-like peptide (GLP), hormones secreted by the gut that augment insulin secretion from β-cells and slow the absorption of nutrients (Nilsson et al. 2004, Jakubowicz and Froy 2012). Moreover, whey protein peptides have been shown to serve as endogenous inhibitors of dipeptidyl peptidase-4 (DPP-4) in the proximal gut, which prevent incretin (e.g., GLP-1) degradation (Jakubowicz and Froy 2012). Whey protein found in dairy is typically rich in leucine, an amino acid that may help combat the poor mitochondrial function that is characteristic of T2D and insulin resistance. It has also been implicated in pathways that reduce oxidative stress, improve insulin sensitivity, and activate fat oxidation (Hirahatake et al. 2014).

4.3.4 Fatty Acids

Dairy products containing fat are thought to contain bioactive lipids that can act in a protective way against cardiometabolic diseases by mediating metabolic and inflammatory pathways (Hirahatake et al. 2014). Total saturated fatty acids (SFA) have historically been thought to be associated with increased diabetes and cardiovascular risk; however, specific fatty acids may possess functional health properties and could predict a lower risk of T2D (Nestel et al. 2014). Furthermore, it has been suggested that dairy fat contributes to the inverse association observed between dairy product consumption and T2D (Ericson et al. 2015). Generally, dietary data based on food records does not permit distinctions between individual fatty acids (Nestel et al. 2014) and reports are based on total SFA intake. More recent comprehensive epidemiological studies, which have conducted analyses measuring individual plasma fatty acids, have detected dairy biomarkers of various chain lengths, including 14:0 (myristic acid), 15:0 (pentadecanoic acid), 17:0 (margaric acid) and t16:1 n-7 (trans-palmitoleate) (Hirahatake et al. 2014, Forouhi et al. 2014). However, these biomarkers only reflect the dairy intake of products containing fat and do not reflect nonfat dairy intake. Nevertheless, incident diabetes was inversely associated with both pentadecanoic acid and margaric acid (which are SFAs that are unique to dairy) in a model that adjusted for diet, energy intake, demographic factors, obesity, and other lifestyle factors. These conclusions not only indicate that not all SFA have a negative impact on metabolic diseases, but also suggest that SFA specific to dairy products may be beneficial to health (Forouhi et al. 2014). The concentration of pentadecanoic and margaric acid are relatively low in blood compared with total plasma fatty acids. Circulating plasma pentadecanoic and margaric acid may be a mere indicator of the intake of dairy food containing fat (Nestel et al. 2014). The SFA pentadecanoic acid is a short-term marker for dairy food intake and has been linked to reduced T2D risk (Santaren et al. 2014) and lower incidence of insulin resistance (Mozaffarian et al. 2010). The fatty acid 17:0 is strongly and positively associated with full-fat dairy intake and insulin sensitivity and inversely associated with insulin resistance in overweight and obese men and women (Nestel et al. 2014). Another 14-carbon SFA, myristic acid, was found to mediate the inverse association between dairy foods and glycemia, insulin, and HbA_{1c} concentrations (Drehmer et al. 2015). A prospective cohort from the Malmo Diet and Cancer study found a decreased risk of incident T2D associated with the highest quintile intakes of short to medium fatty acid chains (4–10 carbons), lauric acid, and myristic acid. Furthermore, robust inverse associations were also observed for intakes of cream and high-fat fermented milk and cheese, but not low-fat dairy (Ericson et al. 2015).

Mozaffarian et al. (2010) have shown in a cohort of 3736 adults from the Cardiovascular Health Study that circulating trans-palmitoleate (principally derived from naturally occurring dairy/ruminant *trans*-fats) is not only associated with higher LDL cholesterol, but also with lower triglycerides, fasting insulin, blood pressure, and incident diabetes (Mozaffarian et al. 2010). It is thought that Mozaffarian's findings may simply reflect trans-palmitoleate as a biomarker of dairy food intake. The evidence on trans-palmitoleate in regard to its potential benefits for cardiometabolic diseases remains under dispute. For example, though red meat is an extremely rich source of trans-palmitoleate, there is little indication that red meat consumption could be protective for T2D. It is possible that factors in the diet, particularly in red meat, not found in dairy may hinder any potential benefits of trans-palmitoleate (Hirahatake et al. 2014). A randomized clinical trial has also demonstrated evidence that high intakes of dairy products reduced insulin sensitivity compared with high intakes of lean red meat in a group of 47 overweight and obese men and women (Turner et al. 2015b). Results from a meta-analysis of intervention studies examining the relationship between dairy intake and insulin sensitivity found that five studies found no relationship, four studies had a positive association, and one study had a negative association, which confirms that additional studies need to be conducted to validate the association between dairy and glucose metabolism (Turner et al. 2015a). At this time, there are no yogurt-specific studies that make any distinction between dairy fats coming from different dairy products.

4.3.5 Fermentation and Ferments

Forouhi's (2015) review suggests that the fermented properties of yogurt may be responsible for the inverse relationship between yogurt and diabetes (Forouhi 2015). Bacterial cultures responsible for the fermentation in yogurt may also be responsible for the stronger inverse relationship noted in fermented dairy and yogurts compared with nonfermented dairy products. Fermentation may generate compounds that could contribute to blood glucose regulation, thereby reducing the risk of T2D. For example, the fermentation of yogurt by LAB may lead to the increased production of bioactive peptides with physiologic effects, such as increased insulin sensitivity and glucose tolerance. Fermentation may also enhance the content of conjugated linoleic acid (CLA), which is thought to promote blood glucose control (Bhattacharya et al. 2006).

Fermentation in yogurt distinguishes it from milk and the importance of dairy ferments may be supported in part by findings in studies such as Chen et al. (2014), who reported that yogurt was significantly associated with a reduced risk of T2D in three pooled cohorts and in an updated meta-analysis, whereas other dairy products were not appreciably associated with T2D risk (Chen et al. 2014). It can therefore be proposed that the strong protective effects of yogurt on T2D go beyond its base ingredients in milk. Other factors that are unique to yogurt may be responsible for the protective relationship consistently observed between yogurt consumption and reduced T2D risk (e.g., lactic acid bacteria or the fermentation process). A review has recently indicated that cultured dairy products (yogurt and doogh) have a beneficial effect on glycemic control and diabetic markers (e.g., HbA_{1c}) (Pasin and Comerford 2015). Additional dairy components such as oligosaccharides may modify the microbiome, which could also have a beneficial impact on host metabolism (Hirahatake et al. 2014). Further research is needed to investigate the impact of yogurt bacteria on gut and host glucose regulation and metabolism.

4.4 CONCLUSIONS

- Prospective studies have shown that the consumption of dairy products, specifically low-fat dairy, has the potential to reduce the risk of T2D.
- An increasing number of meta-analyses of large prospective cohort studies have evaluated the specific impact of yogurt on T2D incidence, demonstrating consistent inverse relationships for the protective effect of yogurt on

T2D. Given that large cohort studies have accounted for lifestyle factors, and that meta-analyses of these studies are still able to find a strong significant inverse relationship between yogurt consumption and T2D incidence, the evidence is extremely promising.
- The insulinotropic effects of yogurt peptides and vitamins and minerals such as vitamin D, calcium, and magnesium could act positively to reduce T2D risk. However, the specific mechanisms by which these nutrients exert their effect are not well known. Moreover, the low glycemic load of yogurt, its content in protein, lipid, and bacteria, and its texture and acidity could also have an impact on satiety and obesity-related mechanisms to lower T2D incidence.
- There is emerging evidence that the consumption of specific dairy fatty acids may be inversely associated with T2D, which warrants closer examination.
- More data is required, particularly from well-controlled clinical studies, to quantify the efficacy of yogurt in modulating the prevention and treatment of T2D. The reduction of postprandial blood glucose responses, long-term blood glucose control, and insulin sensitivity need to be measured using appropriated and recognized biomarkers (e.g., HbA_{1c}) and efficient techniques such as oral glucose tolerance test (OGTT) and hyperinsulinemic-euglycemic clamps.

REFERENCES

Aune, D., T. Norat, P. Romundstad, and L. J. Vatten. 2013. Dairy products and the risk of type 2 diabetes: A systematic review and dose-response meta-analysis of cohort studies. *Am J Clin Nutr* 98 (4):1066–83.

Bhattacharya, A., J. Banu, M. Rahman, J. Causey, and G. Fernandes. 2006. Biological effects of conjugated linoleic acids in health and disease. *J Nutr Biochem* 17 (12):789–810.

Calle, C., B. Maestro, and M. Garcïa-Arencibia. 2008. Genomic actions of 1,25-dihydroxyvitamin D3 on insulin receptor gene expression, insulin receptor number and insulin activity in the kidney, liver and adipose tissue of streptozotocin-induced diabetic rats. *BMC Mol Biol* 9:65.

Candido, F. G., W. T. Ton, and C. Alfenas Rde. 2013. Dairy products consumption versus type 2 diabetes prevention and treatment; a review of recent findings from human studies. *Nutr Hosp* 28 (5):1384–95.

Chen, M., Q. Sun, E. Giovannucci, D. Mozaffarian, J. E. Manson, W. C. Willett, and F. B. Hu. 2014. Dairy consumption and risk of type 2 diabetes: 3 cohorts of U.S. adults and an updated meta-analysis. *BMC Med* 12:215.

Chen, M. J., A. Jovanovic, and R. Taylor. 2010. Utilizing the second-meal effect in type 2 diabetes: Practical use of a soya-yogurt snack. *Diabetes Care* 33 (12):2552–54.

Choi, H. K., W. C. Willett, M. J. Stampfer, E. Rimm, and F. B. Hu. 2005. Dairy consumption and risk of type 2 diabetes mellitus in men: A prospective study. *Arch Intern Med* 165 (9):997–1003.

Committee DGA. 2010. *Report of the Dietary Guidelines Advisory Committee on the Dietary Guidelines for Americans, 2010, to the Secretary of Agriculture and the Secretary of Health and Human Services*. Washington, DC: U.S. Department of Agriculture ARS.

Diaz-López, A., M. Bulló, M. Á. Martínez-González, D. Corella, R. Estruch, M. Fito, E. Gómez-Gracia, et al. 2015. Dairy product consumption and risk of type 2 diabetes in

an elderly Spanish Mediterranean population at high cardiovascular risk. *Eur J Nutr* 55 (1):349–60.
Drehmer, M., M. A. Pereira, M. I. Schmidt, M. D. B. Molina, S. Alvim, P. A. Lotufo, and B. B. Duncan. 2015. Associations of dairy intake with glycemia and insulinemia, independent of obesity, in Brazilian adults: The Brazilian longitudinal study of adult health (ELSA-Brasil). *Am J Clin Nutr* 101 (4):775–82.
Du, H., A. Dl van der, M. M. van Bakel, C. J. van der Kallen, E. E. Blaak, M. M. van Greevenbroek, E. H. Jansen, et al. 2008. Glycemic index and glycemic load in relation to food and nutrient intake and metabolic risk factors in a Dutch population. *Am J Clin Nutr* 87 (3):655–61.
Ericson, U., S. Hellstrand, L. Brunkwall, C. A. Schulz, E. Sonestedt, P. Wallstrom, B. Gullberg, et al. 2015. Food sources of fat may clarify the inconsistent role of dietary fat intake for incidence of type 2 diabetes. *Am J Clin Nutr* 101 (5):1065–80.
Forouhi, N. G. 2015. Association between consumption of dairy products and incident type 2 diabetes-insights from the European Prospective Investigation into Cancer study. *Nutr Rev* 73 (Suppl 1):15–22.
Forouhi, N. G., A. Koulman, S. J. Sharp, F. Imamura, J. Kroger, M. B. Schulze, F. L. Crowe, et al. 2014. Differences in the prospective association between individual plasma phospholipid saturated fatty acids and incident type 2 diabetes: The EPIC-InterAct case-cohort study. *Lancet Diabetes Endocrinol* 2 (10):810–18.
Gagnon, C., Z. X. Lu, D. J. Magliano, D. W. Dunstan, J. E. Shaw, P. Z. Zimmet, K. Sikaris, P. R. Ebeling, and R. M. Daly. 2012. Low serum 25-hydroxyvitamin D is associated with increased risk of the development of the metabolic syndrome at five years: Results from a national, population-based prospective study (the Australian Diabetes, Obesity and Lifestyle Study: AusDiab). *J Clin Endocrinol Metab* 97 (6):1953–61.
Gao, D., N. Ning, C. Wang, Y. Wang, Q. Li, Z. Meng, Y. Liu, and Q. Li. 2013. Dairy products consumption and risk of type 2 diabetes: Systematic review and dose-response meta-analysis. *PLoS One* 8 (9):e73965.
Gijsbers, L., E. L. Ding, V. S. Malik, J. de Goede, J. M. Geleijnse, and S. S. Soedamah-Muthu. 2016. Consumption of dairy foods and diabetes incidence: A dose-response meta-analysis of observational studies. *Am J Clin Nutr* 103 (4):1111–24.
Gogebakan, O., A. Kohl, M. A. Osterhoff, M. A. van Baak, S. A. Jebb, A. Papadaki, J. A. Martinez, et al. 2011. Effects of weight loss and long-term weight maintenance with diets varying in protein and glycemic index on cardiovascular risk factors: The diet, obesity, and genes (DioGenes) study: A randomized, controlled trial. *Circulation* 124 (25):2829–38.
Grantham, N. M., D. J. Magliano, A. Hodge, J. Jowett, P. Meikle, and J. E. Shaw. 2013. The association between dairy food intake and the incidence of diabetes in Australia: The Australian Diabetes, Obesity and Lifestyle Study (AusDiab). *Public Health Nutr* 16 (2):339–45.
Hirahatake, K. M., J. L. Slavin, K. C. Maki, and S. H. Adams. 2014. Associations between dairy foods, diabetes, and metabolic health: Potential mechanisms and future directions. *Metabolism* 63 (5):618–27.
Hoyt, G., M. S. Hickey, and L. Cordain. 2005. Dissociation of the glycaemic and insulinaemic responses to whole and skimmed milk. *Br J Nutr* 93 (2):175–7.
International Diabetes Federation. 2015. *IDF Diabetes Atlas* 7th edition. Brussels: International Diabetes Federation.
Jakubowicz, D., and O. Froy. 2012. Biochemical and metabolic mechanisms by which dietary whey protein may combat obesity and type 2 diabetes. *J Nutr Biochem* 24 (1):1–5.
Kirii, K., T. Mizoue, H. Iso, Y. Takahashi, M. Kato, M. Inoue, M. Noda, and S. Tsugane. 2009. Calcium, vitamin D and dairy intake in relation to type 2 diabetes risk in a Japanese cohort. *Diabetologia* 52 (12):2542–50.

Lacroix, I. M., and E. C. Li-Chan. 2014. Investigation of the putative associations between dairy consumption and incidence of type 1 and type 2 diabetes. *Crit Rev Food Sci Nutr* 54 (4):411–32.

Larsen, T. M., S. M. Dalskov, M. van Baak, S. A. Jebb, A. Papadaki, A. F. Pfeiffer, J. A. Martinez, et al. 2010. Diets with high or low protein content and glycemic index for weight-loss maintenance. *N Engl J Med* 363 (22):2102–13.

Liljeberg, H., and I. Bjorck. 1998. Delayed gastric emptying rate may explain improved glycaemia in healthy subjects to a starchy meal with added vinegar. *Eur J Clin Nutr* 52 (5):368–71.

Lindström, C., A. Voinot, A. Forslund, O. Holst, A. Rascon, R. Öste, and E. Östman. 2015. An oat bran-based beverage reduce postprandial glycaemia equivalent to yoghurt in healthy overweight subjects. *Int J Food Sci Nutr* 66 (6):700–705.

Liu, E., N. M. McKeown, P. K. Newby, J. B. Meigs, R. S. Vasan, P. A. Quatromoni, R. B. D'Agostino, and P. F. Jacques. 2009. Cross-sectional association of dietary patterns with insulin-resistant phenotypes among adults without diabetes in the Framingham Offspring Study. *Br J Nutr* 102 (4):576–83.

Liu, S., H. K. Choi, E. Ford, Y. Song, A. Klevak, J. E. Buring, and J. E. Manson. 2006. A prospective study of dairy intake and the risk of type 2 diabetes in women. *Diabetes Care* 29 (7):1579–84.

Margolis, K. L., F. Wei, I. H. de Boer, B. V. Howard, S. Liu, J. E. Manson, Y. Mossavar-Rahmani, et al. 2011. A diet high in low-fat dairy products lowers diabetes risk in postmenopausal women. *J Nutr* 141 (11):1969–74.

Miller, J. B., E. Pang, and L. Broomhead. 1995. The glycemic index of foods containing sugars: Comparison of foods with naturally-occurring v added sugars. *Br J Nutr* 73 (4):613–23.

Montecucco, F., S. Steffens, and F. Mach. 2008. Insulin resistance: A proinflammatory state mediated by lipid-induced signaling dysfunction and involved in atherosclerotic plaque instability. *Mediators Inflamm* 2008:767623.

Mozaffarian, D., H. Cao, I. B. King, R. N. Lemaitre, X. Song, D. S. Siscovick, and G. S. Hotamisligil. 2010. Trans-palmitoleic acid, metabolic risk factors, and new-onset diabetes in U.S. adults: A cohort study. *Ann Intern Med* 153 (12):790–9.

Nestel, P. 2012. Nutrition and metabolism: The changing face of the dairy-cardiovascular risk paradox. *Curr Opin Lipidol* 23 (1):1–3.

Nestel, P. J., N. Straznicky, N. A. Mellett, G. Wong, D. P. De Souza, D. L. Tull, C. K. Barlow, et al. 2014. Specific plasma lipid classes and phospholipid fatty acids indicative of dairy food consumption associate with insulin sensitivity. *Am J Clin Nutr* 99 (1):46–53.

Nikooyeh, B., T. R. Neyestani, M. Farvid, H. Alavi-Majd, A. Houshiarrad, A. Kalayi, N. Shariatzadeh, et al. 2011. Daily consumption of vitamin D or vitamin D+calcium-fortified yogurt drink improved glycemic control in patients with type 2 diabetes: A randomized clinical trial. *Am J Clin Nutr* 93 (4):764–71.

Nilsson, M., M. Stenberg, A. H. Frid, J. J. Holst, and I. M. Bjorck. 2004. Glycemia and insulinemia in healthy subjects after lactose-equivalent meals of milk and other food proteins: The role of plasma amino acids and incretins. *Am J Clin Nutr* 80 (5):1246–53.

O'Connor, L. M., M. A. Lentjes, R. N. Luben, K. T. Khaw, N. J. Wareham, and N. G. Forouhi. 2014. Dietary dairy product intake and incident type 2 diabetes: A prospective study using dietary data from a 7-day food diary. *Diabetologia* 57 (5):909–17.

Ojuka, E. O. 2004. Role of calcium and AMP kinase in the regulation of mitochondrial biogenesis and GLUT4 levels in muscle. *Proc Nutr Soc* 63 (2):275–78.

Ostman, E. M., H. G. Liljeberg Elmstahl, and I. M. Bjorck. 2001. Inconsistency between glycemic and insulinemic responses to regular and fermented milk products. *Am J Clin Nutr* 74 (1):96–100.

Panagiotakos, D. B., N. Tzima, C. Pitsavos, C. Chrysohoou, E. Papakonstantinou, A. Zampelas, and C. Stefanadis. 2005. The relationship between dietary habits, blood glucose and insulin levels among people without cardiovascular disease and type 2 diabetes; the ATTICA study. *Rev Diabet Stud* 2 (4):208–15.

Pasin, G., and K. B. Comerford. 2015. Dairy foods and dairy proteins in the management of type 2 diabetes: A systematic review of the clinical evidence. *Adv Nutr* 6 (3):245–59.

Pereira, M. A., D. R. Jacobs, Jr., L. Van Horn, M. L. Slattery, A. I. Kartashov, and D. S. Ludwig. 2002. Dairy consumption, obesity, and the insulin resistance syndrome in young adults: The CARDIA study. *JAMA* 287 (16):2081–89.

Pittas, A. G., B. Dawson-Hughes, T. Li, R. M. Van Dam, W. C. Willett, J. E. Manson, and F. B. Hu. 2006. Vitamin D and calcium intake in relation to type 2 diabetes in women. *Diabetes Care* 29 (3):650–56.

Pittas, A. G., J. Lau, F. B. Hu, and B. Dawson-Hughes. 2007. The role of vitamin D and calcium in type 2 diabetes. A systematic review and meta-analysis. *J Clin Endocrinol Metab* 92 (6):2017–29.

Rosolova, H., O. Mayer, Jr., and G. Reaven. 1997. Effect of variations in plasma magnesium concentration on resistance to insulin-mediated glucose disposal in nondiabetic subjects. *J Clin Endocrinol Metab* 82 (11):3783–85.

Santaren, I. D., S. M. Watkins, A. D. Liese, L. E. Wagenknecht, M. J. Rewers, S. M. Haffner, C. Lorenzo, and A. J. Hanley. 2014. Serum pentadecanoic acid (15:0), a short-term marker of dairy food intake, is inversely associated with incident type 2 diabetes and its underlying disorders. *Am J Clin Nutr* 100 (6):1532–40.

Scragg, R., M. Sowers, and C. Bell. 2004. Serum 25-hydroxyvitamin D, diabetes, and ethnicity in the Third National Health and Nutrition Examination Survey. *Diabetes Care* 27 (12):2813–18.

Shab-Bidar, S., T. R. Neyestani, A. Djazayery, M. R. Eshraghian, A. Houshiarrad, A. Gharavi, A. Kalayi, et al. 2011. Regular consumption of vitamin D-fortified yogurt drink (doogh) improved endothelial biomarkers in subjects with type 2 diabetes: A randomized double-blind clinical trial. *BMC Med* 9:125.

Sluijs, I., N. G. Forouhi, J. W. Beulens, Y. T. van der Schouw, C. Agnoli, L. Arriola, B. Balkau, et al. 2012. The amount and type of dairy product intake and incident type 2 diabetes: Results from the EPIC-InterAct Study. *Am J Clin Nutr* 96 (2):382–90.

Snijder, M. B., A. A. van der Heijden, R. M. van Dam, C. D. Stehouwer, G. J. Hiddink, G. Nijpels, R. J. Heine, et al. 2007. Is higher dairy consumption associated with lower body weight and fewer metabolic disturbances? The Hoorn Study. *Am J Clin Nutr* 85 (4):989–95.

Soedamah-Muthu, S. S., G. Masset, L. Verberne, J. M. Geleijnse, and E. J. Brunner. 2012. Consumption of dairy products and associations with incident diabetes, CHD and mortality in the Whitehall II study. *Br J Nutr*:1–9.

Tong, X., J. Y. Dong, Z. W. Wu, W. Li, and L. Q. Qin. 2011. Dairy consumption and risk of type 2 diabetes mellitus: A meta-analysis of cohort studies. *Eur J Clin Nutr* 65 (9):1027–31.

Turner, K. M., J. B. Keogh, and P. M. Clifton. 2015a. Dairy consumption and insulin sensitivity: A systematic review of short- and long-term intervention studies. *Nutr Metab Cardiovasc Dis* 25 (1):3–8.

Turner, K. M., J. B. Keogh, and P. M. Clifton. 2015c. Red meat, dairy, and insulin sensitivity: A randomized crossover intervention study. *Am J Clin Nutr* 101 (6):1173–9.

Van Dam, R. M., F. B. Hu, L. Rosenberg, S. Krishnan, and J. R. Palmer. 2006. Dietary calcium and magnesium, major food sources, and risk of type 2 diabetes in U.S. Black women. *Diabetes Care* 29 (10):2238–43.

Villegas, R., Y. T. Gao, Q. Dai, G. Yang, H. Cai, H. Li, W. Zheng, and X. O. Shu. 2009. Dietary calcium and magnesium intakes and the risk of type 2 diabetes: The Shanghai Women's Health Study. *Am J Clin Nutr* 89 (4):1059–67.

WHO. 2012. WHO diabetes fact sheet n°312. http://www.who.int/mediacentre/factsheets/fs312/en/.

Wright, D. C., K. A. Hucker, J. O. Holloszy, and D. H. Han. 2004. Ca^{2+} and AMPK both mediate stimulation of glucose transport by muscle contractions. *Diabetes* 53 (2):330–35.

Yokota, K. 2005. Diabetes mellitus and magnesium. *Clin Calcium* 15 (2):203–12.

Zeitz, U., K. Weber, D. W. Soegiarto, E. Wolf, R. Balling, and R. G. Erben. 2003. Impaired insulin secretory capacity in mice lacking a functional vitamin D receptor. *FASEB J* 17 (3):509–11.

Zhu, Y., H. Wang, J. H. Hollis, and P. F. Jacques. 2015. The associations between yogurt consumption, diet quality, and metabolic profiles in children in the USA. *Eur J Nutr* 54 (4):543–50.

5 Hypertension

Elevated blood pressure is one of the major independent risk factors for cardiovascular disease (CVD). To prevent hypertension and its adverse outcomes (e.g., stroke, heart, and renal failure), health authorities recommend regular physical activity, moderate alcohol intake, weight control, reduced sodium intake, and increased potassium intake (Appel et al. 2006, Mancia et al. 2009, 2013). A diet rich in fruit, vegetables, and low-fat dairy products and low in saturated and total fat has been reported to lower blood pressure in the Dietary Approaches to Stop Hypertension (DASH) Trial (Appel et al. 1997). The DASH diet includes two to three servings of low-fat or nonfat dairy foods per day (2000 calorie diet). Figure 5.1 illustrates the number of portions recommended for each food group in the DASH diet. In 2010, the Dietary Guidelines Advisory Committee (DGAC), assisted by the U.S. Department of Agriculture (USDA) Nutrition Evidence Library, concluded that there was moderate evidence for an inverse relationship between the intake of milk and milk products and blood pressure (McGrane et al. 2011). A meta-analysis of five cohort studies (nearly 45,000 subjects) was conducted to examine the association between dairy food intake from low- and high-fat dairy, cheese, and fluid dairy food (milk or yogurt), and blood pressure. A reduction of blood pressure was found with low-fat dairy foods and fluid dairy (milk or yogurt) foods (Ralston et al. 2012).

Fermented milk has been marketed as a functional food with putative antihypertensive properties (e.g., United States, Spain, United Kingdom, Finland, Switzerland, Italy, South Korea, Japan, Iceland, and Portugal) (Boelsma and Kloek 2009) and consuming yogurt is considered a common traditional treatment for hypertension in some countries such as Turkey (Toprak and Demir 2007). The next sections will discuss the scientific evidence on yogurt and its potential impact on hypertension.

5.1 STUDIES IN ADULTS

5.1.1 Cross-Sectional Studies

In a cross-sectional cohort of 5,616 adults from the Tehran Lipid and Glucose Study (TLGS), high consumptions of high-fat dairy and nonfermented dairy and milk intake were inversely associated with hypertension. On the other hand, yogurt and cheese were positively associated with hypertension. This finding for yogurt contrasts with other studies that have found either neutral or inverse associations. Authors cite potential residual confounding factors that explain this relationship (Mirmiran et al. 2015).

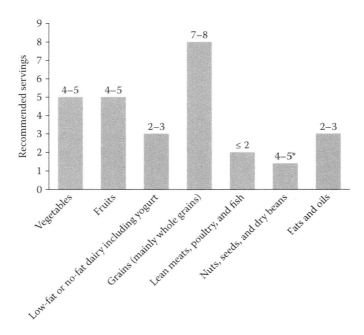

FIGURE 5.1 Daily portions recommended from each food group under the DASH diet, including low-fat or nonfat dairy and yogurt. *Recommendations for nuts, seeds, and dry beans are weekly and not daily.

5.1.2 Prospective Studies

The association between dietary intake and the 15-year incidence of elevated blood pressure was assessed in the Coronary Artery Risk Development in Young Adults (CARDIA) study, which included 4304 participants aged 18–30 years. A plant-based food intake (whole grains, refined grains, fruit, vegetables, nuts, and legumes) was inversely associated with elevated blood pressure. The consumption of milk and dairy desserts was also inversely related to elevated blood pressure. In dairy product subgroup analyses, no association was found for yogurt (p for trend = .14) (Steffen et al. 2005).

Wang et al. (2008) evaluated the associations between the intakes of dairy products, calcium, and vitamin D and the incidence of hypertension in a prospective cohort (28,886 U.S. women aged ≥45 years). The consumption of low-fat dairy products, calcium, and vitamin D was inversely associated with the risk of hypertension in middle-aged and older women. A reduction of 10%–15% in hypertension risk was observed for all four major low-fat dairy products (comparing the highest with the lowest intake category); however, the reduction was statistically significant only for skim milk and yogurt. Multivariate adjustment substantially attenuated the inverse association for yogurt (Wang et al. 2008).

The role of anthropometric characteristics and dietary habits was evaluated in a large cohort of Mediterranean women (10,083 women, 35–64 years) from the

European Prospective Investigation into Cancer and Nutrition–Florence. The consumption of yogurt, vegetables, and eggs was inversely associated with systolic blood pressure. Olive oil was inversely associated with diastolic blood pressure and leafy vegetables, milk, and coffee were inversely associated with both systolic and diastolic blood pressure. Authors also reported that body mass index (BMI) and waist circumference, as well as the intake of processed meat, potatoes, and wine, were directly associated with systolic and diastolic blood pressure. Interestingly, additional analyses performed on nutrients showed an inverse association between blood pressure and calcium, potassium, and micronutrients derived from fruits and vegetables, as well as a positive association between blood pressure and sodium and alcohol (Masala et al. 2008).

Data from the Hoorn Study involving 1,124 elderly Dutch (50–75 years) showed that yogurt consumption was inversely associated with systolic blood pressure. However, once adjusted for various confounding factors, the decrease in systolic blood pressure no longer reached statistical significance (Snijder et al. 2007).

The Prevención con Dieta Mediterránea (Prevention with a Mediterranean Diet [PREDIMED]) study examined metabolic syndrome incidence in relation to yogurt consumption in a cohort of older adults (55–80 years) followed for an average of 3.2 years. Blood pressure was the only metabolic syndrome component that was not inversely associated with total yogurt and low-fat yogurt. There was, however, a significant reduction in the risk of hypertension among participants who had a high consumption of whole-fat yogurt compared with a low consumption, HR = 0.62 (95% CI 0.44, 0.86; $p < .001$) (Babio et al. 2015).

The relationship between incident hypertension, changes in blood pressure, and dairy product consumption was examined in a prospective cohort of 2,636 adults from the Framingham Heart Study Offspring Cohort from 1991 to 2008. Inverse relationships in fully adjusted models were found between smaller annual increments of systolic blood pressure and higher intakes of total dairy, low-fat and nonfat dairy, total milk, low-fat and nonfat milk, yogurt, and fermented dairy, but not high-fat dairy, whole-fat milk, or cheese. Similar inverse relationships were seen between annual increments of diastolic blood pressure with higher intakes of total dairy, low-fat and nonfat dairy, total milk, and low-fat and nonfat milk, but not yogurt, fermented dairy, high-fat dairy, whole-fat milk, or cheese. There was also a significantly reduced risk of incident hypertension during the follow-up period in fully adjusted models for each additional serving of total dairy per day, as well as each additional serving per week, of high-fat dairy, yogurt, fermented milk, low-fat and nonfat dairy, and low-fat and nonfat milk. Sensitivity analyses excluded yogurt from the low-fat group, and the relationship was no longer significant, indicating that perhaps yogurt consumption was driving the inverse relationship in the low-fat dairy group. Each additional serving of yogurt per week was associated with a 5% reduction in risk of incident hypertension, HR = 0.95 (95% CI 0.90, 0.99; $p = .02$) (Wang et al. 2015).

5.1.3 META-ANALYSES AND REVIEWS

Soedamah-Muthu et al. (2012) performed a dose–response meta-analysis of prospective cohort studies on dairy intake and risk of hypertension in the general population.

This meta-analysis showed that the consumption of total dairy, low-fat dairy, and milk was inversely and linearly associated with a lower risk of hypertension. However, total fermented dairy (four studies), yogurt (five studies), cheese (eight studies), and high-fat dairy (six studies) were not significantly associated with hypertension incidence. Stratified analyses (age group, continent, weight status, BMI, and follow-up duration), could not be performed on the impact of yogurt alone because of the limited number of studies (Soedamah-Muthu et al. 2012).

The authors of a Cochrane Review of randomized controlled trials on milk or casein fermented with several bacterial strains do not support the use of fermented milk as a treatment for hypertension or as a lifestyle intervention for prehypertension (Usinger et al. 2012). Indeed, despite the positive effect on blood pressure, the reduction was very modest and limited to systolic blood pressure; furthermore, the studies included were very heterogeneous and several were limited at the methodological level.

5.2 MECHANISMS OF ACTION

5.2.1 Effect of Dairy Proteins and Peptides

Milk is an important source for bioactive peptides, which can be released during the fermentation process and through hydrolysis of milk proteins by microorganism-derived enzymes or digestive enzymes (Rai et al. 2015). The amount of bioactive peptides increases during the fermentation of milk. A study using spontaneously hypertensive rats fed fermented milk + isoleucine-proline-proline (IPP) and valine-proline-proline (VPP) showed significant reductions of systolic blood pressure (Sipola et al. 2001). Moreover, human studies have shown positive effects following treatment with fermented food enriched with bioactive peptides on arterial stiffness (Jauhiainen et al. 2005) and blood pressure in hypertensive subjects (Mizushima et al. 2004, Seppo et al. 2003, Tuomilehto et al. 2004). It has been reported that the magnitude of the fall in blood pressure following dairy peptide consumption is related to baseline blood pressure (de Leeuw et al. 2009). Potential antihypertensive components of yogurt are illustrated in Figure 5.2.

Peptides with the amino acid sequence isoleucine–proline–proline (IPP) and valine–proline–proline (VPP) are the best characterized peptides found in fermented milk (Boelsma and Kloek 2009). Many studies evaluating the role of dairy protein/peptides on hypertension focused on the effect of lactotripeptides (such as IPP and VPP), which have shown angiotensin-converting-enzyme (ACE)-inhibitory effect *in vitro*. ACE is one of the key enzymes in blood pressure regulation, because it generates the vasoconstrictor angiotensin-II and inactivates the vasodilator bradykinin. However, because the action of bioactive peptides depends on their bioavailability, it is difficult to establish a direct relationship between ACE-inhibitory peptides activity detected *in vitro* and hypotensive action *in vivo*. Indeed, because of the intestinal breakdown of the peptides, very effective *in vitro* ACE-inhibitory peptides from α-casein failed to have a positive effect on blood pressure in hypertension models. However, recently, the tripeptide IPP has been shown to selectively escape from intestinal degradation and enter intact in the circulation (Foltz et al. 2007). Fermented

Hypertension

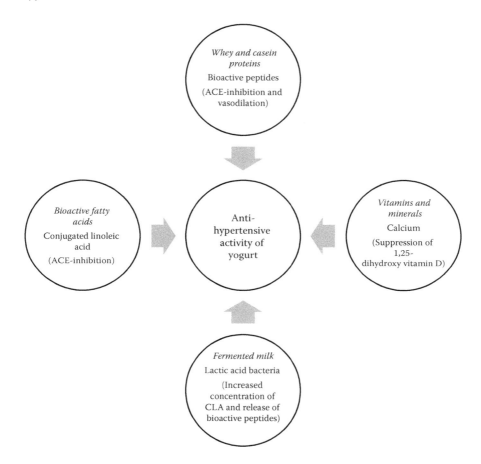

FIGURE 5.2 Yogurt components with potential antihypertensive activity.

dairy products such as yogurt may have ACE-inhibitory peptides and are the best-known dietary sources of these peptides (Rai et al. 2015). Both regular yogurt and a probiotic yogurt were found to have higher levels of ACE-inhibitory action than a UHT milk control (Shakerian et al. 2015). Regular (freeze-dried) yogurt and probiotic yogurt had antihypertensive effects when fed to spontaneously hypertensive rats, significantly lowering systolic and diastolic blood pressure (Ramchandran and Shah 2011). ACE-inhibitory properties in fermented milks have not been clearly demonstrated in humans (Usinger et al. 2012). In addition to ACE inhibition, it has been proposed that lactotripeptides also have an effect on vasoactive substances (e.g., vasoconstrictor endothelin-1, eicosanoids, and nitric oxide) and opioid agonist effects (Boelsma and Kloek 2009).

5.2.2 Effect of Ca, K, Mg, and Lipids

Some studies have reported an inverse association between calcium intake and the risk of hypertension. Dietary calcium is thought to reduce blood pressure, in comparison to those fed skim milk, by suppressing 1,25-dihydroxyvitamin D, which increases vascular smooth muscle intracellular calcium, peripheral vascular resistance, and blood pressure (Zemel 2001). However, a Cochrane Review of calcium supplementation in adults found that evidence of a causal association between calcium supplementation and a reduction in blood pressure was weak (Dickinson et al. 2006). This could be related to the limited quality and heterogeneity of the trials.

In some studies, the relationship between dairy products and lower blood pressure was still significant after adjusting for dietary calcium, suggesting that other nutrients could play a role in mediating this association (Pereira et al. 2002, Ruidavets et al. 2006). Increased potassium intake raises plasma potassium levels and this is related to endothelium-dependent vasodilatation. This vasodilatation is increased by the stimulation of the sodium pump (Na-K ATPase) and the opening of the potassium channels of the Na-K ATPase (Lawes et al. 2008). Some authors observed that calcium, potassium, and magnesium are regularly present simultaneously in foods such as dairy products and that a specific balance between these three minerals seems to be needed for optimal control of blood pressure by the body (Azadbakht et al. 2005).

5.3 CONCLUSIONS

- Available evidence implicating the protective association between yogurt and hypertension is increasingly promising, but remains weak and slightly contradictory. Additional prospective studies in diverse populations are needed.
- The few available randomized controlled trial studies are very heterogeneous and several had questionable methodologies. Yogurt-specific randomized controlled trials are needed to provide more conclusive evidence of a causal relationship between yogurt intake and reduced blood pressure.
- The micronutrient composition of yogurt, together with high protein, bioactive lactotripeptides, and low sodium, could exert additive or synergetic protective effects against hypertension.
- Additional investigation into the potential impact of bioactive yogurt peptides and other constituents such as calcium, potassium, and magnesium on hypertension is warranted.

REFERENCES

Appel, L. J., M. W. Brands, S. R. Daniels, N. Karanja, P. J. Elmer, and F. M. Sacks. 2006. Dietary approaches to prevent and treat hypertension: A scientific statement from the American Heart Association. *Hypertension* 47 (2):296–308.

Appel, L. J., T. J. Moore, E. Obarzanek, W. M. Vollmer, L. P. Svetkey, F. M. Sacks, G. A. Bray, et al. 1997. A clinical trial of the effects of dietary patterns on blood pressure. DASH collaborative research group. *N Engl J Med* 336 (16):1117–24.

Azadbakht, L., P. Mirmiran, A. Esmaillzadeh, and F. Azizi. 2005. Dairy consumption is inversely associated with the prevalence of the metabolic syndrome in Tehranian adults. *Am J Clin Nutr* 82 (3):523–30.

Babio, N., N. Becerra-Tomás, M. A. Martínez-González, D. Corella, R. Estruch, E. Ros, C. Sayón-Orea, et al. 2015. Consumption of yogurt, low-fat milk, and other low-fat dairy products is associated with lower risk of metabolic syndrome incidence in an elderly Mediterranean population. *J Nutr* 145 (10):2308–16.

Boelsma, E., and J. Kloek. 2009. Lactotripeptides and antihypertensive effects: A critical review. *Br J Nutr* 101 (6):776–86.

De Leeuw, P. W., K. van der Zander, A. A. Kroon, R. M. Rennenberg, and M. M. Koning. 2009. Dose-dependent lowering of blood pressure by dairy peptides in mildly hypertensive subjects. *Blood Press* 18 (1–2):44–50.

Dickinson, H. O., D. J. Nicolson, J. V. Cook, F. Campbell, F. R. Beyer, G. A. Ford, and J. Mason. 2006. Calcium supplementation for the management of primary hypertension in adults. *Cochrane Database Syst Rev* (2):CD004639.

Foltz, M., E. E. Meynen, V. Bianco, C. van Platerink, T. M. Koning, and J. Kloek. 2007. Angiotensin converting enzyme inhibitory peptides from a lactotripeptide-enriched milk beverage are absorbed intact into the circulation. *J Nutr* 137 (4):953–58.

Jauhiainen, T., H. Vapaatalo, T. Poussa, S. Kyronpalo, M. Rasmussen, and R. Korpela. 2005. *Lactobacillus helveticus* fermented milk lowers blood pressure in hypertensive subjects in 24-h ambulatory blood pressure measurement. *Am J Hypertens* 18 (12 Pt 1):1600–5.

Lawes, C. M., S. Vander Hoorn, and A. Rodgers. 2008. Global burden of blood-pressure-related disease, 2001. *Lancet* 371 (9623):1513–18.

Mancia, G., R. Fagard, K. Narkiewicz, J. Redon, A. Zanchetti, M. Böhm, T. Christiaens, et al. 2013. 2013 ESH/ESC guidelines for the management of arterial hypertension. *Eur Heart J* 34 (28):2159–19.

Mancia, G., S. Laurent, E. Agabiti-Rosei, E. Ambrosioni, M. Burnier, M. J. Caulfield, R. Cifkova, et al. 2009. Reappraisal of European guidelines on hypertension management: A European Society of Hypertension Task Force document. *J Hypertens* 27 (11):2121–58.

Masala, G., B. Bendinelli, D. Versari, C. Saieva, M. Ceroti, F. Santagiuliana, S. Caini, et al. 2008. Anthropometric and dietary determinants of blood pressure in over 7000 Mediterranean women: The European Prospective Investigation into Cancer and Nutrition-Florence cohort. *J Hypertens* 26 (11):2112–20.

McGrane, M. M., E. Essery, J. Obbagy, J. Lyon, P. Macneil, J. Spahn, and L. Van Horn. 2011. Dairy consumption, blood pressure, and risk of hypertension: An evidence-based review of recent literature. *Curr Cardiovasc Risk Rep* 5 (4):287–98.

Mirmiran, P., M. Golzarand, Z. Bahadoran, S. Mirzaei, and F. Azizi. 2015. High-fat dairy is inversely associated with the risk of hypertension in adults: Tehran lipid and glucose study. *Int Dairy J* 43:22–26.

Mizushima, S., K. Ohshige, J. Watanabe, M. Kimura, T. Kadowaki, Y. Nakamura, O. Tochikubo, and H. Ueshima. 2004. Randomized controlled trial of sour milk on blood pressure in borderline hypertensive men. *Am J Hypertens* 17 (8):701–6.

Pereira, M. A., D. R. Jacobs, Jr., L. Van Horn, M. L. Slattery, A. I. Kartashov, and D. S. Ludwig. 2002. Dairy consumption, obesity, and the insulin resistance syndrome in young adults: The CARDIA study. *JAMA* 287 (16):2081–89.

Rai, A. K., S. Sanjukta, and K. Jeyaram. 2015. Production of angiotensin I converting enzyme inhibitory (ACE-I) peptides during milk fermentation and their role in reducing hypertension. *Crit Rev Food Sci Nutr*. In press. doi:10.1080/10408398.2015.1068736.

Ralston, R. A., J. H. Lee, H. Truby, C. E. Palermo, and K. Z. Walker. 2012. A systematic review and meta-analysis of elevated blood pressure and consumption of dairy foods. *J Hum Hypertens* 26 (1):3–13.

Ramchandran, L., and N. P. Shah. 2011. Yogurt can beneficially affect blood contributors of cardiovascular health status in hypertensive rats. *J Food Sci* 76 (4):H131–36.

Ruidavets, J. B., V. Bongard, C. Simon, J. Dallongeville, P. Ducimetiere, D. Arveiler, P. Amouyel, et al. 2006. Independent contribution of dairy products and calcium intake to blood pressure variations at a population level. *J Hypertens* 24 (4):671–81.

Seppo, L., T. Jauhiainen, T. Poussa, and R. Korpela. 2003. A fermented milk high in bioactive peptides has a blood pressure-lowering effect in hypertensive subjects. *Am J Clin Nutr* 77 (2):326–30.

Shakerian, M., S. H. Razavi, S. A. Ziai, F. Khodaiyan, M. S. Yarmand, and A. Moayedi. 2015. Proteolytic and ACE-inhibitory activities of probiotic yogurt containing non-viable bacteria as affected by different levels of fat, inulin and starter culture. *J Food Sci Technol* 52 (4):2428–33.

Sipola, M., P. Finckenberg, J. Santisteban, R. Korpela, H. Vapaatalo, and M. L. Nurminen. 2001. Long-term intake of milk peptides attenuates development of hypertension in spontaneously hypertensive rats. *J Physiol Pharmacol* 52 (4):745–54.

Snijder, M. B., A. A. van der Heijden, R. M. van Dam, C. D. Stehouwer, G. J. Hiddink, G. Nijpels, R. J. Heine, L. M. Bouter, et al. 2007. Is higher dairy consumption associated with lower body weight and fewer metabolic disturbances? The Hoorn Study. *Am J Clin Nutr* 85 (4):989–95.

Soedamah-Muthu, S. S., L. D. Verberne, E. L. Ding, M. F. Engberink, and J. M. Geleijnse. 2012. Dairy consumption and incidence of hypertension: A dose-response meta-analysis of prospective cohort studies. *Hypertension* 60 (5):1131–37.

Steffen, L. M., C. H. Kroenke, X. Yu, M. A. Pereira, M. L. Slattery, L. Van Horn, M. D. Gross, and D. R. Jacobs, Jr. 2005. Associations of plant food, dairy product, and meat intakes with 15-y incidence of elevated blood pressure in young black and white adults: The Coronary Artery Risk Development in Young Adults (CARDIA) study. *Am J Clin Nutr* 82 (6):1169–77; quiz 1363–64.

Toprak, D., and S. Demir. 2007. Treatment choices of hypertensive patients in Turkey. *Behav Med* 33 (1):5–10.

Tuomilehto, J., J. Lindstrom, J. Hyyrynen, R. Korpela, M. L. Karhunen, L. Mikkola, T. Jauhiainen, et al. 2004. Effect of ingesting sour milk fermented using Lactobacillus helveticus bacteria producing tripeptides on blood pressure in subjects with mild hypertension. *J Hum Hypertens* 18 (11):795–802.

Usinger, L., C. Reimer, and H. Ibsen. 2012. Fermented milk for hypertension. *Cochrane Database Syst Rev* 4:CD008118.

Wang, H., C. S. Fox, L. M. Troy, N. M. McKeown, and P. F. Jacques. 2015. Longitudinal association of dairy consumption with the changes in blood pressure and the risk of incident hypertension: The Framingham Heart Study. *Br J Nutr* 114 (11):1887–99.

Wang, L., J. E. Manson, J. E. Buring, I. M. Lee, and H. D. Sesso. 2008. Dietary intake of dairy products, calcium, and vitamin D and the risk of hypertension in middle-aged and older women. *Hypertension* 51 (4):1073–79.

Zemel, M. B. 2001. Calcium modulation of hypertension and obesity: Mechanisms and implications. *J Am Coll Nutr* 20 (5 Suppl):428S–435S; discussion 440S–442S.

6 Cardiovascular Diseases

Cardiovascular diseases (CVD) encompass a broad range of diseases involving the heart, brain, and blood vessels that together are the leading cause of death worldwide, killing more people around the globe than any other cause of death. Smoking, overweight, hypertension, high plasma cholesterol levels, and diabetes mellitus are risk factors for CVD (Mendis et al. 2011). Pathogenic pathways activated by an unhealthy diet and unfavorable lifestyles that could lead to CVD are illustrated in Figure 6.1.

Elevated serum low-density lipoprotein (LDL) cholesterol is a recognized risk factor for coronary heart disease (CHD) and systolic blood pressure is a recognized risk factor for both CHD and stroke. As such, according to the European Food Safety Authority, health claims can be made with regard to the reduction of LDL cholesterol and the reduced risk of CHD or reduced blood pressure and the reduced risk of CHD or stroke. While maintenance of normal high-density lipoprotein (HDL) cholesterol, triglyceride, and homocysteine levels are thought to be beneficial for cardiovascular health, human nutritional invention studies on CHD risk are needed to validate specific associations between disease risk and the reduction of triglycerides and homocysteine or the increase in HDL cholesterol before health claims regarding these variables can be substantiated (EFSA Panel of Dietetic Products 2011). Endpoints of disease risk accepted by the National Institutes of Health and/or the Food and Drug Administration's (FDA) Center for Drug Evaluation and Research for CVD include serum LDL cholesterol, total serum cholesterol, and blood pressure (FDA 2009, Perk et al. 2012).

Cornerstone recommendations for the prevention of CVD include a healthy diet, which is characterized by limiting energy intake to levels needed to maintain or obtain a healthy body mass index (BMI) (≤ 25 kg/m^2); <10% of total energy intake from saturated fatty acids (SFA) (replacement by polyunsaturated fatty acids); limit trans-unsaturated fatty acids to as little as possible; <5 g/day of salt; 30–45 g/day of fiber; two to three servings/day of fruit; two to three servings/day of vegetables; ≥ 2 servings/week of fish (one of which should fatty fish); limit alcohol consumption to two glasses/day for men and one glass/day for women. These key concepts of a healthy diet are supported by a class 1 recommendation (general agreement and/or evidence of benefit), level B evidence (single randomized clinical trials or large nonrandomized studies), and high-quality evidence. To lower total and LDL cholesterol, recommendations for dairy intake include promoting moderate consumption of nonfat or low-fat milk, yogurt, cheese, or other dairy products and limiting the consumption of regular cheese, cream, whole-fat milk, and whole-fat yogurt (Reiner et al. 2011, Perk et al. 2012). However, a study suggested that individuals who have high consumption of any type of milk (including whole fat) are less likely to develop CVDs (stroke and ischemic heart disease) than those who have a low intake of milk (Elwood et al. 2004). This indicates that components other than SFA in dairy food could preserve or improve cardiometabolic health (Lamarche 2008). The Multi-Ethnic Study of Atherosclerosis followed 45–84-year-old subjects ($n=5,209$) from

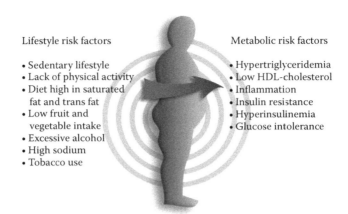

FIGURE 6.1 Lifestyle and metabolic risk factors for cardiovascular disease. (Adapted from Després, J.P., *Circulation*, 126, no. 10, 1301–1313, 2012.)

2000 to 2010 and concluded that the associations between saturated fat consumption and health may be dependent on food-specific fatty acids or other nutrient constituents in foods that contain saturated fat (de Oliveira Otto et al. 2012). A review of observational studies did not support the hypothesis that dairy fat or high-fat dairy foods contribute to obesity or cardiometabolic risk. The authors of the review stated that high-fat dairy consumption within typical dietary patterns is inversely associated with obesity risk (Kratz et al. 2013). Furthermore, not all SFAs have a negative impact on CVD and the food matrix in which they are found may also play a role in mediating some of the known negative properties of certain SFAs (Rozenberg et al. 2015).

A dietary intervention conducted on Australian adults with habitually low dairy intakes (in the absence of energy restriction) showed that the recommended intakes of low-fat dairy products (four servings per day of reduced fat dairy) could be incorporated into their diet without negative impacts on cardiometabolic health (Crichton et al. 2012). Moreover, a meta-analysis of prospective studies indicates that milk intake is not associated with total mortality (eight studies) and may be inversely associated with overall CVD risk (four studies) (Soedamah-Muthu et al. 2011). At present, the majority of observational studies have failed to find a positive association between the intake of dairy products and risk of CVD, CHD, and stroke, regardless of milk fat levels (Huth and Park 2012). An essential component of the Mediterranean diet is fermented foods, such as yogurt and cheese, and there is increasing evidence that these foods are implicated in dietary protection against CVD (Tapsell 2015). While not as well researched and established, the prudent diet, which includes yogurt, has been implicated in reducing markers of visceral fat and inflammation in individuals with high LDL cholesterol levels (Adamsson et al. 2015). Furthermore, the consumption of items from the dairy food group was characteristic of adolescents identified with low cardiovascular risk (Moreno et al. 2015) and adult patients admitted to hospital with acute ischemic stroke consumed less yogurt than control patients (Rodriguez-Campello et al. 2014). Other observational studies and some randomized trials support the inverse association between the consumption of yogurt and other dairy foods and CVD (Astrup 2014b). Results from numerous studies have consistently demonstrated that milk, cheese, and yogurt do not contribute to CVD risk (Rice 2014). While it appears that the consumption of dairy products is not related to an increased risk of CVD, particularly low-fat dairy (Rozenberg et al. 2015), more research is needed to elucidate the specific impact of high-fat dairy versus low-fat dairy, dairy protein versus dairy fat, different dairy subgroups, fermented dairy, and specific SFAs on CVD (Givens 2015). The following sections will discuss in detail studies investigating the relationship between yogurt consumption and CVD risk.

6.1 STUDIES IN ADOLESCENTS

The relationship between dairy intake and CVD risk was evaluated in a cross section of adolescents (12.5–17.5 years) from eight European cities participating in the Healthy Lifestyle in Europe by Nutrition in Adolescence (HELENA) study (2006–2007). Dairy consumption was inversely associated with CVD risk in girls. Moreover, in both genders, waist circumference and sum of skin folds were inversely associated with the consumption of yogurt and milk and milk- and yogurt-based beverages and a positive association was observed with cardiorespiratory fitness (Bel-Serrat et al. 2014).

In a cross section of 494 adolescents (15–18 years old), the intake of dairy products was examined in relation to cardiometabolic risk factors. Adolescents who had appropriate milk intakes, defined as >483 g/day, had a significantly lower risk of having a high cardiometabolic risk score than those with low milk intakes. No significant associations were found between appropriate intakes of total dairy, yogurt, or cheese and cardiometabolic risk scores. Appropriate intakes were based on median intakes of each dairy group for the entire population (Abreu et al. 2014).

As part of the Sydney Childhood Eye Study, a cross-sectional study of 824 adolescents (17 years old) had retinal photographs taken and provided dairy intake data from a food frequency questionnaire. Yogurt was the only dairy food that was associated with retinal vessel caliber, indicating a beneficial association between high yogurt intake and retinal microvascular signs, which is indicative of future CVD events (Gopinath et al. 2014).

6.2 STUDIES IN ADULTS

6.2.1 Cross-Sectional Studies

In a cross section of Italian adults (378 men and 129 women), significant lower odds (OR = 0.55; CI 0.32–0.95) for acute myocardial infarction were observed for adults consuming less than seven yogurts per week compared with nonconsumers. Importantly, yogurt was the only dairy product (among different types of milk and cheese) to have a significant cardioprotective effect (Tavani et al. 2002).

Amani et al. (2010) performed a case-control study designed to assess the link between dietary pattern and coronary artery disease (CAD) risk factors in 108 patients (mean age: 50 years). In this study, the consumption of hydrogenated fats and full-fat yogurt (fat content >2.5%) was associated with a higher coronary artery disease risk, while the consumption of fish, tea, and vegetable oils had protective effects (Amani et al. 2010).

The relation between yogurt, milk, and cheese intake and common carotid artery intima-media thickness (CCA-IMT), a well-known marker of CHD risk, was investigated in 1080 white women >70 years. Subjects consuming >100 g yogurt/day (all types combined) had a significantly lower CCA-IMT than subjects with a lower consumption (after adjustment for baseline, dietary, and lifestyle risk factors). No association was found for total dairy product, milk, or cheese consumption (Ivey et al. 2011).

6.2.2 Prospective Studies

Moss and Freed (2003) correlated European food consumption in 1989 to CHD deaths of older men (65–74 years) in 1993. Yogurt was not correlated with CHD death rates. However, milk, ice cream, cream, jams and preserves, and butter were significantly and positively correlated with CHD death rates (Moss and Freed 2003).

Larsson et al. (2009) examined, within the Alpha-Tocopherol, Beta-Carotene Cancer Prevention Study (mean follow-up of 13.6 years; 26,556 Finnish male smokers aged 50–69 years), the association between the intake of different types of dairy foods and the risk of stroke subtypes. Positive associations between yogurt intake and subarachnoid hemorrhage (RR = 1.83 for the highest vs. lowest quintile of intake; 95% CI = 1.20–2.80) and between whole milk intake and risk of intracerebral hemorrhage were observed. No strong relationships were found between the intakes of total dairy milk, sour milk, cheese, ice cream, or butter and the risk of any stroke subtypes (Larsson et al. 2009).

The association between the intake of different types of dairy products (fermented milk, milk, cheese, cream, and butter) and the incidence of CVD was also evaluated in the Swedish Malmö Diet and Cancer cohort with a mean follow-up of 12 years (44–74 years; 62% females). The overall consumption of dairy products was inversely associated with risk of CVD. Among the specific dairy products, a statistically significant inverse relationship was observed for fermented milk only (yogurt and cultured sour milk). When compared with subjects with the lowest intake, the highest consumption of fermented milk was associated with a 15% reduction in incidence of CVD ($p = .003$). The authors concluded that it is important to examine dairy products separately when investigating their health effects (Sonestedt et al. 2011).

The association between dairy product consumption and the risk of mortality from all causes, ischemic heart disease (IHD), and stroke was assessed using the Netherlands Cohort Study (NLCS) (120,852 men and women aged 55–69 years at baseline). After a 10-year follow-up, both butter and dairy fat intake showed a slightly increased risk of all-cause and IHD mortality in women only. Fermented full-fat milk, which mainly included full-fat yogurt, was inversely associated with all-cause mortality and nonsignificantly with stroke mortality in men and women (Goldbohm et al. 2011).

In a prospective study of community-dwelling older adults (50–93 years old), the relationship between dairy foods and CHD incidence was investigated in men

($n = 751$) and women ($n = 1{,}008$) over an average follow-up of 16.2 years. No significant associations were found in this population between whole milk, nonfat milk, yogurt, or cheese intake and CHD. There was, however, a significantly increased risk of incident CHD among women who consumed low-fat cheese and nonfat milk sometimes or often versus never or rarely (Avalos et al. 2013).

A follow-up study of the European Prospective Investigation into Cancer and Nutrition—Netherlands (EPIC-NL) cohort sought to further investigate fermented dairy products. No significant associations between total fermented foods (dairy products, cheese, vegetables, and meat), total fermented dairy (yogurt, buttermilk and quark, but no cheese), yogurt, or cheese with CVD mortality were observed (Praagman et al. 2015a). Similarly, in a prospective cohort of Dutch older adults (≥ 55 years) from the Rotterdam Study, no significant associations between total dairy, low-fat dairy, milk, fermented dairy, cheese, or yogurt and incident or fatal stroke were found. There was, however, a significant inverse relationship between high-fat dairy and fatal stroke. There were no associations between total dairy or dairy subgroups and incident CHD or fatal CHD (Praagman et al. 2015b).

6.2.3 Clinical Studies

Some studies examined the hypocholesterolemic effect of yogurt. This cholesterol-lowering effect of yogurt was noted for the first time in a study of Maasai tribes (Mann 1974). These findings were confirmed a few years later. A reduction of serum cholesterol was observed following 1 week of yogurt supplementation (3×240 mL/day), and this reduction was greater with yogurt than with milk containing 2% butterfat. The amount of fat given each day by either yogurt or milk was equivalent (Hepner et al. 1979). Moreover, Bazzare et al. (1986) found that 1 week of yogurt supplementation resulted in a significant decrease in total cholesterol and an increase in HDL cholesterol in normo-cholesterolemic women. However, other interventions did not report significant effects of yogurt on cholesterol levels even at very high concentrations. During a 10-week study, the effect of different dairy products (skim milk, 2% milk, whole milk, sweet acidophilus milk, buttermilk, or 1.8% yogurt) on serum cholesterol was evaluated in 68 healthy adults. The study failed to observe any significant difference in total, LDL, or HDL cholesterol. However, significant weight gain was seen in subjects consuming yogurt and there was an increase in triglyceride levels in this group (Thompson et al. 1982). Rossouw et al. (1981) and Massey (1984) found no effect of yogurt consumption (2 L/day and 480 mL/day, respectively) on total cholesterol or LDL cholesterol values in adolescent schoolboys and college students. McNamara et al. (1989) also demonstrated that yogurt (2 L/day) has no effects on plasma cholesterol levels in normolipidemic males.

The effects of consuming yogurt for 1 year on lipid profiles were evaluated in two populations; young adults and seniors. Live-culture yogurt, pasteurized fermented milk, and a control (no yogurt) were given (200 g/day). Seniors in the control group showed an increase in both total and LDL cholesterol, whereas the lipid profile in the yogurt-consuming groups remained stable during the study (Van de Water et al. 1999).

A clinical trial tested the hypothesis that circulating inflammatory and atherogenic biomarkers would be influenced by full-fat dairy food according to their fermentation status. Five single breakfast test meals containing control low-fat milk or 45 g of fat from yogurt, butter, cream, or cheese were given to 13 subjects over 3 weeks. Interleukin (IL)-6, IL-1β, tumor necrosis factor-α, high-sensitive C-reactive protein, monocyte chemoattractant protein-1, macrophage inflammatory protein-1α, intercellular adhesion molecule-1, and vascular cell adhesion molecule-1 were obtained from plasma 3 and 6 hours after the meal. Between-group analysis showed no differences between the five meals. There were no significant differences in fasting biomarker concentrations between nonfermented and fermented dairy diets (Nestel et al. 2012).

Low-grade systemic inflammation is considered a key etiologic factor in the development and progression of CVD. A systematic review of randomized controlled nutrition intervention studies in overweight and obese adults was performed to evaluate the impact of dairy products on biomarkers of inflammation. This review showed that dairy product consumption does not exert adverse effects on biomarkers of inflammation in overweight or obese adults. Moreover, it was not possible to distinguish between the effects of specific dairy products (milk, yogurt, and cheese, or low-fat dairy and high-fat dairy products) on inflammation. Major factors limiting the interpretation of results were the heterogeneity of dairy products and the lack of details regarding the type and content of fat in these products (Labonte et al. 2013).

A crossover study design was used to test the hypocholesterolemic effects of a symbiotic yogurt compared with a conventional yogurt in 29 German women. The consumption of 300 g of yogurt/day for 7 weeks did not reduce total or LDL cholesterol. However, the consumption of yogurt (either conventional or symbiotic) over the entire treatment period (21 weeks) did result in an increase in HDL cholesterol, suggesting that regular long-term consumption of yogurt may lead to a more favorable LDL:HDL cholesterol ratio (Kiessling et al. 2002). In another study, 33 Austrian women were asked to consume either 100 g of a probiotic or conventional yogurt daily for 2 weeks, followed by 200 g of the same product for an additional 2 weeks. Significant reductions in LDL cholesterol were seen over the 4 weeks in both yogurt groups, resulting in a more favorable LDL:HDL cholesterol ratio (Fabian and Elmadfa 2006).

In a randomized clinical trial, the effects of probiotic yogurt, conventional yogurt, and a control on hypercholesterolemia were examined. No significant differences in lipid profiles between the three groups were observed. There were, however, significant decreases in cholesterol and the total:HDL cholesterol ratio from baseline to post-intervention in both groups compared with the control. The results suggest that yogurt may possess antihyperlipidemic properties with or without an added probiotic, which can be attributed to the consumption of fermented milk (Sadrzadeh-Yeganeh et al. 2010).

6.2.4 META-ANALYSES AND SYSTEMATIC REVIEWS

A meta-analysis of 26 publications reviewed the data of foods high in saturated fat in relation to the risk of mortality. High intakes of yogurt, milk, cheese, and butter were not associated with an increased risk of mortality compared with low intakes, whereas high intakes of meat were significantly associated with an increased risk of mortality. Associations varied according to the food group and population. The authors proposed that this could be explained by factors beyond the saturated fat content of individual foods (O'Sullivan et al. 2013).

A meta-analysis of 22 prospective cohort studies examined the relationship between dairy consumption and the risk of stroke, CHD, and CVD. Three studies on yogurt and stroke were identified and five for yogurt and CHD; no significant associations were found. Overall, total dairy consumption reduced the risk for stroke and CVD, but not CHD (Qin et al. 2015).

6.3 MECHANISMS OF ACTION

6.3.1 Effect of Lipids and Other Nutrients

Universal nutrition recommendations to reduce SFA intake (limiting foods such as meats, dairy, and eggs) have been undermined by increasingly convincing evidence, including a meta-analysis of observational and randomized clinical trials, that do not support these guidelines (Astrup 2014a). SFAs have been shown to increase blood LDL cholesterol concentration in comparison with carbohydrates, which have a neutral effect on LDL cholesterol (EFSA Panel of Dietetic Products 2011). Thus, it has been proposed that SFAs have an independent role in increasing LDL cholesterol concentration (EFSA Panel of Dietetic Products 2011) and increased LDL cholesterol has been linked to the development of CVD, which forms the basis for the recommendation to limit SFA intake to less than 10% of total energy intake (Perk et al. 2012).

A review on dietary fats and CHD stated that modest reductions in CHD rates are possible by reducing saturated fat intake through replacement with a combination of poly- and mono-unsaturated fat (Willett 2012). Other groups have pointed out that some food sources high in saturated fat (such as dairy products) contain different types of saturated and unsaturated fatty acids, each of which could act in different ways on lipid metabolism. Moreover, yogurt and other dairy products make a significant contribution to intakes of other nutrients, which may have an impact on CVD risk (Huth and Park 2012, Nestel 2012). For example, in the Prevención con Dieta Mediterránea (Prevention with a Mediterranean Diet [PREDIMED]) study, high intakes of whole-fat yogurt were inversely associated with both hypertriglyceridemia and low HDL cholesterol (Babio et al. 2015) and a short-term diet containing low-fat dairy did not result in more favorable CVD risk biomarkers compared with a full-fat fermented dairy diet (Nestel et al. 2013). Furthermore, research to elucidate the mechanisms by which other fatty acids in yogurt and milk, such as oleic acid, naturally occurring rumenic acid, and *trans*-palmitoleic acid, act on CVD risk is needed. Small clinical studies have been performed to establish cause-and-effect relationships between different sources of trans-fatty acids and risk factors of CVD and inconclusive results have emerged. This may be due to insufficient statistical power in some studies, whereas others have used doses of ruminant trans-fatty acids that are not realistically attainable via the diet (Gebauer et al. 2011).

Other studies have evaluated the effect of different types of dairy fats on CVD incidence. It has been shown that plasma phospholipid 15:0, a biomarker of dairy fat intake, was inversely associated with incident CVD and CHD (de Oliveira Otto et al. 2013). Moreover, circulating trans-palmitoleate has been associated with higher LDL cholesterol, as well as lower triglycerides, fasting insulin, blood pressure, and incident diabetes in a U.S. cohort (2617 adults; the Multi-Ethnic Study of Atherosclerosis) (Mozaffarian et al. 2013). The association between 14:0, 15:0, 17:0, t16:1n-7 and stroke was evaluated in two large cohorts from the Health Professionals Follow-up Study (18,225) and the Nurse's Health Study (32,826). After adjustment for demographic, lifestyle, and cardiovascular risk factors, no significant associations between circulating biomarkers of dairy fat (15:0, 17:0, and t16:1n-7), 14:0, and stroke were observed. The authors conclude that the inability to find any associations may be due to the limited biological impacts of SFA on stroke, insufficient statistical power, or measurement error (Yakoob et al. 2014).

A meta-analysis of 19 prospective cohort studies investigated the relationship between dietary fatty acid intake and coronary outcomes. No significant associations were found between total SFA, total monounsaturated fatty acid (MUFA), total long-chain omega-3 fatty acids, or total omega-6 fatty acids and coronary outcomes. There was a significantly increased risk associated with total trans-fatty acid intake and a significantly reduced risk associated with alpha-linoleic intake. Among individual SFA, palmitic acid and stearic acid were positively associated with coronary outcomes and myristic, pentadecanoic, and margaric acid were inversely associated with coronary outcomes, but only margaric acid reached significance based on four studies (Chowdhury et al. 2014). Following the consumption of 250 g of full-fat yogurt or 60 g of camembert cheese for 5 weeks during a randomized clinical trial, there were no negative effects on the serum lipid of blood pressure, indicating that full-fat dairy products have a neutral effect on health (Schlienger et al. 2014).

The beneficial effect on CVD observed in some studies following the consumption of yogurt may also be attributable to other nutrients, such as proteins, vitamin D, calcium, magnesium, and potassium (Cam and de Mejia 2012), or the combination of these (Rice et al. 2011). Dietary calcium intake was found to be associated with a reduced incidence of stroke among middle-aged Japanese (especially calcium from dairy products) (Umesawa et al. 2008). However, it should be mentioned that epidemiological data has shown that serum calcium levels in the upper limit of the normal range can represent a risk factor for vascular disease (Reid et al. 2010). For example, in one study the death rate for subjects with serum calcium levels between 2.45 and 2.5 mmol/L was 1.3 times higher than those with baseline calcium between 2.3 and 2.45 mmol/L (Leifsson and Ahren 1996).

6.3.2 Effect of Bacteria on Cholesterol

Yogurt's protective effects on CVD are based on the assumption that its consumption would result in the establishment of adequate microbial populations within the gut that are capable of producing short-chain fatty acids (SCFA). These SCFA can reduce cholesterol synthesis or increase bile acid resorption. However, these mechanisms have not been validated in yogurt consumers (Nestel 2008). Cholesterol is a natural component of milk fat (around 100 mg/L). *In vitro* studies have shown that some strains of bifidobacteria and lactobacilli can assimilate cholesterol (Klaver and van der Meer 1993). It has been demonstrated that the fermentation of milk by the symbiosis of *Streptococcus thermophilus* and *Lactobacillus bulgaricus* leads to a reduction of cholesterol content in milk (Juskiewicz and Panfil-Kuncewicz 2003). Moreover, bacteria can assimilate cholesterol directly from the gut or by deconjugating bile salts and can impact on cholesterol absorption (St-Onge et al. 2000). Live bacteria can also ferment indigestible food–derived carbohydrates and produce SCFA in the gastrointestinal tract. This can cause a reduction in plasma total cholesterol concentrations either by inhibiting hepatic cholesterol synthesis or by redistributing cholesterol from plasma to the liver (Pereira and Gibson 2002). Given that yogurt bacteria do not colonize the intestine, the daily consumption of yogurt is necessary for any long-term effect on metabolism (St-Onge et al. 2000).

6.4 CONCLUSIONS

- Interventional trials reported conflicting results regarding the effects of yogurt on serum cholesterol concentrations. However, different methodologies have been used in trials (dose of yogurt administered, % of fat in yogurt, baseline blood cholesterol concentrations, type/presence of placebo, etc.), which has led to variable results.
- Most of the interventional trials failed to report adverse effects of yogurt intake on cholesterol levels and CVD risk, despite high consumption or its contribution of SFA to the diet.
- Observational studies examining the effect of different dairy products on CVD risk have observed that yogurt consumption may reduce CVD risk and CVD biomarkers compared with other dairy foods, but this relationship has not been consistently demonstrated.
- As emerging evidence indicates that not all dairy fats may be adverse to health, more studies are needed to clarify the effects of specific dairy fatty acids on different markers of CVD health.
- CVD involve many pathogenic pathways that could be activated by an unhealthy diet. Yogurt consumption may have cardiovascular benefits that could extend beyond its potential effect on blood cholesterol. More clinical trials are needed to carefully assess the effect of yogurt or specific yogurt nutrients on blood cholesterol as well as other CVD risk factors such as blood pressure, insulin resistance/type 2 diabetes, visceral/ectopic fat, and inflammation to fully determine causal relationships between dietary yogurt consumption and CVD risk.

REFERENCES

Abreu, S., P. Moreira, C. Moreira, J. Mota, I. Moreira-Silva, P. C. Santos, et al. 2014. Intake of milk, but not total dairy, yogurt, or cheese, is negatively associated with the clustering of cardiometabolic risk factors in adolescents. *Nutr Res* 34 (1):48–57.

Adamsson, V., A. Reumark, M. Marklund, A. Larsson, and U. Riserus. 2015. Role of a prudent breakfast in improving cardiometabolic risk factors in subjects with hypercholesterolemia: A randomized controlled trial. *Clin Nutr* 34 (1):20–26.

Amani, R., M. Noorizadeh, S. Rahmanian, N. Afzali, and M. H. Haghighizadeh. 2010. Nutritional related cardiovascular risk factors in patients with coronary artery disease in Iran: A case-control study. *Nutr J* 9:70.

Astrup, A. 2014a. A changing view on saturated fatty acids and dairy: From enemy to friend. *Am J Clin Nutr* 100 (6):1407–8.

Astrup, A. 2014b. Yogurt and dairy product consumption to prevent cardiometabolic diseases: Epidemiologic and experimental studies. *Am J Clin Nutr* 99 (5 Suppl):1235S–42S.

Avalos, E. E., E. Barrett-Connor, D. Kritz-Silverstein, D. L. Wingard, J. N. Bergstrom, and W. K. Al-Delaimy. 2013. Is dairy product consumption associated with the incidence of CHD? *Public Health Nutr* 16 (11):2055–63.

Babio, N., N. Becerra-Tomás, M. A. Martínez-González, D. Corella, R. Estruch, E. Ros, C. Sayón-Orea, et al. 2015. Consumption of yogurt, low-fat milk, and other low-fat dairy products is associated with lower risk of metabolic syndrome incidence in an elderly Mediterranean population. *J Nutr* 145 (10):2308–16.

Bazzarre, T. L., S. L. Wu, and J. A. Yuhas. 1986. Total and HDL-cholesterol concentrations following yogurt and calcium supplementation. *Nutr Rep Int* 28:1225–32.

Bel-Serrat, S., T. Mouratidou, D. Jiménez-Pavón, I. Huybrechts, M. Cuenca-García, L. Mistura, F. Gottrand, et al. 2014. Is dairy consumption associated with low cardiovascular disease risk in European adolescents? Results from the HELENA study. *Pediatr Obes* 9 (5):401–10.

Cam, A., and E. G. de Mejia. 2012. Role of dietary proteins and peptides in cardiovascular disease. *Mol Nutr Food Res* 56 (1):53–66.

Chowdhury, R., S. Warnakula, S. Kunutsor, F. Crowe, H. A. Ward, L. Johnson, O. H. Franco, et al. 2014. Association of dietary, circulating, and supplement fatty acids with coronary risk: A systematic review and meta-analysis. *Ann Intern Med* 160 (6):398–406.

Crichton, G. E., P. R. C. Howe, J. D. Buckley, A. M. Coates, and K. J. Murphy. 2012. Dairy consumption and cardiometabolic health: Outcomes of a 12-month crossover trial. *Nutr Metab (Lond)* 9:19.

De Oliveira Otto, M. C., D. Mozaffarian, D. Kromhout, A. G. Bertoni, C. T. Sibley, D. R. Jacobs, Jr., and J. A. Nettleton. 2012. Dietary intake of saturated fat by food source and incident cardiovascular disease: The multi-ethnic study of atherosclerosis. *Am J Clin Nutr* 96 (2):397–404.

De Oliveira Otto, M. C., J. A. Nettleton, R. N. Lemaitre, L. M. Steffen, D. Kromhout, S. S. Rich, Y. M. Tsai, et al. 2013. Biomarkers of dairy fatty acids and risk of cardiovascular disease in the multi-ethnic study of atherosclerosis. *J Am Heart Assoc* 2 (4):e000092.

EFSA Panel of Dietetic Products, Nutrition and Allergies. 2011. Guidance on the scientific requirements for health claims related to antioxidants, oxidative damage and cardiovascular health. *EFSA Journal* 9 (12):2474.

Elwood, P. C., J. E. Pickering, J. Hughes, A. M. Fehily, and A. R. Ness. 2004. Milk drinking, ischaemic heart disease and ischaemic stroke II. Evidence from cohort studies. *Eur J Clin Nutr* 58 (5):718–24.

Fabian, E., and I. Elmadfa. 2006. Influence of daily consumption of probiotic and conventional yoghurt on the plasma lipid profile in young healthy women. *Ann Nutr Metab* 50 (4):387–93.

FDA. 2009. Guidance for industry: Evidence-based review system for the scientific evaluation of health claims: Final. Edited by U.S. Department of Health and Human Services. Center for Food Safety and Applied Nutrition. College Park, MD: FDA.

Gebauer, S. K., J. M. Chardigny, M. U. Jakobsen, B. Lamarche, A. L. Lock, S. D. Proctor, and D. J. Baer. 2011. Effects of ruminant trans fatty acids on cardiovascular disease and cancer: A comprehensive review of epidemiological, clinical, and mechanistic studies. *Adv Nutr* 2 (4):332–54.

Givens, D. I. 2015. Dairy products: Good or bad for cardiometabolic disease? *Am J Clin Nutr* 101 (4):695–96.

Goldbohm, R. A., A. M. Chorus, F. Galindo Garre, L. J. Schouten, and P. A. van den Brandt. 2011. Dairy consumption and 10-y total and cardiovascular mortality: A prospective cohort study in the Netherlands. *Am J Clin Nutr* 93 (3):615–27.

Gopinath, B., V. M. Flood, G. Burlutsky, J. C. Louie, L. A. Baur, and P. Mitchell. 2014. Dairy food consumption, blood pressure and retinal microcirculation in adolescents. *Nutr Metab Cardiovasc Dis* 24 (11):1221–27.

Hepner, G., R. Fried, S. St Jeor, L. Fusetti, and R. Morin. 1979. Hypocholesterolemic effect of yogurt and milk. *Am J Clin Nutr* 32 (1):19–24.

Huth, P. J., and K. M. Park. 2012. Influence of dairy product and milk fat consumption on cardiovascular disease risk: A review of the evidence. *Adv Nutr* 3 (3):266–85.

Ivey, K. L., J. R. Lewis, J. M. Hodgson, K. Zhu, S. S. Dhaliwal, P. L. Thompson, and R. L. Prince. 2011. Association between yogurt, milk, and cheese consumption and common carotid artery intima-media thickness and cardiovascular disease risk factors in elderly women. *Am J Clin Nutr* 94 (1):234–39.

Juskiewicz, M., and H. Panfil-Kuncewicz. 2003. Reduction of cholesterol content in milk with dairy thermophilic cultures application. *Milchwissenschaft* 58:370–3.

Kiessling, G., J. Schneider, and G. Jahreis. 2002. Long-term consumption of fermented dairy products over 6 months increases HDL cholesterol. *Eur J Clin Nutr* 56 (9):843–49.

Klaver, F. A., and R. van der Meer. 1993. The assumed assimilation of cholesterol by lactobacilli and bifidobacterium bifidum is due to their bile salt-deconjugating activity. *Appl Environ Microbiol* 59 (4):1120–24.

Kratz, M., T. Baars, and S. Guyenet. 2013. The relationship between high-fat dairy consumption and obesity, cardiovascular, and metabolic disease. *Eur J Nutr* 52 (1):1–24.

Labonte, M. E., P. Couture, C. Richard, S. Desroches, and B. Lamarche. 2013. Impact of dairy products on biomarkers of inflammation: A systematic review of randomized controlled nutritional intervention studies in overweight and obese adults. *Am J Clin Nutr* 97 (4):706–17.

Lamarche, B. 2008. Review of the effect of dairy products on non-lipid risk factors for cardiovascular disease. *J Am Coll Nutr* 27 (6):741S–46S.

Larsson, S. C., S. Mannisto, M. J. Virtanen, J. Kontto, D. Albanes, and J. Virtamo. 2009. Dairy foods and risk of stroke. *Epidemiology* 20 (3):355–60.

Leifsson, B. G., and B. Ahren. 1996. Serum calcium and survival in a large health screening program. *J Clin Endocrinol Metab* 81 (6):2149–53.

Mann, G. V. 1974. Studies of a surfactant and cholesteremia in the Maasai. *Am J Clin Nutr* 27 (5):464–69.

Massey, L. K. 1984. Effect of changing milk and yogurt consumption on human nutrient intake and serum lipoproteins. *J Dairy Sci* 67 (2):255–62.

McNamara, D. J., A. E. Lowell, and J. E. Sabb. 1989. Effect of yogurt intake on plasma lipid and lipoprotein levels in normolipidemic males. *Atherosclerosis* 79 (2–3):167–71.

Mendis, S., P. Puska, and B. Norrving, eds. 2011. *Global Atlas on Cardiovascular Disease Prevention and Control*. Geneva: World Health Organization.

Moreno, L., S. Bel-Serrat, A. Santaliestra Pasías, and G. Bueno. 2015. Dairy products, yogurt consumption, and cardiometabolic risk in children and adolescents. *Nutrition Reviews* 73 (Suppl 1):8–14.

Moss, M., and D. Freed. 2003. The cow and the coronary: Epidemiology, biochemistry and immunology. *Int J Cardiol* 87 (2–3):203–16.

Mozaffarian, D., M. C. de Oliveira Otto, R. N. Lemaitre, A. M. Fretts, G. Hotamisligil, M. Y. Tsai, D. S. Siscovick, et al. 2013. Trans-palmitoleic acid, other dairy fat biomarkers, and incident diabetes: The Multi-Ethnic Study of Atherosclerosis (MESA). *Am J Clin Nutr* 97 (4):854–61.

Nestel, P. 2012. Nutrition and metabolism: The changing face of the dairy-cardiovascular risk paradox. *Curr Opin Lipidol* 23 (1):1–3.

Nestel, P. J. 2008. Effects of dairy fats within different foods on plasma lipids. *J Am Coll Nutr* 27 (6):735S–40S.

Nestel, P. J., N. Mellett, S. Pally, G. Wong, C. K. Barlow, K. Croft, T. A. Mori, et al. 2013. Effects of low-fat or full-fat fermented and non-fermented dairy foods on selected cardiovascular biomarkers in overweight adults. *Br J Nutr* 110 (12):2242–49.

Nestel, P. J., S. Pally, G. L. MacIntosh, M. A. Greeve, S. Middleton, J. Jowett, and P. J. Meikle. 2012. Circulating inflammatory and atherogenic biomarkers are not increased following single meals of dairy foods. *Eur J Clin Nutr* 66 (1):25–31.

O'Sullivan, T. A., K. Hafekost, F. Mitrou, and D. Lawrence. 2013. Food sources of saturated fat and the association with mortality: A meta-analysis. *Am J Public Health* 103 (9):e31–42.

Pereira, D. I., and G. R. Gibson. 2002. Effects of consumption of probiotics and prebiotics on serum lipid levels in humans. *Crit Rev Biochem Mol Biol* 37 (4):259–81.

Perk, J., G. De Backer, H. Gohlke, I. Graham, Z. Reiner, W. M. Verschuren, C. Albus, et al. 2012. European guidelines on cardiovascular disease prevention in clinical practice (version 2012): The fifth joint task force of the European Society of Cardiology and other societies on cardiovascular disease prevention in clinical practice (constituted by representatives of nine societies and by invited experts). *Int J Behav Med* 19 (4):403–88.

Praagman, J., G. W. Dalmeijer, Y. T. van der Schouw, S. S. Soedamah-Muthu, W. M. Monique Verschuren, H. Bas Bueno-de-Mesquita, J. M. Geleijnse, et al. 2015. The relationship between fermented food intake and mortality risk in the European Prospective Investigation into Cancer and Nutrition-Netherlands cohort. *Br J Nutr* 113 (3):498–506.

Praagman, J., O. H. Franco, M. A. Ikram, S. S. Soedamah-Muthu, M. F. Engberink, F. J. van Rooij, A. Hofman, et al. 2015. Dairy products and the risk of stroke and coronary heart disease: The Rotterdam Study. *Eur J Nutr* 54 (6):981–90.

Qin, L. Q., J. Y. Xu, S. F. Han, Z. L. Zhang, Y. Y. Zhao, and I. M. Szeto. 2015. Dairy consumption and risk of cardiovascular disease: An updated meta-analysis of prospective cohort studies. *Asia Pac J Clin Nutr* 24 (1):90–100.

Reid, I. R., M. J. Bolland, and A. Grey. 2010. Does calcium supplementation increase cardiovascular risk? *Clin Endocrinol (Oxf)* 73 (6):689–95.

Reiner, Z., A. L. Catapano, G. De Backer, I. Graham, M. R. Taskinen, O. Wiklund, S. Agewall, et al. 2011. ESC/EAS Guidelines for the management of dyslipidaemias. *Rev Esp Cardiol* 64 (12):1168 e1–e60.

Rice, B. H. 2014. Dairy and cardiovascular disease: A review of recent observational research. *Curr Nutr Rep* 3:130–38.

Rice, B. H., C. J. Cifelli, M. A. Pikosky, and G. D. Miller. 2011. Dairy components and risk factors for cardiometabolic syndrome: Recent evidence and opportunities for future research. *Adv Nutr* 2 (5):396–407.

Rodríguez-Campello, A., J. Jiménez-Conde, Á. Ois, E. Cuadrado-Godia, E. Giralt-Steinhauer, H. Schroeder, G. Romeral, et al. 2014. Dietary habits in patients with ischemic stroke: A case-control study. *PLoS One* 9 (12):e114716.

Rossouw, J. E., E. M. Burger, P. Van der Vyver, and J. J. Ferreira. 1981. The effect of skim milk, yoghurt, and full cream milk on human serum lipids. *Am J Clin Nutr* 34 (3):351–56.

Rozenberg, S., J. J. Body, O. Bruyere, P. Bergmann, M. L. Brandi, C. Cooper, J. P. Devogelaer, et al. 2015. Effects of dairy products consumption on health: Benefits and beliefs-a commentary from the Belgian Bone Club and the European Society for Clinical and Economic Aspects of Osteoporosis, Osteoarthritis and Musculoskeletal Diseases. *Calcif Tissue Int*.

Sadrzadeh-Yeganeh, H., I. Elmadfa, A. Djazayery, M. Jalali, R. Heshmat, and M. Chamary. 2010. The effects of probiotic and conventional yoghurt on lipid profile in women. *Br J Nutr* 103 (12):1778–83.

Schlienger, J. L., F. Paillard, J. M. Lecerf, M. Romon, C. Bonhomme, B. Schmitt, Y. Donazzolo, et al. 2014. Effect on blood lipids of two daily servings of camembert cheese. An intervention trial in mildly hypercholesterolemic subjects. *Int J Food Sci Nutr* 65 (8):1013–18.

Soedamah-Muthu, S. S., E. L. Ding, W. K. Al-Delaimy, F. B. Hu, M. F. Engberink, W. C. Willett, and J. M. Geleijnse. 2011. Milk and dairy consumption and incidence of cardiovascular diseases and all-cause mortality: Dose-response meta-analysis of prospective cohort studies. *Am J Clin Nutr* 93 (1):158–71.

Sonestedt, E., E. Wirfalt, P. Wallstrom, B. Gullberg, M. Orho-Melander, and B. Hedblad. 2011. Dairy products and its association with incidence of cardiovascular disease: The Malmö diet and cancer cohort. *Eur J Epidemiol* 26 (8):609–18.

St-Onge, M. P., E. R. Farnworth, and P. J. Jones. 2000. Consumption of fermented and nonfermented dairy products: Effects on cholesterol concentrations and metabolism. *Am J Clin Nutr* 71 (3):674–81.

Tapsell, L. C. 2015. Fermented dairy food and CVD risk. *Br J Nutr* 113 Suppl 2:S131–35.

Tavani, A., S. Gallus, E. Negri, and C. La Vecchia. 2002. Milk, dairy products, and coronary heart disease. *J Epidemiol Community Health* 56 (6):471–72.

Thompson, L. U., D. J. Jenkins, M. A. Amer, R. Reichert, A. Jenkins, and J. Kamulsky. 1982. The effect of fermented and unfermented milks on serum cholesterol. *Am J Clin Nutr* 36 (6):1106–11.

Umesawa, M., H. Iso, J. Ishihara, I. Saito, Y. Kokubo, M. Inoue, and S. Tsugane. 2008. Dietary calcium intake and risks of stroke, its subtypes, and coronary heart disease in Japanese: The JPHC Study Cohort I. *Stroke* 39 (9):2449–56.

Van de Water, J., C. L. Keen, and M. E. Gershwin. 1999. The influence of chronic yogurt consumption on immunity. *J Nutr* 129 (7 Suppl):1492S–5S.

Willett, W. C. 2012. Dietary fats and coronary heart disease. *J Intern Med* 272 (1):13–24.

Yakoob, M. Y., P. Shi, F. B. Hu, H. Campos, K. M. Rexrode, E. J. Orav, W. C. Willett, et al. 2014. Circulating biomarkers of dairy fat and risk of incident stroke in U.S. men and women in 2 large prospective cohorts. *Am J Clin Nutr* 100 (6):1437–47.

7 Metabolic Syndrome

The metabolic syndrome (MetS) or the "insulin resistance syndrome" was described by G. M. Reaven in the late 1980s, but scientists had already identified various coexisting components of this syndrome as early as the 1920s (Sarafidis and Nilsson 2006). Today, several definitions of MetS exist, causing confusion as to whether they identify the same individuals or evaluate a surrogate of risk factors (Kassi et al. 2011). According to the International Diabetes Federation (IDF), MetS diagnostic criteria include abdominal obesity and two of the following four factors: raised triglycerides (TG), reduced high-density lipoprotein (HDL) cholesterol, raised blood pressure, and raised fasting plasma glucose (Huang 2009). Recently, other factors also linked to the syndrome have been identified, such as chronic pro-inflammatory and pro-thrombotic states, nonalcoholic fatty liver disease, and sleep apnea (Kassi et al. 2011). Factors leading to the development of MetS are illustrated in Figure 7.1.

Observational studies have evaluated the impact of dairy product intake on MetS. Mennen et al. (2000) performed one of the first large studies, Data from an Epidemiological Study in the Insulin Resistance Syndrome (DESIR), evaluating the relationship between different foods and the presence of MetS in a cohort of 4,976 adults (30–64 years). The authors found a lower prevalence of MetS in men, but not women, who consumed more than one portion of dairy per day compared with less than one portion per day. In women, there was only an inverse association between diastolic blood pressure and high dairy intake of more than four portions per day, whereas in men there were inverse associations between dairy consumption and TG, HDL cholesterol, diastolic blood pressure, and fasting glucose (Mennen et al. 2000). In a subsequent study, the DESIR cohort was followed for 9 years and incident MetS (defined according to IDF criteria) was inversely associated with dairy intake and dietary calcium in all adults (Fumeron et al. 2011). Similar observations of reductions in the risk of having MetS with higher intakes of dairy were observed in populations of Tehranian adults (Azadbakht et al. 2005) and in middle-aged and older American women (Liu et al. 2005). In these studies, the relationship seemed to be attributed, at least in part, to calcium. In other studies, total dairy intake during adolescence and young adulthood was not associated with being overweight or having MetS in adulthood (te Velde et al. 2011), or with the baseline intake of dairy in French adults (28–60 years) and 5-year changes in MetS-related variables (Samara et al. 2013). The absence of significant associations in this study compared with the studies of Azadbakht et al. (2005) and Liu et al. (2005) might be related to factors such as the young and relatively healthy population involved, the longitudinal design, the high baseline dairy intake of the subjects, and lifestyle variables other than those included in the analyses.

A systematic review assessed the effects of dairy consumption on the risk of developing MetS. Dairy intake was inversely associated with MetS in 7 out of the 13 cross-sectional and prospective cohort studies identified. However, the

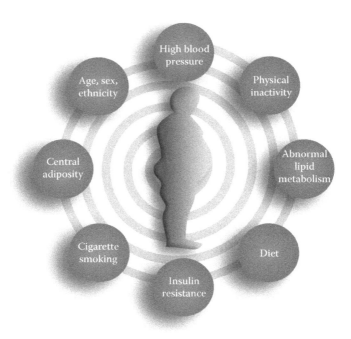

FIGURE 7.1 Dietary, lifestyle and metabolic risk factors involved in the development of the MetS. (From Steele, R. M. et al., *J Appl Phys,* 105 (1), 342–51, 2008; Standl, E., *Eur Heart J,* Suppl 7 (D), D10–13, 2005.)

generalizability of the conclusions is limited by the different sets of criteria used to diagnose MetS and the lack of evidence from prospective cohort studies and clinical trials (Crichton et al. 2011). The impact of yogurt on individual components of MetS and the potential mechanisms of action have been discussed in the previous sections. Thus, the following paragraphs will discuss the studies evaluating the influence of yogurt consumption on the overall impact of this disorder. Definitions of different MetS diagnostic criteria that are utilized in the following studies are described in Table 7.1.

7.1 STUDIES IN ADOLESCENTS

A cross-sectional study of a cohort of 785 adolescents (10–19 years old) from the Tehran Lipid and Glucose Study examined the relationship between dairy food intake and MetS. The prevalence of MetS in the Iranian adult population is known to be much higher than elsewhere in the word. In this young sample, the prevalence of MetS, based on the Ferranti criteria (Table 7.1), was also very high at 22%. Total dairy, low-fat dairy, high-fat dairy, milk, yogurt, and cheese consumption were not significantly associated with MetS in this population (Ghotboddin Mohammadi et al. 2015).

TABLE 7.1
Different criteria used to diagnose MetS in adults and adolescents

Criteria	Definition	Reference
International Diabetes Federation (IDF)	Central obesity (waist circumference >94 cm for men and >80 cm for women) and any two of the following four criteria: hyperglycemia (≥ 100 mg/dL) or diagnosis of diabetes; hypertriglyceridemia (≥ 150 mg/dL) or treatment; low HDL cholesterol (<40 mg/dL for men and <50 mg/dL for women) or treatment; high systolic or diastolic blood pressure (systolic >130 and/or diastolic $\geq$ 85 mm Hg) or treatment for hypertension.	(Huang 2009)
National Cholesterol Education Program Expert Panel and Adult Treatment Panel III (NCEP/ATP III)	Three or more of the following five criteria: central obesity (>102 cm for men and >89 cm for women); hyperglycemia (≥ 100 mg/dL) or treatment; hypertriglyceridemia (≥ 150 mg/dL) or treatment; low HDL cholesterol (<40 mg/dL for men and <50 mg/dL for women) or treatment; high systolic or diastolic blood pressure (systolic > 130 and/or diastolic $\geq$ 85 mm Hg).	(Huang 2009)
Harmonized criteria	Three or more of the following five criteria: high waist circumference (population and country specific cut-offs); hypertriglyceridemia (≥ 150 mg/dL); low HDL (<40 mg/dL for men and <50 mg/dL for women); hypertension (systolic > 130 and/or diastolic $\geq$ 85 mm Hg); hyperglycemia (≥ 100 mg/dL).	(Alberti et al. 2009)
Metabolic risk score	A mean of z scores of metabolic risk factors: waist circumference, systolic blood pressure, HDL cholesterol, TG, and fasting glucose	(Drehmer et al. 2016)
Ferranti criteria (adolescents)	Three or more of the following five criteria: hyperglycemia (≥ 110 mg/dL); hypertriglyceridemia (≥ 100 mg/dL); low HDL (<50 mg/dL for girls and <45 mg for boys); central obesity for age (>75th percentile for age and sex); high blood pressure (>90th percentile for age, sex and height).	(Ghotboddin et al. 2015)

7.2 STUDIES IN ADULTS

7.2.1 Cross-Sectional Studies

The effects of different types of dairy products on MetS were evaluated in a cross section of 2,064 Dutch older adults (50–75 years) who had participated in the Hoorn Study. There was an inverse association between yogurt consumption and systolic blood pressure, but no other MetS variables, and the association was attenuated in fully adjusted models (Snijder et al. 2007).

A cross-sectional study assessed the association between the consumption of a variety of dairy products, MetS, and obesity in adults from the National Health and

Nutrition Examination Survey. Significant inverse associations were found between metabolic disorders and intakes of yogurt, whole milk, calcium, and magnesium. The odds ratio for each 100 g daily serving of yogurt and MetS was 0.40 (95% CI: 0.18, 0.89). However, the relationship was attenuated following adjustment for other dietary components. In this study, calcium appeared to account for the protective effect of yogurt on the risk of MetS (Beydoun et al. 2008).

A cross-sectional study of American adults participating in the Framingham Heart Study Offspring Cohort (1998–2001) and Third Generation (2002–2005) cohorts was conducted to evaluate whether yogurt consumption was associated with a better metabolic profile and diet quality assessed by the Dietary Guidelines Adherence Index (DGAI) score. Dietary intake was assessed with a validated food frequency questionnaire. Yogurt was generalized in the database as being low fat and with fruit. Yogurt consumption was inversely associated with levels of TG, glucose, insulin resistance, and systolic blood pressure ($p < .05$). However, the relationships with TG and insulin were no longer statistically significant after additional adjustments for body mass index (BMI) were made. Yogurt consumers also had a higher DGAI score and a greater intake of some nutrients (e.g., potassium) than nonconsumers (Wang et al. 2013).

A cross-sectional study was conducted among 460 Japanese adults aged 21–67 years to evaluate the association between major dietary patterns and the prevalence of MetS. MetS was defined according to the modified National Cholesterol Education Program ATP III criteria. A Westernized breakfast pattern (high intakes of milk and yogurt, bread, and confectionaries; low intakes of rice and alcoholic beverages) was inversely associated with the prevalence of MetS and high blood pressure (Akter et al. 2013).

The association between different types of dairy food consumption and the risk of MetS was investigated in 4,862 Korean adults. The MetS was defined according to the joint interim statement of the IDF and the American Heart Association/National Heart, Lung, and Blood Institute. The prevalence of MetS was significantly lower in subjects with higher yogurt or milk consumption. Moreover, the adjusted odds ratios (ORs) for lower HDL cholesterol was 28% lower among subjects in the highest category of yogurt intake compared with subjects in the lowest category (Kim 2013).

In a cross-sectional analysis of 9,835 adults (35–74 years old) from the Brazilian Longitudinal Study of Adult Health, the relationship between dairy food intake and MetS was once again examined. A MetScore was computed from mean z-scores of MetS components: waist circumference, systolic blood pressure, HDL cholesterol, fasting TG, and fasting glucose. After controlling for covariates in the fully adjusted model, such as demographics, BMI, lifestyle factors, and dietary intake, MetScores were inversely associated with total dairy and full-fat dairy, but not low-fat dairy. In subgroup analyses, yogurt and butter were significantly and inversely associated with MetScores. Additional analyses adjusting for saturated fatty acids (SFAs) in dairy revealed that they may be potentially responsible for mediating the relationship between full-fat dairy and MetScores (Drehmer et al. 2016).

7.2.2 Prospective Cohort Studies

The CARDIA study examined the association between different types of dairy products and the incidence of MetS. This 10-year prospective study involved 3,157 black and white young adults from U.S. metropolitan areas. No significant reductions in the risk of MetS or its components were associated with daily yogurt consumption. However, in this particular study, yogurt consumption was low in comparison with other dairy products (around 1.8% of total dairy products). Total dairy consumption was inversely associated with the incidence of several MetS components (e.g., obesity, impaired glucose homeostasis, hypertension, and dyslipidemia) among individuals who were overweight at baseline. These associations were similar across race and gender (Pereira et al. 2002).

A follow-up study of Snijder et al. (2007) was carried out with 1,124 older Dutch adults (50–75 years old) from the Hoorn Study on the relationship between dairy intake and 6.4-year changes in weight, adiposity, and metabolic risk factors (glycemia, lipids, and blood pressure). The highest quartile of dairy intake was significantly associated with a higher BMI, weight, and waist circumference and lower HDL levels in subjects with a BMI <25 kg/m². Similar to the previous cross-sectional study (Snijder et al. 2007), yogurt and other individual dairy subgroups were still not associated with any metabolic or body composition parameters (Snijder et al. 2008).

The relationship between yogurt consumption and risk of developing MetS (defined by harmonized criteria) was investigated in a prospective cohort from the Seguimiento Universidad de Navarra (SUN) project in Spain. The study followed a cohort of 8063 adults for 6 years with a mean age of 36.4 (SD 11.6) who developed 306 incident cases of MetS. Associations between total yogurt, whole-fat yogurt, and MetS incidences were observed in crude models only. When models were adjusted for covariates, all associations between yogurt and MetS were attenuated. It was observed, however, that a high concomitant yogurt and fruit consumption was inversely associated with MetS risk (Sayón-Orea et al. 2015).

In a prospective cohort of 1868 older Spanish adults (55–80 years), recruited from 2003 to 2009 and followed for a median of 3.2 years, the relationship between dairy food consumption and incident MetS was examined and defined according to harmonized criteria. In this cohort of older Spanish adults, there was a greater incidence of MetS than in the previous study by Sayón-Orea et al. (2015). A significantly lower risk of incident MetS was observed in subjects with the highest tertile of low-fat yogurt and whole-fat yogurt intake compared with the lowest tertile in all models, and a significant linear trend for reduced risk according to tertiles of yogurt consumption. In the fully adjusted model (age, sex, lifestyle factors, dietary components, and baseline MetS components), the HR for total yogurt, low-fat yogurt, and whole-fat yogurt were 0.77 (0.65, 0.91), 0.73 (0.62, 0.86), and 0.78 (0.66, 0.92), respectively. High cheese consumption was associated with a higher risk for MetS, whereas low-fat milk was associated with a lower risk. Total yogurt, low-fat yogurt, and high-fat yogurt consumption were also associated with a lower risk for each individual component of MetS (abdominal obesity, hypertriglyceridemia, low HDL, high blood pressure, and high fasting plasma glucose), except high blood pressure in total yogurt and low-fat yogurt groups. There were significant linear trends in the reduction of risk for all MetS components with an increased consumption of whole-fat yogurt. Results from the Prevención con Dieta Mediterránea (Prevention with a Mediterranean Diet [PREDIMED]) study strongly suggest that all types of yogurt were associated with a lower incidence of MetS, but that the relationship may be particularly strong for whole-fat yogurt (Babio et al. 2015).

7.3 MECHANISMS OF ACTION

Low-grade inflammation underlies the metabolic disorders that define MetS (Da Silva and Rudkowska 2014). Dairy product consumption is suggested to be associated with improvements in systemic inflammation, although results are inconsistent (Labonte et al. 2013). A randomized study compared low-fat dairy consumption (10 oz 1% milk, 6 oz nonfat yogurt, and 4 oz 2% cheese) to a carbohydrate-based control diet (1.5 oz granola bar and 12 oz 100% juice) on systemic inflammation in patients with MetS. The authors concluded that three servings of dairy resulted in improving systemic inflammation in the test group (Dugan et al. 2015). It can be hypothesized that dairy consumption, particularly low-fat dairy such as yogurt (yogurt is often low in fat compared with cheese), is implicated in MetS by reducing systemic inflammation and oxidative stress markers (Da Silva and Rudkowska 2014). This relationship may also be indirect due to yogurt's association with healthy dietary patterns.

A cross-sectional study among young adults (23–25 years old) was conducted to investigate the association between dairy food intake, MetS, and its components, defined according to IDF criteria. Higher dairy product consumption was inversely associated with the prevalence of MetS and abdominal obesity. These associations, however, were attenuated when controlling for calcium (Martins et al. 2015). The results from this study suggest that calcium may play a role in modulating MetS development. The specific mechanisms involved are the same as those proposed to be involved in weight maintenance, for example, attenuating calcium deficiencies and increasing fecal fat excretion (Dugan and Fernandez 2014).

In addition to calcium, a review by Abedini et al. (2015) specified the role of fat and protein in mechanisms for the development of MetS. Protein may be implicated in MetS by increasing satiety (reduced energy intake), improving lipoprotein profiles compared with carbohydrates, providing precursors for angiotensin-converting-enzyme (ACE)-inhibitory peptide contributing to blood pressure control, and enhancing calcium absorption (Abedini et al. 2015). Leucine and branched-chain amino acids from dairy products may be involved in decreasing plasma glucose levels by modulating insulin (Dugan and Fernandez 2014). It has also been postulated that specific SFAs found in dairy foods in moderate amounts may contribute to modulating the relationship seen between whole-fat dairy products and MetS (Drehmer et al. 2016).

7.4 CONCLUSIONS

- Many studies have suggested that yogurt and dairy products may have protective effects on most of the individual MetS components; however, results are inconsistent.
- There are methodological differences among studies (such as different MetS diagnostic criteria or the age of the population studied), which make

it difficult to draw clear conclusions about the present evidence. Moreover, some of the available studies were not designed to assess the specific effect of yogurt consumption on MetS.
- At present, there are no meta-analyses or randomized clinical trials to provide a strong level of evidence validating the benefits of yogurt on MetS. High-quality randomized controlled trials are needed to evaluate the impact of yogurt and yogurt nutrients consumption on MetS risk within a balanced diet.

REFERENCES

Abedini, M., E. Falahi, and S. Roosta. 2015. Dairy product consumption and the metabolic syndrome. *Diabetes Metab Syndr* 9 (1):34–37.

Akter, S., A. Nanri, N. M. Pham, K. Kurotani, and T. Mizoue. 2013. Dietary patterns and metabolic syndrome in a Japanese working population. *Nutr Metab (Lond)* 10 (1):30.

Alberti, K. G. M. M., R. H. Eckel, S. M. Grundy, et al. 2009. Harmonizing the metabolic syndrome: A joint interim statement of the International Diabetes Federation Task Force on Epidemiology and Prevention; National Heart, Lung, and Blood Institute; American Heart Association; World Heart Federation; International Atherosclerosis Society; and International Association for the Study of Obesity. *Circulation* 120:1640.

Azadbakht, L., P. Mirmiran, A. Esmaillzadeh, and F. Azizi. 2005. Dairy consumption is inversely associated with the prevalence of the metabolic syndrome in Tehranian adults. *Am J Clin Nutr* 82 (3):523–30.

Babio, N., N. Becerra-Tomás, M. A. Martínez-González, D. Corella, R. Estruch, E. Ros, C. Sayón-Orea, et al. 2015. Consumption of yogurt, low-fat milk, and other low-fat dairy products is associated with lower risk of metabolic syndrome incidence in an elderly Mediterranean population. *J Nutr* 145 (10):2308–16.

Beydoun, M. A., T. L. Gary, B. H. Caballero, R. S. Lawrence, L. J. Cheskin, and Y. Wang. 2008. Ethnic differences in dairy and related nutrient consumption among U.S. adults and their association with obesity, central obesity, and the metabolic syndrome. *Am J Clin Nutr* 87 (6):1914–25.

Crichton, G. E., J. Bryan, J. Buckley, and K. J. Murphy. 2011. Dairy consumption and metabolic syndrome: A systematic review of findings and methodological issues. *Obesity Reviews* 12 (5):e190–201.

Da Silva, M. S., and I. Rudkowska. 2014. Dairy products on metabolic health: Current research and clinical implications. *Maturitas* 77 (3):221–28.

Drehmer, M., M. A. Pereira, M. I. Schmidt, S. Alvim, P. A. Lotufo, V. C. Luft, and B. B. Duncan. 2016. Total and full-fat, but not low-fat, dairy product intakes are inversely associated with metabolic syndrome in adults. *J Nutr Biochem* 146 (1):81–89.

Dugan, C. E., D. Aguilar, Y. K. Park, J. Y. Lee, and M. L. Fernandez. 2015. Dairy consumption lowers systemic inflammation and liver enzymes in typically low-dairy consumers with clinical characteristics of metabolic syndrome. *J Am Coll Nutr* 35 (2):1–7.

Dugan, C. E., and M. L. Fernandez. 2014. Effects of dairy on metabolic syndrome parameters: A review. *Yale J Biol Med* 87 (2):135–47.

Fumeron, F., A. Lamri, N. Emery, N. Bellili, R. Jaziri, I. Porchay-Baldérelli, O. Lantieri, et al. 2011. Dairy products and the metabolic syndrome in a prospective study, DESIR. *J Am Coll Nutr* 30 (5 Suppl 1):454S–63S.

Ghotboddin Mohammadi, S., P. Mirmiran, Z. Bahadoran, Y. Mehrabi, and F. Azizi. 2015. The association of dairy intake with metabolic syndrome and its components in adolescents: Tehran lipid and glucose study. *Int J Endocrinol Metab* 13 (3):e25201.

Huang, P. L. 2009. A comprehensive definition for metabolic syndrome. *Dis Model Mech* 2 (5–6):231–37.
Kassi, E., P. Pervanidou, G. Kaltsas, and G. Chrousos. 2011. Metabolic syndrome: Definitions and controversies. *BMC Med* 9:48.
Kim, J. 2013. Dairy food consumption is inversely associated with the risk of the metabolic syndrome in Korean adults. *J Hum Nutr Diet* 26 (Suppl 1):171–79.
Labonte, M. E., P. Couture, C. Richard, S. Desroches, and B. Lamarche. 2013. Impact of dairy products on biomarkers of inflammation: A systematic review of randomized controlled nutritional intervention studies in overweight and obese adults. *Am J Clin Nutr* 97 (4):706–17.
Liu, S., Y. Song, E. S. Ford, J. E. Manson, J. E. Buring, and P. M. Ridker. 2005. Dietary calcium, vitamin D, and the prevalence of metabolic syndrome in middle-aged and older U.S. women. *Diabetes Care* 28 (12):2926–32.
Martins, M. L., G. Kac, R. A. Silva, H. Bettiol, M. A. Barbieri, V. C. Cardoso, and A. A. Silva. 2015. Dairy consumption is associated with a lower prevalence of metabolic syndrome among young adults from Ribeirao Preto, Brazil. *Nutrition* 31 (5):716–21.
Mennen, L. I., L. Lafay, E. J. M. Feskens, M. Novak, P. Lépinay, and B. Balkau. 2000. Possible protective effect of bread and dairy products on the risk of the metabolic syndrome. *Nutr Res* 20 (3):335–47.
Pereira, M. A., D. R. Jacobs, Jr., L. Van Horn, M. L. Slattery, A. I. Kartashov, and D. S. Ludwig. 2002. Dairy consumption, obesity, and the insulin resistance syndrome in young adults: The CARDIA study. *JAMA* 287 (16):2081–89.
Samara, A., B. Herbeth, N. C. Ndiaye, F. Fumeron, S. Billod, G. Siest, and S. Visvikis-Siest. 2013. Dairy product consumption, calcium intakes, and metabolic syndrome-related factors over 5 years in the STANISLAS study. *Nutrition* 29 (3):519–24.
Sarafidis, P. A., and P. M. Nilsson. 2006. The metabolic syndrome: A glance at its history. *J Hypertens* 24 (4):621–26.
Sayón-Orea, C., M. Bes-Rastrollo, A. Marti, A. M. Pimenta, N. Martin-Calvo, and M. A. Martínez-González. 2015. Association between yogurt consumption and the risk of metabolic syndrome over 6 years in the SUN study. *BMC Public Health* 15:170.
Snijder, M. B., R. M. van Dam, C. D. Stehouwer, G. J. Hiddink, R. J. Heine, and J. M. Dekker. 2008. A prospective study of dairy consumption in relation to changes in metabolic risk factors: The Hoorn Study. *Obesity* 16 (3):706–9.
Snijder, M. B., A. A. van der Heijden, R. M. van Dam, C. D. Stehouwer, G. J. Hiddink, G. Nijpels, R. J. Heine, et al. 2007. Is higher dairy consumption associated with lower body weight and fewer metabolic disturbances? The Hoorn Study. *Am J Clin Nutr* 85 (4):989–95.
Standl, E. 2005. Aetiology and consequences of the metabolic syndrome. *Eur Heart J* Suppl 7 (D):D10–13.
Steele, R. M., S. Brage, K. Corder, N. J. Wareham, and U. Ekelund. 2008. Physical activity, cardiorespiratory fitness, and the metabolic syndrome in youth. *J Appl Phys* 105 (1):342–51.
Te Velde, S. J., M. B. Snijder, A. E. van Dijk, J. Brug, L. L. Koppes, W. van Mechelen, and J. W. Twisk. 2011. Dairy intake from adolescence into adulthood is not associated with being overweight and metabolic syndrome in adulthood: The Amsterdam Growth and Health Longitudinal Study. *J Hum Nutr Diet* 24 (3):233–44.
Wang, H., K. A. Livingston, C. S. Fox, J. B. Meigs, and P. F. Jacques. 2013. Yogurt consumption is associated with better diet quality and metabolic profile in American men and women. *Nutr Res* 33 (1):18–26.

Section III

Yogurt and Other Health Conditions

8 Yogurt and Gut Health

8.1 LACTOSE DEFICIENCY, MALABSORPTION, AND INTOLERANCE

Lactose is the primary carbohydrate in milk. To be digested, lactose must be hydrolyzed in the intestinal brush border by an enzyme, lactase, into two monosaccharides, glucose and galactose, which are rapidly absorbed in the small intestine (Paige 2005). Lactose is the most important energy source for infants and supplies one of the few sources of galactose in the human diet. Once past the weaning stage, humans' ability to secrete lactase diminishes, leading to the development of lactase deficiency (or lactase nonpersistence) (Silanikove et al. 2015). Lactase deficiency can lead to undigested lactose reaching the colon (lactose malabsorption) and possibly lactose intolerance (lactose malabsorption accompanied by gastrointestinal symptoms). Due to inconsistent definitions and use of the term *lactose intolerance*, in 2010, the National Institutes of Health (NIH) developed a consensus statement on a formal definition of lactose intolerance: "the onset of gastrointestinal symptoms following a blinded single-dose challenge of ingested lactose by an individual with lactose malabsorption, which are not observed when an individual ingests an indistinguishable placebo" (Suchy et al. 2010). Despite this consensus definition, it should be noted that the terms *lactase deficiency*, *lactose malabsorption*, and *lactose intolerance* are still used interchangeably and inconsistently, which continues to cause confusion about the true prevalence of lactose intolerance versus lactase deficiency. The difference between lactose absorption and lactase malabsorption is illustrated in Figure 8.1 and the difference between lactose malabsorption and lactose intolerance is illustrated in Figure 8.2.

As much as 75% of the adult population worldwide is estimated to be lactose deficient and it remains an important cause of lactose malabsorption when physiologic doses (>12 g) are consumed. Over the centuries, humans have adapted to digest and absorb lactose (Silanikove et al. 2015) through such developments as genetic mutations that have resulted in lactase persistence, allowing certain populations (e.g., Northern Europeans and some tribes in Africa that herd cattle) to become lactose absorbers (Smith et al. 2008, Misselwitz et al. 2013); the development of products reduced in lactose content, such as cheese and yogurt, which allow lactose-intolerant individuals to better tolerate milk-based products (Silanikove et al. 2015); and it has been argued that regular intake of lactose by those with lactose deficiency may lead to a more favorable microbiome, resulting in colonic adaptations and an improved tolerance of dairy foods (Szilagyi 2015).

There are four main forms of lactose deficiency: congenital lactase deficiency, primary hypolactasia, secondary hypolactasia, and developmental lactase deficiency (Amiri et al. 2015). Congenital lactase deficiency is an extremely rare disease that occurs during infancy and is a severe form of the deficiency in which lactase activity

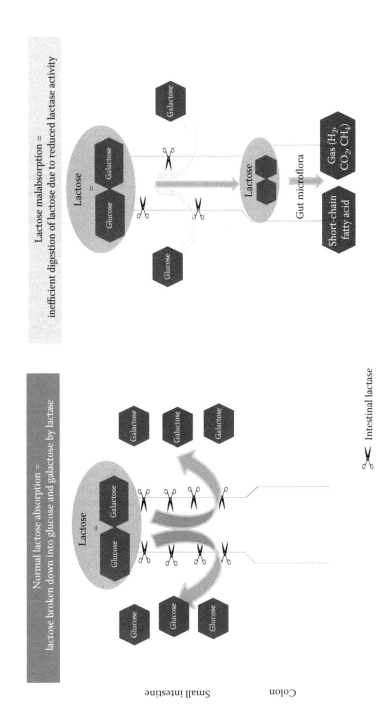

FIGURE 8.1 Comparison between normal lactose absorption and lactose malabsorption. (Reprinted with permission from Danone Research.)

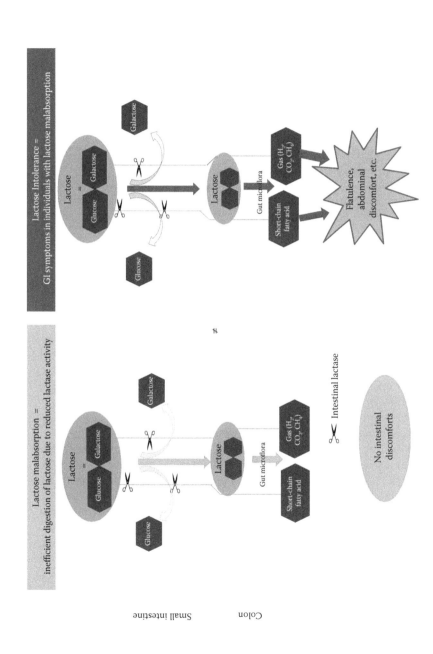

FIGURE 8.2 Comparison between lactose malabsorption and lactose intolerance; lactose malabsorption does not always equal lactose intolerance. (Reprinted with permission from Danone Research.) Note: The development of symptoms associated with lactose intolerance is highly variable and can depend on the amount of lactose consumed, low levels of intestinal lactase activity, the consumption of other foods with lactose, fermentation of lactose by colonic flora, and individual responsiveness to the by-products of lactose fermentation (H_2, CO_2, and CH_4 gases and short-chain fatty acids) Suchy, F.J. et al., *NIH Consens State Sci Statements*, 27(2), 1–27, 2010.

is very low or absent in the intestinal epithelium (Robayo-Torres and Nichols 2007). In contrast, primary lactase deficiency or hypolactasia is a very common, genetically determined, and irreversible phenomenon characterized by the down-regulation of lactase activity, which occurs soon after weaning in most ethnic groups and manifests as lactase deficiency in adulthood (Robayo-Torres and Nichols 2007, Amiri et al. 2015). Secondary hypolactasia or acquired lactase deficiency can be the consequence of an intestinal disease or injury (Amiri et al. 2015), meaning any condition that damages the small-intestinal mucosa brush border. It is transient and reversible with the correction of the underlying disease (Montalto et al. 2006). Secondary hypolactasia may be caused by conditions such as Crohn's disease, celiac sprue, short bowel syndrome, or bacterial and parasitic infections (Adolfsson et al. 2004). Developmental lactase deficiency occurs in preterm infants born less than 34 weeks of gestation, before the lactase enzyme is fully developed (Amiri et al. 2015).

Lactose intolerance only occurs when lactose malabsorption is associated with clinical symptoms: bloating, flatulence, abdominal pain, and diarrhea (Deng et al. 2015). This occurs when undigested lactose present in the intestinal lumen causes increased osmolarity, drawing water and salt into the small intestine and thereby decreasing transit time (Piaia et al. 2003). Once undigested lactose reaches the large intestine, it is processed by colonic bacteria into hydrogen, carbon dioxide, methane, and short-chain fatty acids. The gasses produced result in flatulence and abdominal discomfort, while short-chain fatty acids induce an osmotic load, leading to diarrhea. However, malabsorbed lactose in the colonic lumen does not always result in gastrointestinal symptoms. A standard 100 mL portion of milk contains approximately 7 g of lactose (Solomons 2002); generally, small amounts of milk products can be tolerated without causing symptoms in individuals who have not benefited from the genetic adaptation of lactase persistence. The degree of lactase deficiency, the frequency of consumption, the dose of lactose ingested, the specificity of the individual intestinal flora, gastrointestinal motility, and the sensitivity of the gastrointestinal tract to by-products of microbial lactose digestion all influence the clinical manifestations (Heyman 2006, Deng et al. 2015).

A diagnosis of lactose intolerance is sometimes complicated by the nonspecific nature of the clinical symptoms and perceptions about dairy product consumption. Lactose intolerance can be easily diagnosed with high sensitivity and specificity using a hydrogen breath test following the ingestion of a standard dose of lactose (25–50 g); however, this test may also produce false negatives. Other tests with high accuracies are also available to diagnose lactase activity or the presence of a lactase persistence gene; however, these tests do not provide any indications regarding potential clinical manifestations (Mattar et al. 2012). Many individuals self-report lactose intolerance without actually being diagnosed. It is thought that the symptoms experienced could be related to other components of the milk products ingested or gastrointestinal conditions such as irritable bowel syndrome (Pal et al. 2015, Suchy et al. 2010). For true lactose malabsorbers, lactose intolerance can be well managed and is easy to treat (Paige 2005, National Medical Association 2009).

It is possible to consume yogurt and dairy products despite having maldigestion or lactose intolerance. Most individuals diagnosed with lactose intolerance or lactose maldigestion can tolerate up to 12 g of lactose in a single dose with few or no symptoms and can tolerate even higher amounts if intake is spread throughout the day (20–24 g) (Wilt et al. 2010, EFSA Panel on Dietetic Products, Nutrition and Allergies 2010a). Subjective observations from a small clinical trial (10 individuals) suggested that lactose-intolerant young adults may tolerate up to 200 mL (9.6 g of lactose) of yogurt served in one meal (Mądry et al. 2012). Moreover, gradually increasing lactose in the diet is an effective strategy for managing lactose intolerance (National Medical Association 2009). Many lactose-intolerant individuals have traditionally consumed yogurt without experiencing any digestive discomfort (Savaiano 2014).

According to the NIH, many individuals with real or perceived lactose intolerance avoid dairy and ingest inadequate amounts of calcium and vitamin D, which may predispose them to decreased bone accrual, osteoporosis, and other adverse health outcomes (Suchy et al. 2010). Indeed, studies performed in different countries (Parsons et al. 1997, Du et al. 2002, Rockell et al. 2005, Black et al. 2002) demonstrated that children who followed dairy-free diets had reduced bone mineral content and bone mineral density. The primary nutritional concern for a lactose exclusion diet is its positive association with lower intakes of calcium and vitamin D (Wilt et al. 2010), which could lead to idiopathic osteoporosis in women (Rozenberg et al. 2015). Symptomatic lactose-intolerant individuals have lower calcium intake than lactose-tolerant individuals as well as nonsymptomatic lactose-intolerant groups (Di Stefano et al. 2002); this is likely due to lactose avoidance diets that exclude dairy consumption. Furthermore, Di Stefano et al. (2002) showed that there was a significantly higher prevalence of osteopenia in symptomatic lactose-intolerant individuals, which was attributed to lower calcium intakes (Di Stefano et al. 2002). Additionally, there is evidence supporting the role of lactose as a dietary prebiotic in lactose nonpersistent individuals; *in vitro* and *in vivo* animal models and human clinical studies have consistently shown the ability of lactose to favorably alter colonic microbiota (Szilagyi 2015). The NIH suggest that educational programs and behavioral approaches for individuals and their health-care providers should be validated and developed to improve the nutrition and symptoms of individuals with lactose intolerance and dairy avoidance. Lactose malabsorbers can tolerate up to one cup of fluid milk with no or few symptoms and additional lactose can be tolerated if it is eaten with a meal or spread in small amounts throughout the day (Suchy et al. 2010). In fact, the 2010 Dietary Guidelines for Americans suggest that individuals suffering from lactose intolerance consume yogurt or cheese, smaller portions of milk, or select lactose-free varieties of dairy products (USDA Agriculture 2010). Given that there are viable alternatives for individuals who are lactose intolerant, there is a general consensus that it is not necessary to avoid all dairy products (Rozenberg et al. 2015), particularly yogurt (Heaney 2013). These studies will be discussed in the following sections.

8.1.1 STUDIES IN CHILDREN

Few studies have compared the effect of yogurt on lactose intolerance in pediatric populations. In children, lactose maldigestion is most often the consequence of other acute conditions such as infectious diarrhea rather than primary lactase deficiency, and lactose intolerance may in fact be overdiagnosed in this group (Grimheden et al. 2012).

Shermak et al. (1995) compared typical servings of milk, pasteurized yogurt, and yogurt containing active live culture in 14 lactose-malabsorbing children. Breath hydrogen concentration values and symptoms were recorded for 8 hours after the ingestion of 12 g of lactose served in milk or yogurt. Lactose-maldigesting children experienced significantly fewer symptoms after consuming yogurt with live cultures than after milk ($p < .005$). Pasteurized yogurt showed an intermediate effect. The lower effect of pasteurized products could be due to both the decrease in live bacteria and/or the decrease in bacterial lactase content. However, lactose from yogurt was not better digested than lactose from milk, as indicated by similar areas under the curve in the breath hydrogen concentration test (Shermak et al. 1995). Montes et al. (1995) observed a decrease in the symptoms of 20 lactose-maldigesting children following the ingestion of yogurt with live bacteria.

8.1.2 Studies in Adults

The responses to ingesting a physiological dose of lactose (12–15.7 g) from various types of products—milk (control), heated yogurt, yogurt and lactose, heated yogurt and lactase, sweet acidophilus milk (*Lactobacillus acidophilus*), and sweet acidophilus milk/sonicated cells—were tested in 14 healthy adults. Lactose intolerance was determined if breath hydrogen concentrations were over 20 ppm after ingesting 250 mL of milk containing 15.7 g of lactose. No evidence of lactose malabsorption was noted following the ingestion of a 250 mL glass of milk, based on the breath hydrogen test. Breath hydrogen values following yogurt ingestion were on average 81% lower than those of the control milk. These results are significant, because even when yogurt was inactivated by heat the mean breath hydrogen value (14.9 ± 1.9 SD) was significantly lower than the mean value for the control milk (28.7 ± 2.7). Even in the lactose-supplemented yogurt, the breath hydrogen value remained lower (15.5 ± 2.7) than the control milk. The lower breath hydrogen values indicated a better tolerance for yogurt compared with milk, which can be attributed to the reduction of lactose through fermentation and increased lactase activity with the presence of indigenous bacterial lactase (McDonough et al. 1987).

A subsequent study tested the effectiveness of commercial plain yogurt, sweet acidophilus milk (*L. acidophilus*), hydrolyzed-lactose milk, and a lactase tablet against a whole-milk control in 10 lactose-intolerant black individuals. The findings demonstrated that plain yogurt was as effective as the lactose-hydrolyzed milk in reducing lactose malabsorption symptoms; however, it also received the least acceptable score in the sensory assessment. Furthermore, yogurt lactase was superior to exogenous lactase in alleviating symptoms associated with lactose malabsorption (Onwulata et al. 1989).

Marteau et al. (1990) measured breath hydrogen concentration in eight lactase-deficient volunteers who ingested 18 g of lactose in the form of milk, yogurt, and heated yogurt (450 g/day). An intestinal perfusion technique was used. Interestingly, approximately one-fifth of the lactase activity contained in yogurt reached the terminal ileum. These findings indicated that more than 90% of the lactose in yogurt was digested in the small intestine of lactase-deficient subjects. The authors suggested that both the slow orocecal transit time (OCTT) and the lactase activity contained in the viable starter culture were responsible for the efficient absorption (Marteau et al. 1990).

Pelletier et al. (2001) compared the effect of different dairy products and the impact of heat treatment on lactose intolerance. Using a double-blind, randomized crossover study in 24 male lactose malabsorbers, the effects of ingesting milk, yogurt, heat-treated yogurt, and two products obtained by the dilution of yogurt with heat-treated products were evaluated. Each product contained approximately the same amount of lactose, but the amount of bacteria varied. Hydrogen production and adverse events were followed for 8 hours after the ingestion of the products. To have a double-blind design, the milk used was acidified and thickened prior to the study and looked like yogurt. The results demonstrated that the breath hydrogen excretion and complaints for digestive events after yogurt ingestion were reduced compared with other products. Changing the texture of the milk had no effects on the results (which were similar to those of conventional milk). This study highlighted the importance of having a high population of live bacteria in the product (Pelletier et al. 2001).

In a double-blind crossover study, 22 lactose maldigesters experienced more effective lactose digestion and less severe gastrointestinal symptoms after fresh yogurt intake compared with heat-treated yogurt (500 mL/day). The OCTT was shorter following heated yogurt ingestion compared with fresh yogurt ingestion (Labayen et al. 2001).

Using a double-blind, randomized 3×3 Latin-square design, 45 healthy adults received yogurt, heat-treated yogurt, and acidified jellified milk, all containing 20 g of lactose. Hydrogen concentrations in breath samples were analyzed by gas chromatography. Compared with the heat-treated yogurt and acidified jellified milk, the peak hydrogen concentration (Cmax) of yogurt and the hydrogen concentration area under the curve (AUC) were both significantly decreased. The authors concluded that the live bacteria in dairy products could improve lactose digestion in male adult lactose malabsorbers (He et al. 2004).

Several studies have compared the effect of the consumption of fresh yogurt with live cultures to pasteurized yogurt with reduced or no live cultures on intestinal lactose utilization (Savaiano et al. 1984, Dewit 1988, Lerebours et al. 1989, Pochart et al. 1989, Rizkalla et al. 2000). Each of these studies observed an improvement in lactose digestion with fresh yogurt compared with pasteurized yogurt. It may be particularly important to improve lactose digestion in the elderly, since lactase activity declines with age. A Spanish team observed that lactose digestion in healthy institutionalized elderly was improved considerably with a yogurt with live cultures, whereas pasteurized yogurt did not induce the same effect (Varela-Moreiras et al. 1992).

Many studies in different population and age groups have shown that yogurt consumption improves lactose digestion. Based on 14 human studies, the European Food Safety Authority (EFSA) panel concluded that a cause and effect relationship has been established between the consumption of live cultures in yogurt and improved lactose digestion in individuals with lactose maldigestion. The EFSA found that there was sufficient evidence to permit the claim that "Live yogurt cultures in yogurt improve digestion of lactose in yogurt in individuals with lactose maldigestion." However, the yogurt should contain at least 10^8 CFU per gram of live starter microorganisms, specifically *L. bulgaricus* and *Streptococcus thermophilus* (EFSA Panel on Dietetic Products, Nutrition and Allergies 2010b).

8.1.3 Mechanisms of Action

8.1.3.1 Activity of Yogurt Bacteria

The symptoms of lactose intolerance can be influenced by the amount of lactose ingested, small-intestinal lactase activity, transit time, and colonic processing of lactose (Vesa 2000, Vonk et al. 2003, He et al. 2006, 2008). Even though yogurt generally contains similar amounts of lactose as milk, it has been shown to be better tolerated by lactose-intolerant individuals (Savaiano 2014).

The first hypothesis proposing the mechanism of lactose tolerance following yogurt ingestion came from a 1976 study in rats that suggested that yogurt bacteria remained viable up to 3 hours after feeding, which could contribute to lactose digestion in the gastrointestinal tract (Goodenough and Kleyn 1976). This hypothesis was later confirmed by Kolars et al. (1984), who suggested that lactose hydrolysis was possible through bacteria-derived lactase in yogurt (Savaiano 2014). Lactose in yogurt could be better tolerated than lactose in other dairy products, partly because of the activity of microbial β-galactosidase, which digests lactose (Martini et al. 1991, Montalto et al. 2006). It has been shown that *L. bulgaricus* and *S. thermophilus* contain high β-galactosidase activity (Hartley and Denariaz 1993). This lactase activity works optimally at a pH of 7, coinciding with the proximal small intestine and small terminal ileum, and is further activated in the presence of bile (Savaiano 2014). This particularity may explain the superiority of yogurt compared with other dairy products in improving lactose maldigestion (yogurt should contain at least 10^8 CFU per serving of live starter microorganisms) (EFSA Panel on Dietetic Products, Nutrition and Allergies 2010b). The bacterial cell wall is a mechanical protection for lactase during gastric transit and the release of the enzyme into the small intestine is a determinant of efficiency (de Vrese et al. 2001). Bacterial lactase seems to be protected from gastric acidity and appears to be delivered in its active form into the small intestine. Drouault et al. (2002) applied a bacterial luciferase to monitor the gene expression of *S. thermophilus* in the digestive tract of germ-free mice. The microorganism was able to produce *de novo* active β-galactosidase enzyme in the digestive tract, although *S. thermophilus* did not multiply during gastrointestinal transit. The enzyme production was enhanced when lactose (the inducer) was added to the diet. This study demonstrated that *S. thermophilus* could produce β-galactosidase during its gastrointestinal transit in mice and that this enzyme reduces the lactose content in the digestive tract (Drouault et al. 2002). This buffering capacity protects yogurt bacteria from the acidic gastric environment. The slower gastrointestinal transit time of yogurt compared with milk also assists lactose digestion (Savaiano 2014). However, the effectiveness of yogurts could differ according to the variety. For example, plain yogurt may be more effective on lactose digestion than sweetened yogurt (Onwulata et al. 1989). It was also observed that after ingestion of fresh yogurt by lactose malabsorbers, viable starter cultures could reach the duodenum and contain lactase activity (Pochart et al. 1989). However, other studies found that yogurt consumption could not stimulate the endogenous (brush border) lactase activity in the small intestine of lactase-deficient subjects (Lerebours et al. 1989, He et al. 2008).

8.1.3.2 Colonic Processing of Lactose and Adaptation

Colonic metabolism of lactose has been suggested to play an important role in lactose tolerance. The lactose in yogurt can be considered as a prebiotic for people with lactose maldigestion (Szilagyi 2004), since not all the lactose in yogurt is digested in those individuals and could serve as a substrate for fermentation by the colonic microbiota, which produces gas and other by-products of fermentation such as short-chain fatty acids. The different impact of lactose on microbiota could also depend on the genetic lactase status (Szilagyi et al. 2010). Moreover, the regular consumption of lactose is likely to lead to colonic adaptation, decreased symptoms, and further increased intake and tolerability (Hertzler and Savaiano 1996, Szilagyi 2015, Pribila et al. 2000).

8.1.3.3 Physical Properties

The high osmolality and energy density of yogurt could also play a role. Compared with milk, yogurt delays gastric emptying and increases intestinal transit time, causing a slower delivery of lactose along the intestine (Marteau et al. 1990, Labayen et al. 2001). The slower transit optimizes the action of β-galactosidase in the small bowel, which decreases the osmotic load of lactose (Labayen et al. 2001, de Vrese et al. 2001). The gastrointestinal transit time could also be increased by the low pH in fermented milk, which delays the gastric emptying from the stomach into the small intestine (de Vrese et al. 2001).

Vonk et al. (2003) observed that the gastric emptying was similar between fresh and heated yogurt, while the OCTT of fresh yogurt was markedly longer than that of heated yogurt. Furthermore, there was a strong inverse correlation between gastrointestinal symptoms and OCTT, suggesting that when intestinal transit time increases, lactose digestion and tolerance may improve. However, the improved lactose digestion and tolerance of fresh yogurt was mainly attributed to the presence of living bacteria (Vonk et al. 2003). More studies are needed to investigate the mechanism by which fermentation processes and lactose metabolites could influence the development of symptoms in individuals with lactose intolerance (He et al. 2006). Future research priorities include: determining whether colonic adaptation is universal among all individuals with lactase nonpersistence; determining the frequency of complete asymptomatic adaptation; quantifying the amount of dairy food intake needed for adaptation; identifying any potential differences in the genome between lactase-persistent individuals, lactase-persistent dairy food consumers, lactase-non-persistent individuals, and lactase-non-persistent dairy food consumers; and determining whether disease outcomes are modified in lactase-non-persistent dairy food consumers (Szilagyi 2015).

8.1.4 CONCLUSIONS

- Lactose is the most important energy source for infants; however, there is a genetically determined down-regulation of lactase activity, which occurs soon after weaning in most ethnic groups, resulting in lactase deficiency.
- Lactase deficiency can result in the delivery of undigested lactose to the colon, resulting in lactose malabsorption. Lactose intolerance occurs when lactose malabsorption causes gastrointestinal symptoms (gas, bloating, diarrhea, pain, and discomfort).
- Lactase deficiency, lactose malabsorption, and lactose intolerance are inconsistently used in the literature. The gold-standard definition for lactose intolerance as defined by the NIH is: "the onset of gastrointestinal symptoms following a blinded single-dose challenge of ingested lactose by an individual with lactose malabsorption, which are not observed when an individual ingests an indistinguishable placebo."
- Lactose intolerance is not well correlated with lactose malabsorption and has been shown to be very subjective. In children, lactose maldigestion could be overdiagnosed and is most often the consequence of diseases other than primary lactase deficiency.
- A high population of live bacteria in yogurt seems to be important to improve lactose digestion in lactose malabsorbers. Indeed, the consumption of heat-treated fermented milks results in a lesser improvement in lactose digestion than the consumption of live yogurt in most studies. The EFSA panel concluded in 2010 that a cause and effect relationship has been established between the consumption of live yogurt cultures in yogurt and improved lactose digestion in individuals with lactose maldigestion.
- Different mechanisms, including β-galactosidase activity, colonic processing of lactose, and yogurt's physical properties, could explain the beneficial effect of yogurt on lactose intolerance digestion compared with milk.

8.2 TREATMENT OF DIARRHEA

Diarrhea is a leading cause of malnutrition in children under 5 years old and is still a major cause of childhood morbidity and mortality. It is usually a symptom of an infection in the intestinal tract, which can be caused by a variety of bacterial, viral, and parasitic organisms. Individuals with diarrhea experience imbalances in electrolytes and water movement across the gut, which can lead to abdominal pain, dehydration, malnutrition, weight loss, and so on. Diarrhea is defined by at least three episodes of liquid feces per 24-hour period (or more frequent passage than is normal) (WHO 2009). Osmotic diarrhea could be the cause of a nonabsorbable compound (e.g., lactose), whereas secretory diarrhea is often associated with viral (e.g., Rotavirus) or bacterial enteritis (e.g., *Salmonella, Shigella, Vibrio cholerae,* or *Escherichia coli*). WHO (1988) defines acute diarrhea as less than 14 days in duration and persistent diarrhea as 14 days or longer. Antibiotic treatment is often accompanied by diarrhea and other gastrointestinal side effects. Some studies have shown that antibiotic-associated diarrhea occurs in around 11%–26% of children given antibiotics in an outpatient setting (Turck et al. 2003, Vanderhoof et al. 1999, Arvola et al. 1999).

Foods suitable for a child with diarrhea are usually the same as those consumed by healthy children and they should be easy to digest. WHO (2005) states that, in case of acute diarrhea, "Recommended foods should be culturally acceptable, readily available, have a high content of energy and provide adequate amounts of essential micronutrients. They should be well cooked, and mashed or ground to make them easy to digest; fermented foods are also easy to digest." Moreover, it has been stated in a recent update on persistent diarrhea in children that yogurt-based or amino acid–based diets may accelerate their recovery and that zinc supplementation reduces the severity and duration of diarrhea (Moore 2011).

Over the last two decades, more studies on the effect of the microbiota and pre- and probiotics and their impact on health have emerged, providing greater rationale for the use of bacteria-fermented products in the prevention and treatment of diarrhea (de Vrese and Marteau 2007). The World Gastroenterology Organization affirms that controlled clinical intervention studies and meta-analyses support the use of specific probiotic strains and products in the treatment and prevention of Rotavirus diarrhea in infants. However, because significant differences in the effects have been reported between closely related strains, the effect on diarrhea needs to be verified for each specific strain in humans (WGO 2008). Until now, the majority of studies on the use of probiotics in the prevention and treatment of diarrhea have been performed in children and few studies have been performed in healthy adults (Pereg et al. 2005). The following paragraphs will focus on the evidence regarding the effect of regular yogurt and its microorganisms on the treatment of different types of diarrhea.

8.2.1 Treatment of Acute Diarrhea

Niv et al. (1963) were the first to conduct a study on the effects of yogurt on diarrhea in children. Despite a small ($n = 45$) and heterogeneous group, the authors noted a faster recovery from diarrhea in the "yogurt group" than in the "Neomycin-kaolin-pectin group," an antibiotic acting on *E. coli*, *Enterobacter*, *Campylobacter*, and *Klebsiella* (Niv et al. 1963).

The effect of yogurt, compared with milk, on acute diarrhea was evaluated in malnourished children aged 4–47 months with acute noncholera diarrhea. Children were randomly assigned to receive small frequent feedings of milk formula or yogurt formula (made by adding a combination of *S. thermophilus* and *L. bulgaricus* starter cultures to milk formula) at a dose of 120 mL/kg body weight. The children in the milk group had a significantly higher median percent weight gain at the end of the study (after 72 hours) and at recovery. In this study, yogurt treatment did not result in any significant clinical benefit compared with milk (Bhatnagar et al. 1998).

Boudraa et al. (2001) performed a controlled clinical trial on 112 well-nourished young children aged 3–24 months with acute watery diarrhea. Children consumed either an infant formula or yogurt. The two treatments were comparable in terms of lactose concentration, pH, flavor, and texture. The presence of sugars in the stool was used as a marker of carbohydrate malabsorption. The cessation of diarrhea and the appropriate weight gain after 7 days was similar in both groups. Moreover, in children with reduced sugars in stools, the rate of recovery was similar in milk and yogurt groups, but children who consumed yogurt had a significantly and clinically relevant decrease in stool frequency as well as duration of diarrhea (Boudraa et al. 2001).

A meta-analysis of controlled trials on acute infectious diarrhea performed by Van Niel et al. (2002) demonstrated a reduction in diarrhea duration of about 0.7 days with the intake of yogurt including *L.* bacteria in children. Moreover, there was a reduction in diarrhea frequency of 1.6 stools on the second day of treatment in the yogurt groups. Sub-analyses suggested a dose–response relationship (Van Niel et al. 2002).

Children aged 6–24 months with acute nonbloody and nonmucoid diarrhea (for less than 4 days) were included in a randomized clinical trial. The yogurt group received at least 15 mL/kg/day of pasteurized yogurt plus routine hospital treatment, whereas the control group received routine hospital treatment only. Children in the yogurt group had a reduced mean hospitalization days ($p = .035$) and diarrhea frequency ($p = .049$) and an increased weight gain ($p = .017$) compared with children in the control group (Pashapour and Iou 2006).

8.2.2 Treatment of Persistent Diarrhea

A clinical trial evaluated the effect of milk compared with yogurt in nine Algerian boys, aged 7–29 months, with chronic diarrhea, jejunal villous atrophy, and lactase deficiency. The children received a diagnostic load of lactose, and on the following days, in random order, milk or yogurt. Lactose malabsorption and fecal output were decreased after the ingestion of yogurt compared with milk. These results show that the absorption of lactose is better after ingesting yogurt than milk and suggest that diarrhea may be improved by substituting milk with yogurt (Dewit 1987).

A randomized clinical trial was performed to evaluate the clinical efficacy of substituting yogurt for milk in the diet of 78 children aged 3–36 months with confirmed persistent diarrhea. Children consumed either milk (infant formula) or yogurt (infant formula fermented with *L. bulgaricus* and *S. thermophilus*). Weight loss greater than 5% in a single day or persistent diarrhea for 5 days was significantly decreased in children who consumed yogurt compared with children who consumed milk. The beneficial effects of yogurt consumption were apparent within 48 hours in $67 \pm 8\%$ of children (Touhami et al. 1992).

An intervention was conducted to test the effect of yogurt supplementation on different parameters in 402 Chinese children aged 3–5 years whose height for age and/or weight for age were less than the reference level. Children in the yogurt group consumed 125 g/day of yogurt 5 day per week for a period of 10 months in addition to their usual diet, whereas the control group continued to consume their usual diet. In the yogurt group, the intake of calcium, zinc, and vitamin B2 was significantly higher than that in the control group and they observed a decrease in the incidence and duration of diarrhea and upper respiratory infection (He et al. 2005).

De Mattos et al. (2009) tested the effect of consuming three different lactose-free diets (soy-based formula, hydrolyzed protein-based formula, and amino acid–based formula) and a yogurt-based formula on the stool output and duration of diarrhea in children. The diets were administered to 154 male infants aged 1–30 months with persistent diarrhea. Children who were fed the yogurt-based diet or the amino acid–based diet had a significant reduction in stool output and in the duration of diarrhea compared with other test diets. The authors recommended the use of an inexpensive and readily available yogurt-based diet as the first choice for the nutritional management of mild to moderate persistent diarrhea. The benefits observed in the yogurt group may have resulted from the intake of vitamin A and zinc that was two- and threefold higher, respectively, than in the other three treatment groups. A more complex amino acid–based diet could be used for more severe cases of diarrhea (de Mattos et al. 2009).

8.2.3 ANTIBIOTIC-ASSOCIATED DIARRHEA

8.2.3.1 Studies in Children

Conway et al. (2007) evaluated whether eating yogurt could prevent antibiotic-associated diarrhea in children over 1 year of age who were prescribed a 1-week course of antibiotics. The consumption of 150 mL of yogurt (12-day follow-up period) did not prevent antibiotic-associated diarrhea compared with the other test groups. Indeed, the rates of diarrhea were not statistically different: 14% of children in the no-yogurt control group versus 11% and 7% in the commercial yogurt group and bio yogurt, respectively. The weaknesses of this study included the absence of a placebo and the fact that the authors did not take into account in their analysis that different antibiotic agents cause diarrhea at a different rate (Conway et al. 2007). It would have been interesting to evaluate the outcomes for patients using small- versus broad-spectrum antibiotics in the different groups (Overeem et al. 2008).

Pediatric patients ($n = 76$) aged 5 months to 6 years treated with antibiotics (amoxycillin or co-amoxiclav) were randomized into a test group (yogurt treatment) and a control group (no treatment). The test group was fed 75 mL of yogurt each morning for the first 3 days of their antibiotic treatment. A significantly lower proportion of patients developed diarrhea in the test group (5.4%) compared with the control group (27%). The authors therefore concluded that broad-spectrum antibiotic-associated diarrhea could effectively be reduced with a prophylactic treatment of yogurt. Yogurt prophylaxis was thought to be cost appropriate, easily administered, and culturally acceptable (Ranasinghe et al. 2007).

A randomized, double-blind, placebo-controlled clinical trial was conducted in which 70 children (1–12 years old) being treated with antibiotics were given 200 g/day of either a probiotic yogurt (*L. rhamnosus* and *L. acidophilus*) or a pasteurized yogurt (placebo) throughout the course of their treatment. Results showed that the probiotic yogurt performed significantly better than the pasteurized yogurt in reducing the incidence of antibiotic-associated diarrhea. While the study did not have a nonyogurt control, it was suggested that the use of yogurt as a vehicle for probiotic delivery likely had the added benefit of providing energy and nutrients that would not otherwise be contained in a probiotic capsule (Fox et al. 2015).

A systematic review and meta-analysis of yogurt treatment for antibiotic-associated diarrhea was conducted by Patro-Golab et al. (2015b) citing only two articles that met inclusion criteria: Ranasinghe et al. (2007) and Conway et al. (2007). Despite the promising results of these two studies, they were considered low in methodological quality. A fixed effects model ($n = 314$) found a borderline significant reduced risk of diarrhea associated with yogurt consumption. However, the significance was entirely lost in a random effects model and the authors concluded that there was a paucity of evidence to support the use of yogurt in antibiotic-associated diarrhea prevention (Patro-Golab et al. 2015b). A subsequent meta-analysis by the same authors investigating the use of yogurt in the treatment of acute gastroenteritis in hospital settings had similar conclusions based on four studies. Yogurt was not found to have a significant effect on stool volume and its effects on the duration of diarrhea and stool frequency were inconsistent. However, yogurt was reported to have a positive effect on weight gain (Patro-Golab et al. 2015a). Despite the lack of evidence regarding efficacy in the treatment and management of antibiotic-associated diarrhea or acute gastroenteritis, yogurt is not likely to cause any harm and is a food that is well tolerated, widely accepted, and has excellent nutritional value for children experiencing acute gastrointestinal illnesses.

8.2.3.2 Studies in Adults

Shapiro (1960) evaluated the effect of yogurt on antibiotic treatment side effects. Following the administration of tetracycline, 15 patients received yogurt as a dietary supplement after gastrointestinal disturbances. In patients receiving antimicrobial drugs over a long period, yogurt was helpful in lessening the symptoms of antibiotic side effects and in maintaining nutritional status. The most efficient way was to give the yogurt 1 hour after the antibiotic (Shapiro 1960).

Beniwal et al. (2003) performed a clinical trial to test the effect of yogurt consumption on the prevention of antibiotic-associated diarrhea. Around 230 g of yogurt was administered to hospitalized patients receiving oral or intravenous antibiotics and they were followed for 8 days. The mean age of the study group was 70 years and 43% were male. Patients receiving yogurt reported less frequent diarrhea (12% vs. 24%; $p = .04$), and significantly fewer total days of diarrhea (23% vs. 60%). The authors concluded that dietary supplementation with yogurt is a simple, effective, and safe treatment that decreases the incidence and duration of antibiotic-associated diarrhea (Beniwal et al. 2003).

8.2.4 MECHANISMS OF ACTION

Yogurt is an easily digested food and its high essential nutrient content may help restore the nutritional status and act positively on diarrhea. Few studies have evaluated the mechanisms of action of traditional yogurt strains on different types of diarrhea. Indeed, lactic bacteria have strain-specific effects, some of which could be particularly efficient in the treatment of diarrhea. A meta-analysis of randomized controlled studies using different *Lactobacillus* strains has indicated that they offer a safe and effective means of treating acute infectious diarrhea in children (Van Niel et al. 2002).

Lactase, secreted by yogurt bacteria, improves the absorption of lactose and yogurt, slowing down the intestinal transit, which could facilitate the action of residual intestinal lactase and regulate intestinal motility. Moreover, the passage of yogurt bacteria through the gut could contribute to the elimination of pathogenic enteric bacteria by the production of acid, hydrogen peroxide, or antimicrobial substances (Heyman 2000, Rohde et al. 2009). They could also reinforce the intestinal barrier capacity by competing with pathogenic bacteria for adhesion to the enterocytes and nutrients (Adolfsson et al. 2004, Heyman 2000, de Vrese and Marteau 2007).

The beneficial effects of yogurt on diarrhea are often described in the presence of live bacteria, but inactive bacteria may also have preventive or curative capacities (Heyman 2000). Interestingly, different yogurt matrices (e.g., with added fruits) have been shown to be suitable for probiotic bacteria, which can shorten the duration of antibiotic-associated diarrhea (de Vrese et al. 2011).

Lactic acid bacteria (LAB) have also been described as reinforcing the nonspecific immune defense (such as phagocytosis and cytokine production) and specific immunity, particularly the secretory immune system mediated by secretory Immunoglobin A (IgA) or Immunoglobin M (IgM) in response to infectious antigens and perhaps to soluble food antigens. Other possible mechanisms include a trophic role on the intestinal epithelium, down-regulatory activity in cow's milk, allergy, and anti-inflammatory effects (Heyman 2000).

8.2.5 Conclusions

- Yogurt is a nutrient-dense food that is easy to digest, making it a recommended food for acute diarrhea.
- A meta-analysis of controlled trials has indicated that yogurt is safe and effective in reducing the duration and frequency of acute diarrhea in children. Furthermore, there is indication that the beneficial effects may be dose dependent.
- Treating persistent diarrhea with yogurt in young children may enhance or replenish nutritional status, which is particularly important in developing countries where the rates of lactose malabsorption and malnutrition are high.
- Evidence is too sparse to determine whether yogurt prophylaxis or treatments are effective in reducing antibiotic-associated diarrhea incidence or the severity of symptoms. However, it remains a widely accepted, low-cost, nutrient-dense food, which can lead to weight gain in ill patients taking antibiotics.
- The effect of yogurt and its clinical efficacy when compared with milk could be due, at least in part, to the decrease in lactose malabsorption symptoms.
- Mechanisms of actions can include the ability of yogurt bacteria to potentially compete with pathogenic bacteria during their passage through the gastrointestinal system, as well as the possible reinforcement of nonspecific immune responses.
- More yogurt-specific studies are needed to evaluate the effects on prevention and treatment of different types of diarrhea. Since almost all clinical studies on yogurt and diarrhea have been conducted on children, it would be interesting to know more about the effects on adults.

8.3 THE MICROBIOTA

There are numerous knowledge gaps regarding the mechanisms by which yogurt microorganisms modulate various physiological functions and affect the composition of human intestinal microbiota. However, in recent years there has been a sharp increase in the number of publications addressing the intestinal microbiota. The importance of the gut microbiome is now established in numerous systemic disease states such as obesity and cardiovascular disease and in intestinal conditions such as inflammatory bowel disease (Kinross et al. 2011).

According to a crossover design study in which healthy participants consumed fresh and heat-treated yogurt for 15 days, the main change in human microbiota observed after yogurt consumption was an increase in the density of LAB and *Clostridium perfringens* to the detriment of *Bacteroides*. Interestingly, bacterial changes were not different after the consumption of fresh and heat-treated yogurt. This suggests that changes in microbiota may not require bacterial viability. The authors conclude that even if probiotic effects cannot be established for specific yogurt strains, yogurt should also be considered a prebiotic food, although this concept must be confirmed by more studies (García-Albiach et al. 2008).

The consumption of yogurt may confer beneficial changes to the balance and metabolic activities of the indigenous microbiota (Alvaro et al. 2007, García-Albiach et al. 2008) independently of yogurt bacteria viability (García-Albiach et al. 2008). While causal effects between the microbiome and common diseases are not yet defined, epidemiological evidence suggests associations between gut bacterial colonization and diseases such as obesity. The ability of probiotics, prebiotics, and fermented foods to modulate the microbiota is not fully understood and needs to be further investigated to be optimized (Goulet 2015). Daily yogurt consumption is thought to help decrease pathogens in the gut (Fisberg and Machado 2015).

8.3.1 CONCLUSIONS

- The possible effect of yogurt bacteria on the composition of human intestinal microbiota has not been sufficiently explored. Most of the studies have evaluated the recovery of bacteria in feces, which might not reflect local changes in microbiota composition in specific niches of the gastrointestinal tract. Understanding the interactions between diet, microbiome, and host is essential to the development of future health-care strategies.

8.4 VIABILITY OF YOGURT BACTERIA

It has been observed that although the standard yogurt bacteria, *S. thermophilus* and *L. bulgaricus*, provide some benefits to the host, their effects could be minor compared with specific probiotic strains, because they poorly resist passage through the gastrointestinal system (Lin et al. 1991). *S. thermophilus* have been shown to survive and to adhere poorly to intestinal epithelial cells (Conway et al. 1987), but could have competitive and growth advantages over *L. bulgaricus* (Ben-Yahia et al. 2012). Yogurt bacterial cell viability may also differ according to the concentration of ingested cells and specific strains (Morelli 2014). Nevertheless, *S. thermophilus* have been found in viable quantities in fecal matter, thereby demonstrating their capacity to remain viable during digestion (Uriot et al. 2016). Furthermore, complex food matrices such as milk play a role in protecting bacteria during passage through the gastrointestinal system and enhancing the delivery of viable bacteria (Bove et al. 2013). Using a dynamic TNO gastrointestinal model simulation, it was found that *S. thermophiles* LMD9 had improved viability in a fermented milk matrix rather than in a regular milk matrix, suggesting that the pre-exposure to an acid medium can make bacterial cells more resistant to passage through the gastrointestinal system (Uriot et al. 2016). An animal model has shown that some protective effects of probiotics, such as immunostimulation, are mediated by their own DNA rather than by their ability to resist passage through the gastrointestinal tract (Rachmilewitz et al. 2004). Further studies have demonstrated the immunomodulatory, antioxidant, and colonization resistance properties of *S. thermophiles* both *in vivo* and *in vitro* (Uriot et al. 2016). Any beneficial health properties of yogurt bacteria are likely to be strain specific. Specific strains can enhance the vitamin content of yogurt, whereas others can confer immune action. Investigating the strain-specific properties of traditional yogurt cultures (*S. thermophilus* and *L. delbrueckii* ssp. *bulgaricus*) would help exploit their full potential health benefits (Morelli 2014).

Traditional yogurt bacteria have nonhuman origins. Their presence in the intestine comes mostly from the ingestion of fermented products. Indeed, *L. delbrueckii* ssp. *bulgaricus* is found in large quantities in yogurt, kefir, fermented milk products, and various cheeses. Studies performed on humans tested the viability of yogurt strains after the consumption of yogurt by checking the presence of bacteria in different compartments of the digestive tract or in feces. The fate of yogurt bacteria in the digestive tract was studied in children. The survival of both yogurt starters in children's feces by conventional microbiology for up to 5 days after yogurt consumption was reported. A subsequent study has also shown that *L. bulgaricus* and *S. thermophilus* can survive transit in the digestive tract in a healthy population (Bianchi-Salvadori et al. 1978). The authors suggested that the bacteria in yogurt survive transit both in adults and in children and that casein and fat can protect the yogurt bacteria during their passage through the upper digestive tract.

Robins-Browne and Levine (1981) cultured aspirates of gastric and intestinal juices to study the gastrointestinal survival of *L. bulgaricus* and *L. acidophilus* (freeze-dried commercial preparations dissolved in milk) in seven volunteers. They noted an increase in lactobacilli in the stomach and small intestine for 3–6 hours after ingestion; after this period, the viable counts of lactobacilli returned to baseline. This study indicated that *L. bulgaricus* could survive in the stomach and small intestine but did not colonize the small intestine and that *L. acidophilus* may be more resistant to intestinal passage (Robins-Browne and Levine 1981). Pochart et al. (1989) evaluated the bacterial enzymes' activity in the gastrointestinal tracts of lactase-deficient subjects. During their transit, bacteria demonstrated β-galactosidase activity; however, in this study yogurt bacteria were not detected in stools (Pochart et al. 1989).

The survival of *S. thermophilus* and *L. bulgaricus* during the gastrointestinal transit of healthy volunteers consuming yogurt was assessed by Mater et al. (2005)

using culture on selective media. Yogurt contained rifampin and streptomycin-resistant strains of *S. thermophilus* and *L. bulgaricus*. Over a 12-day period of fresh yogurt intake, out of 39 samples recovered from 13 healthy subjects, 32 contained viable *S. thermophilus* and 37 samples contained *L. bulgaricus* (Mater et al. 2005).

The majority of studies have evaluated the recovery of bacteria in feces; however, this method only gives a general idea of the viability and survival of the organisms in the intestine. Molecular biology techniques have also been used to identify yogurt bacteria in feces. The quantitative real-time polymerase chain reaction (PCR) technique offers the possibility of analyzing the quantitative changes within a particular bacterial group (Malinen et al. 2005). However, PCR-amplified DNA detection does not distinguish between live, damaged, or dead cells (Bae and Wuertz 2009).

In a study in humans, a combination of classic and molecular techniques to detect yogurt bacteria after yogurt consumption was used. Using conventional methods, *L. bulgaricus* was detected in 6 subjects out of 10 at day 7. *S. thermophilus* was not detected at any time as non-*S. thermophilus* cocci were too numerous in readable plates. Molecular methods were used to confirm that strains found in feces were the specific yogurt strains. At day 0, there were no detectable *S. thermophilus* or *L. bulgaricus*, whereas at day 7, *L. bulgaricus* was detected in 9 out of 10 subjects and *S. thermophilus* in 7 out of 10 subjects (Callegari 2004).

Using PCR techniques, Brigidi et al. (2003) fed five healthy subjects with a diet containing 250 g of yogurt/day or a pharmaceutical preparation (containing viable, lyophilized bacteria: *S. thermophilus*, *Bifidobacteriums* spp., and *Lactobacillus* spp.) for 10 days. They demonstrated that *S. thermophilus* could be detected in fecal samples from subjects. The concentration of these bacteria remained constant for 10 days following yogurt treatment and then slowly decreased below the detection limit of direct PCR analysis (Brigidi et al. 2003).

Using PCR primers for species- and strain-specific identification of orally administered strains, Elli et al. (2006) showed that yogurt bacteria, especially *L. bulgaricus*, can be detected in the feces of 20 healthy individuals after a few days of ingestion of 250 g/day of a plain yogurt. In this study, *S. thermophilus* was detected in only one subject on day 7 (Elli et al. 2006).

In a double-blind prospective study in 114 healthy young volunteers, the presence of yogurt microorganisms in human feces after repeated oral yogurt intake (15 days) was determined by PCR and DNA hybridization of total fecal DNA. DNA of yogurt bacteria was found in only 10 of 96 individuals after the consumption of fresh yogurt and in 2 of 96 individuals after the consumption of pasteurized yogurt (del Campo et al. 2005).

Ballesta et al. (2008) also found that the gastrointestinal tract affected the survival of *L. bulgaricus* and *S. thermophilus* after giving fresh or pasteurized yogurt over 75 days to healthy adults. *L. bulgaricus* was isolated in 0.7% of the fecal samples analyzed and DNA from lactic bacteria was detected in only 12.5% of the samples analyzed. *S. thermophilus* was not found in any sample (Bae and Wuertz 2009, Ballesta et al. 2008).

Despite the fact that there are still controversial results in the literature showing the viability of yogurt starters bacteria following their ingestion in humans, consumption of yogurt may ensure some changes to the balance and metabolic activities of the indigenous microbiota, as recently shown by some authors (Zhong et al. 2006, García-Albiach et al. 2008, Alvaro et al. 2007).

8.4.1 Conclusions

- It is not entirely clear whether the yogurt cultures *L. bulgaricus* and *S. thermophilus* can sufficiently survive the passage through the human intestine. It seems that yogurt bacteria partly survive transit in humans and could confer beneficial effects to the host, but cannot colonize the gut. The bacteria present in yogurt are not substantially represented in the natural human intestinal microbiota and the survival of yogurt bacteria has been shown to be less important than that of some other probiotic strains.

REFERENCES

Adolfsson, O., S. N. Meydani, and R. M. Russell. 2004. Yogurt and gut function. *Am J Clin Nutr* 80 (2):245–56.

Alvaro, E., C. Andrieux, V. Rochet, L. Rigottier-Gois, P. Lepercq, M. Sutren, P. Galan, Y. Duval, C. Juste, and J. Doré. 2007. Composition and metabolism of the intestinal microbiota in consumers and non-consumers of yogurt. *Br J Nutr* 97 (1):126–33.

Amiri, M., L. Diekmann, M. von Köckritz-Blickwede, and H. Y. Naim. 2015. The diverse forms of lactose intolerance and the putative linkage to several cancers. *Nutrients* 7 (9):7209–30.

Arvola, T., K. Laiho, S. Torkkeli, H. Mykkanen, S. Salminen, L. Maunula, and E. Isolauri. 1999. Prophylactic Lactobacillus GG reduces antibiotic-associated diarrhea in children with respiratory infections: A randomized study. *Pediatrics* 104 (5):e64.

Bae, S., and S. Wuertz. 2009. Discrimination of viable and dead fecal *Bacteroidales* bacteria by quantitative PCR with propidium monoazide. *Appl Environ Microbiol* 75 (9):2940–4.

Ballesta, S., C. Velasco, M. V. Borobio, F. Argüelles, and E. J. Perea. 2008. Fresh versus pasteurized yogurt: Comparative study of the effects on microbiological and immunological parameters, and gastrointestinal comfort. *Enferm Infecc Microbiol Clin* 26 (9):552–57.

Beniwal, R. S., V. C. Arena, L. Thomas, S. Narla, T. F. Imperiale, R. A. Chaudhry, and U. A. Ahmad. 2003. A randomized trial of yogurt for prevention of antibiotic-associated diarrhea. *Dig Dis Sci* 48 (10):2077–82.

Ben-Yahia, L., C. Mayeur, F. Rul, and M. Thomas. 2012. Growth advantage of *Streptococcus thermophilus* over *Lactobacillus bulgaricus in vitro* and in the gastrointestinal tract of gnotobiotic rats. *Benef Microbes* 3 (3):211–19.

Bhatnagar, S., K. D. Singh, S. Sazawal, S. K. Saxena, and M. K. Bhan. 1998. Efficacy of milk versus yogurt offered as part of a mixed diet in acute noncholera diarrhea among malnourished children. *J Pediatr* 132 (6):999–1003.

Bianchi-Salvadori, B., M. Gotti, F. Brughera, and V. Polinelli. 1978. Etude sur les variations de la flore lactique et bifide intestinale par rapport à l'administration des cellules lactiques du yaourt. *Le Lait* 58 (571–572):17–42.

Black, R. E., S. M. Williams, I. E. Jones, and A. Goulding. 2002. Children who avoid drinking cow milk have low dietary calcium intakes and poor bone health. *Am J Clin Nutr* 76 (3):675–80.

Boudraa, G., M. Benbouabdellah, W. Hachelaf, M. Boisset, J. F. Desjeux, and M. Touhami. 2001. Effect of feeding yogurt versus milk in children with acute diarrhea and carbohydrate malabsorption. *J Pediatr Gastroenterol Nutr* 33 (3):307–13.

Bove, P., P. Russo, V. Capozzi, A. Gallone, G. Spano, and D. Fiocco. 2013. *Lactobacillus plantarum* passage through an oro-gastro-intestinal tract simulator: Carrier matrix effect and transcriptional analysis of genes associated to stress and probiosis. *Microbiol Res* 168 (6):351–59.

Brigidi, P., E. Swennen, B. Vitali, M. Rossi, and D. Matteuzzi. 2003. PCR detection of Bifidobacterium strains and Streptococcus thermophilus in feces of human subjects after oral bacteriotherapy and yogurt consumption. *Int J Food Microbiol* 81 (3):203–9.

Callegari, M. L., L. Morelli, S. Ferrari, J. M. Coba-Sanz, and J. M. Antoine. 2004. Yogurt symbiosis survived in human gut after ingestion. *FASEB J* 18(4–5):A129.

Conway, P. L., S. L. Gorbach, and B. R. Goldin. 1987. Survival of lactic acid bacteria in the human stomach and adhesion to intestinal cells. *J Dairy Sci* 70 (1):1–12.

Conway, S., A. Hart, A. Clark, and I. Harvey. 2007. Does eating yogurt prevent antibiotic-associated diarrhoea? A placebo-controlled randomised controlled trial in general practice. *Br J Gen Pract* 57 (545):953–59.

Del Campo, R., D. Bravo, R. Cantón, P. Ruiz-Garbajosa, R. García-Albiach, A. Montesi-Libois, F. J. Yuste, et al. 2005. Scarce evidence of yogurt lactic acid bacteria in human feces after daily yogurt consumption by healthy volunteers. *Appl Environ Microbiol* 71 (1):547–49.

De Mattos, A. P., T. C. Ribeiro, P. S. Mendes, S. S. Valois, C. M. Mendes, and H. C. Ribeiro, Jr. 2009. Comparison of yogurt, soybean, casein, and amino acid-based diets in children with persistent diarrhea. *Nutr Res* 29 (7):462–69.

Deng, Y. Y., B. Misselwitz, N. Dai, and M. Fox. 2015. Lactose intolerance in adults: Biological mechanism and dietary management. *Nutrients* 7 (9):8020–35.

De Vrese, M., H. Kristen, P. Rautenberg, C. Laue, and J. Schrezenmeir. 2011. Probiotic lactobacilli and bifidobacteria in a fermented milk product with added fruit preparation reduce antibiotic associated diarrhea and *Helicobacter pylori* activity. *J Dairy Res* 78 (4):396–403.

De Vrese, M., and P. R. Marteau. 2007. Probiotics and prebiotics: Effects on diarrhea. *J Nutr* 137 (3 Suppl 2):803S–11S.

De Vrese, M., A. Stegelmann, B. Richter, S. Fenselau, C. Laue, and J. Schrezenmeir. 2001. Probiotics: Compensation for lactase insufficiency. *Am J Clin Nutr* 73 (2 Suppl):421S–29S.

Dewit, O., Boudraa, G., Touhami, M., Desjeux, J.F. 1987. Breath hydrogen test and stools characteristics after ingestion of milk and yogurt in malnourished children with chronic diarrhoea and lactase deficiency. *J Trop Pediatr* 33:177–80.

Dewit, O., Pochart, P., Desjeux, J.F. 1988. Breath hydrogen concentration and plasma glucose, insulin and free fatty acid levels after lactose, milk, fresh or heated yogurt ingestion by healthy young adults with or without lactose malabsorption. *Nutrition* 2 (4):131–35.

Di Stefano, M., G. Veneto, S. Malservisi, L. Cecchetti, L. Minguzzi, A. Strocchi, and G. R. Corazza. 2002. Lactose malabsorption and intolerance and peak bone mass. *Gastroenterology* 122 (7):1793–99.

Drouault, S., J. Anba, and G. Corthier. 2002. Streptococcus thermophilus is able to produce a beta-galactosidase active during its transit in the digestive tract of germ-free mice. *Appl Environ Microbiol* 68 (2):938–41.

Du, X. Q., H. Greenfield, D. R. Fraser, K. Y. Ge, Z. H. Liu, and W. He. 2002. Milk consumption and bone mineral content in Chinese adolescent girls. *Bone* 30 (3):521–28.

EFSA Panel on Dietetic Products, Nutrition and Allergies. 2010a. Scientific opinion on lactose thresholds in lactose intolerance and galactosemia. *EFSA Journal* 8 (9):1777.

EFSA Panel on Dietetic Products, Nutrition and Allergies. 2010b. Scientific opinion on the substantiation of health claims related to live yogurt cultures and improved lactose digestion. *EFSA Journal* 8 (10):1763.

Elli, M., M. L. Callegari, S. Ferrari, E. Bessi, D. Cattivelli, S. Soldi, L. Morelli, et al. 2006. Survival of yogurt bacteria in the human gut. *Appl Environ Microbiol* 72 (7):5113–7.

Fisberg, M., and R. Machado. 2015. History of yogurt and current patterns of consumption. *Nutr Rev* 73 Suppl 1:4–7.

Fox, M. J, K. D. K. Ahuja, I. K. Robertson, M. J. Ball, and R. D. Eri. 2015. Can probiotic yogurt prevent diarrhoea in children on antibiotics? A double-blind, randomised, placebo-controlled study. *BMJ Open* 5 (1):e006474.

García-Albiach, R., M. J. Pozuelo de Felipe, S. Angulo, M. I. Morosini, D. Bravo, F. Baquero, and R. del Campo. 2008. Molecular analysis of yogurt containing *Lactobacillus delbrueckii* subsp. *bulgaricus* and *Streptococcus thermophilus* in human intestinal microbiota. *Am J Clin Nutr* 87 (1):91–96.

Goodenough, E. R., and D. H. Kleyn. 1976. Influence of viable yogurt microflora on digestion of lactose by the rat. *J Dairy Sci* 59 (4):601–6.

Goulet, O. 2015. Potential role of the intestinal microbiota in programming health and disease. *Nutr Rev* 73 Suppl 1:32–40.

Grimheden, P., B. M. Anderlid, M. Gåfvels, J. Svahn, and L. Grahnquist. 2012. Lactose intolerance in children is an overdiagnosed condition. Risk of missing intestinal diseases such as IBD and celiac disease. *Lakartidningen* 109 (5):218–21.

Hartley, D. L., and G. Denariaz. 1993. The role of lactic acid bacteria in yogurt fermentation. *International-journal-of-immunotherapy* 9 (1):3–17.

He, M., J. M. Antoine, Y. Yang, J. Yang, J. Men, and H. Han. 2004. Influence of live flora on lactose digestion in male adult lactose-malabsorbers after dairy products intake. *Wei Sheng Yan Jiu* 33 (5):603–5.

He, M., Y. X. Yang, H. Han, J. H. Men, L. H. Bian, and G. D. Wang. 2005. Effects of yogurt supplementation on the growth of preschool children in Beijing suburbs. *Biomed Environ Sci* 18 (3):192–97.

He, T., M. G. Priebe, H. J. Harmsen, F. Stellaard, X. Sun, G. W. Welling, and R. J. Vonk. 2006. Colonic fermentation may play a role in lactose intolerance in humans. *J Nutr* 136 (1):58–63.

He, T., M. G. Priebe, Y. Zhong, C. Huang, H. J. Harmsen, G. C. Raangs, J. M. Antoine, G. W. Welling, and R. J. Vonk. 2008. Effects of yogurt and bifidobacteria supplementation on the colonic microbiota in lactose-intolerant subjects. *J Appl Microbiol* 104 (2):595–604.

Heaney, R. P. 2013. Dairy intake, dietary adequacy, and lactose intolerance. *Adv Nutr* 4 (2):151–56.

Hertzler, S. R., and D. A. Savaiano. 1996. Colonic adaptation to daily lactose feeding in lactose maldigesters reduces lactose intolerance. *Am J Clin Nutr* 64 (2):232–36.

Heyman, M. 2000. Effect of lactic acid bacteria on diarrheal diseases. *J Am Coll Nutr* 19 (2 Suppl):137S-146S.

Heyman, M. B. 2006. Lactose intolerance in infants, children, and adolescents. *Pediatrics* 118 (3):1279–86.

Kinross, J. M., A. W. Darzi, and J. K. Nicholson. 2011. Gut microbiome-host interactions in health and disease. *Genome Med* 3 (3):14.

Kolars, J. C., M. D. Levitt, M. Aouji, and D. A. Savaiano. 1984. Yogurt: An autodigesting source of lactose. *N Engl J Med* 310 (1):1–3.

Labayen, I., L. Forga, A. González, I. Lenoir-Wijnkoop, R. Nutr, and J. A. Martínez. 2001. Relationship between lactose digestion, gastrointestinal transit time and symptoms in lactose malabsorbers after dairy consumption. *Aliment Pharmacol Ther* 15 (4):543–49.

Lerebours, E., C. N'Djitoyap Ndam, A. Lavoine, M. F. Hellot, J. M. Antoine, and R. Colin. 1989. Yogurt and fermented-then-pasteurized milk: Effects of short-term and long-term ingestion on lactose absorption and mucosal lactase activity in lactase-deficient subjects. *Am J Clin Nutr* 49 (5):823–27.

Lin, M. Y., D. Savaiano, and S. Harlander. 1991. Influence of nonfermented dairy products containing bacterial starter cultures on lactose maldigestion in humans. *J Dairy Sci* 74 (1):87–95.

Mądry, E., B. Krasińska, and M. Woźniewicz. 2012. Yogurt: A potential strategy for overcoming lactose intolerance: The significance of the dose. *Przegląd Gastroenterologiczny* 7 (2):81–86.

Malinen, E., T. Rinttilä, K. Kajander, J. Mättö, A. Kassinen, L. Krogius, M. Saarela, et al. 2005. Analysis of the fecal microbiota of irritable bowel syndrome patients and healthy controls with real-time PCR. *Am J Gastroenterol* 100 (2):373–82.

Marteau, P., B. Flourie, P. Pochart, C. Chastang, J. F. Desjeux, and J. C. Rambaud. 1990. Effect of the microbial lactase (EC 3.2.1.23) activity in yoghurt on the intestinal absorption of lactose: An *in vivo* study in lactase-deficient humans. *Br J Nutr* 64 (1):71–79.

Martini, M. C., E. C. Lerebours, W. J. Lin, S. K. Harlander, N. M. Berrada, J. M. Antoine, and D. A. Savaiano. 1991. Strains and species of lactic acid bacteria in fermented milks (yogurts): Effect on *in vivo* lactose digestion. *Am J Clin Nutr* 54 (6):1041–46.

Mater, D. D. G., L. Bretigny, O. Firmesse, M. J. Flores, A. Mogenet, J. L. Bresson, and G. Corthier. 2005. *Streptococcus thermophilus* and *Lactobacillus delbrueckii* subsp. *bulgaricus* survive gastrointestinal transit of healthy volunteers consuming yogurt. *Fems Microbiol Letts* 250 (2):185–87.

Mattar, R., D. F. de Campos Mazo, and F. J. Carrilho. 2012. Lactose intolerance: Diagnosis, genetic, and clinical factors. *Clin Exp Gastroenterol* 5:113–21.

McDonough, F. E., A. D. Hitchins, N. P. Wong, P. Wells, and C. E. Bodwell. 1987. Modification of sweet acidophilus milk to improve utilization by lactose-intolerant persons. *Am J Clin Nutr* 45 (3):570–74.

Misselwitz, B., D. Pohl, H. Fruehauf, M. Fried, S. R. Vavricka, and M. Fox. 2013. Lactose malabsorption and intolerance: Pathogenesis, diagnosis and treatment. *United European Gastroenterol J* 1 (3):151–59.

Montalto, M., V. Curigliano, L. Santoro, M. Vastola, G. Cammarota, R. Manna, A. Gasbarrini, and et al. 2006. Management and treatment of lactose malabsorption. *World J Gastroenterol* 12 (2):187–91.

Montes, R. G., T. M. Bayless, J. M. Saavedra, and J. A. Perman. 1995. Effect of milks inoculated with *Lactobacillus acidophilus* or a yogurt starter culture in lactose-maldigesting children. *Journal of Dairy Science* 78 (8):1657–64.

Moore, S. R. 2011. Update on prolonged and persistent diarrhea in children. *Curr Opin Gastroenterol* 27 (1):19–23.

Morelli, L. 2014. Yogurt, living cultures, and gut health. *Am J Clin Nutr* 99 (5):1248S–50S.

National Medical Association. 2009. Lactose intolerance and African Americans: Implications for the consumption of appropriate intake levels of key nutrients. Executive summary. *J Natl Med Assoc* 101 (10):5S–23S.

Niv, M., W. Levy, and N. M. Greenstein. 1963. Yogurt in the treatment of infantile diarrhea. *Clin Pediatr* 2(7):407–11.

Onwulata, C. I., D. R. Rao, and P. Vankineni. 1989. Relative efficiency of yogurt, sweet acidophilus milk, hydrolyzed-lactose milk, and a commercial lactase tablet in alleviating lactose maldigestion. *Am J Clin Nutr* 49 (6):1233–7.

Overeem, K., G. van Soest, and N. Blankenstein. 2008. Antibiotic-associated diarrhoea. *Br J Gen Pract* 58 (549):283–4.

Paige, D.M. 2005. Lactose intolerance. In *Encyclopedia of Human Nutrition.*, edited by M. J. Sadler. Elsevier. Oxford.

Pal, S., K. Woodford, S. Kukuljan, and S. Ho. 2015. Milk intolerance, beta-casein and lactose. *Nutrients* 7 (9):7285–97.

Parsons, T. J., M. van Dusseldorp, M. van der Vliet, K. van de Werken, G. Schaafsma, and W. A. van Staveren. 1997. Reduced bone mass in Dutch adolescents fed a macrobiotic diet in early life. *J Bone Miner Res* 12 (9):1486–94.

Pashapour, N., and S. G. Iou. 2006. Evaluation of yogurt effect on acute diarrhea in 6-24-month-old hospitalized infants. *Turk J Pediatr* 48 (2):115–8.

Patro-Golab, B., R. Shamir, and H. Szajewska. 2015a. Yogurt for treating acute gastroenteritis in children: Systematic review and meta-analysis. *Clin Nutr* 34 (5):818–24.

Patro-Golab, B., R. Shamir, and H. Szajewska. 2015b. Yogurt for treating antibiotic-associated diarrhea: Systematic review and meta-analysis. *Nutrition* 31 (6):796–800.

Pelletier, X., S. Laure-Boussuge, and Y. Donazzolo. 2001. Hydrogen excretion upon ingestion of dairy products in lactose-intolerant male subjects: Importance of the live flora. *Eur J Clin Nutr* 55 (6):509–12.

Pereg, D., O. Kimhi, A. Tirosh, N. Orr, R. Kayouf, and M. Lishner. 2005. The effect of fermented yogurt on the prevention of diarrhea in a healthy adult population. *Am J Infect Control* 33 (2):122–25.

Piaia, M., J. M. Antoine, J. A. Mateos-Guardia, A. Leplingard, and I. Lenoir-Wijnkoop. 2003. Assessment of the benefits of live yogurt: Methods and markers for *in vivo* studies of the physiological effects of yogurt cultures. *Microbial Ecology in Health and Disease* 15 (2–3):79–87.

Pochart, P., O. Dewit, J. F. Desjeux, and P. Bourlioux. 1989. Viable starter culture, beta-galactosidase activity, and lactose in duodenum after yogurt ingestion in lactase-deficient humans. *Am J Clin Nutr* 49 (5):828–31.

Pribila, B. A., S. R. Hertzler, B. R. Martin, C. M. Weaver, and D. A. Savaiano. 2000. Improved lactose digestion and intolerance among African-American adolescent girls fed a dairy-rich diet. *J Am Diet Assoc* 100 (5):524–8; quiz 529–30.

Rachmilewitz, D., K. Katakura, F. Karmeli, T. Hayashi, C. Reinus, B. Rudensky, S. Akira, et al. 2004. Toll-like receptor 9 signaling mediates the anti-inflammatory effects of probiotics in murine experimental colitis. *Gastroenterology* 126 (2):520–28.

Ranasinghe, J. G., G. R. R. D. K Gamlath, S. Samitha, and A. S. Abeygunawardena. 2007. Prophylactic use of yoghurt reduces antibiotic induced diarrhoea in children. *Sri Lanka J Child Health* 36:53–56.

Rizkalla, S. W., J. Luo, M. Kabir, A. Chevalier, N. Pacher, and G. Slama. 2000. Chronic consumption of fresh but not heated yogurt improves breath-hydrogen status and short-chain fatty acid profiles: A controlled study in healthy men with or without lactose maldigestion. *Am J Clin Nutr* 72 (6):1474–79.

Robayo-Torres, C. C., and B. L. Nichols. 2007. Molecular differentiation of congenital lactase deficiency from adult-type hypolactasia. *Nutr Rev* 65 (2):95–98.

Robins-Browne, R. M., and M. M. Levine. 1981. The fate of ingested lactobacilli in the proximal small intestine. *Am J Clin Nutr* 34 (4):514–19.

Rockell, J. E., S. M. Williams, R. W. Taylor, A. M. Grant, I. E. Jones, and A. Goulding. 2005. Two-year changes in bone and body composition in young children with a history of prolonged milk avoidance. *Osteoporos Int* 16 (9):1016–23.

Rohde, C. L., V. Bartolini, and N. Jones. 2009. The use of probiotics in the prevention and treatment of antibiotic-associated diarrhea with special interest in clostridium difficile-associated diarrhea. *Nutr Clin Pract* 24 (1):33–40.

Rozenberg, S., J. J. Body, O. Bruyere, P. Bergmann, M. L. Brandi, C. Cooper, J. P. Devogelaer, et al. 2015. Effects of dairy products consumption on health: Benefits and beliefs-a commentary from the Belgian Bone Club and the European Society for Clinical and Economic Aspects of Osteoporosis, Osteoarthritis and Musculoskeletal Diseases. *Calcif Tissue Int* 98 (1):1–17.

Savaiano, D. A., 2014. Lactose digestion from yogurt: Mechanism and relevance. *Am J Clin Nutr* 99 (5):1251S–55S.

Savaiano, D. A., A. AbouElAnouar, D. E. Smith, and M. D. Levitt. 1984. Lactose malabsorption from yogurt, pasteurized yogurt, sweet acidophilus milk, and cultured milk in lactase-deficient individuals. *Am J Clin Nutr* 40 (6):1219–23.

Shapiro, S. 1960. Control of antibiotic-induced gastrointestinal symptoms with yogurt. *Clin Med* 7:295–99.

Shermak, M. A., J. M. Saavedra, T. L. Jackson, S. S. Huang, T. M. Bayless, and J. A. Perman. 1995. Effect of yogurt on symptoms and kinetics of hydrogen production in lactose-malabsorbing children. *Am J Clin Nutr* 62 (5):1003–6.

Silanikove, N., G. Leitner, and U. Merin. 2015. The interrelationships between lactose intolerance and the modern dairy industry: Global perspectives in evolutional and historical backgrounds. *Nutrients* 7 (9):7312–31.

Smith, G. D., D. A. Lawlor, N. J. Timpson, J. Baban, M. Kiessling, I. N. M. Day, and S. Ebrahim. 2008. Lactase persistence-related genetic variant: Population substructure and health outcomes. *Eur J Hum Genet* 17 (3):357–67.

Solomons, N. W. 2002. Fermentation, fermented foods and lactose intolerance. *Eur J Clin Nutr* 56:S50–S55.

Suchy, F. J., P. M. Brannon, T. O. Carpenter, J. R. Fernandez, V. Gilsanz, J. B. Gould, K. Hall, et al. 2010. NIH consensus development conference statement: Lactose intolerance and health. *NIH Consens State Sci Statements* 27 (2):1–27.

Szilagyi, A. 2004. Redefining lactose as a conditional prebiotic. *Can J Gastroenterol* 18 (3):163–67.

Szilagyi, A. 2015. Adaptation to lactose in lactase non persistent people: Effects on intolerance and the relationship between dairy food consumption and evalution of diseases. *Nutrients* 7 (8):6751–79.

Szilagyi, A., I. Shrier, D. Heilpern, J. Je, S. Park, G. Chong, C. Lalonde, et al. 2010. Differential impact of lactose/lactase phenotype on colonic microflora. *Can J Gastroenterol* 24 (6):373–79.

Touhami, M., G. Boudraa, J. Y. Mary, R. Soltana, and J. F. Desjeux. 1992. Clinical consequences of replacing milk with yogurt in persistent infantile diarrhea. *Ann Pediatr (Paris)* 39 (2):79–86.

Turck, D., J. P. Bernet, J. Marx, H. Kempf, P. Giard, O. Walbaum, A. Lacombe, et al. 2003. Incidence and risk factors of oral antibiotic-associated diarrhea in an outpatient pediatric population. *J Pediatr Gastroenterol Nutr* 37 (1):22–26.

U.S. Department of Agriculture. 2010. *Dietary Guidelines for Americans*. Washington, DC: USDA.

Uriot, O., W. Galia, A. A. Awussi, C. Perrin, S. Denis, S. Chalancon, E. Lorson, et al. 2016. Use of the dynamic gastro-intestinal model TIM to explore the survival of the yogurt bacterium *Streptococcus thermophilus* and the metabolic activities induced in the simulated human gut. *Food Microbiol* 53 (Pt A):18–29.

Vanderhoof, J. A., D. B. Whitney, D. L. Antonson, T. L. Hanner, J. V. Lupo, and R. J. Young. 1999. *Lactobacillus* GG in the prevention of antibiotic-associated diarrhea in children. *J Pediatr* 135 (5):564–8.

Van Niel, C. W., C. Feudtner, M. M. Garrison, and D. A. Christakis. 2002. *Lactobacillus* therapy for acute infectious diarrhea in children: A meta-analysis. *Pediatrics* 109 (4):678–84.

Varela-Moreiras, G., J. M. Antoine, B. Ruiz-Roso, and G. Varela. 1992. Effects of yogurt and fermented-then-pasteurized milk on lactose absorption in an institutionalized elderly group. *J Am Coll Nutr* 11 (2):168–71.

Vesa, T. H., Marteau, P., Korpela, R. 2000. Lactose intolerance. *J Am Coll Nutr* 19:165S–75S.

Vonk, R. J., M. G. Priebe, and H. A. Koetse. 2003. Lactose intolerance: Analysis of underlying factors. *Eur J Clin Invest* 33:70–75.
WGO. 2008. World Gastroenterology Organisation practice guideline: Acute diarrhea. Milwaukee, WI: World Gastroenterology Organisation.
WHO. 1988. Persistent diarrhoea in children in developing countries: Memorandum from a who meeting. *Bull World Health Organ* 66 (6):709–17.
WHO. 2005. The treatment of diarrhoea: A manual for physicians and other senior health workers. Geneva: World Health Organization.
WHO. 2009. Diarrhoeal disease: Fact sheet n°330. http://www.who.int/mediacentre/factsheets/fs330/en/index.html.
Wilt, T. J., A. Shaukat, T. Shamliyan, B. C. Taylor, R. MacDonald, J. Tacklind, I. Rutks,et al. 2010. Lactose intolerance and health. *Evid Rep Technol Assess (Full Rep)* (192):1–410.
Zhong, Y., C. Y. Huang, T. He, and H. M. Harmsen. 2006. Effect of probiotics and yogurt on colonic microflora in subjects with lactose intolerance. *Wei Sheng Yan Jiu* 35 (5):587–91.

9 Immune Responses

The immune system protects the body against environmental pathogens and is divided into two subclasses: the innate (nonspecific) and the adaptive immune system. The adaptive or acquired immune system is characterized by specific responses toward each antigen and by enhanced responses after repeated antigen encounters (immune memory). Lymphocytes (T and B cells) are the main effector cells of the adaptive immune system. B cells are responsible for antibody production (humoral response), whereas helper T cells and T regulatory cells either directly destroy pathogens (cytotoxic T cells, i.e., $CD8^+$ T lymphocytes) or control the function of other cell types (helper T cells, i.e., $CD4^+$ T lymphocytes). Helper T cells can produce different cytokines, such as interferon-gamma (IFN-γ), tumor necrosis factor (TNF-α), and interleukins IL-4 and IL-5 (Meydani and Ha 2000).

In the gut, the microbiota, epithelium and immune systems can react directly against a pathogen and also interact with each other (Antoine 2010). Immune cells within the gut represent about 70% of the total immune cells of the body and are referred to as gut-associated lymphoid tissue (GALT). The antigens are trapped by immune cells in Peyer's patches in the small intestine and many cells are involved in this type of immune response (mainly macrophages, dendritic cells, and B and T lymphocytes). B cells within the GALT secrete a large amount of secretory immunoglobulin A (sIgA) (de Moreno de LeBlanc et al. 2008).

Once in the intestine, lactic acid bacteria (LAB) can modulate specific immune responses or nonspecific associated lymphoid tissue in both animals and humans (Perdigón et al. 1999, Vitini et al. 2000, de Moreno de LeBlanc et al. 2008, Solis Pereyra et al. 1997). Moreover, some peptides (e.g., opioid-like peptides) present in yogurt may maintain or restore intestinal homeostasis and could play an important role in protecting against damaging agents in the intestinal lumen (Plaisancié et al. 2013). There is some evidence that yogurt-induced immune enhancement may be associated with a decreased incidence of conditions such as gastrointestinal disorders, allergic symptoms, and cancer (de Moreno de Leblanc and Perdigón 2004). Metabolites produced during the fermentation of milk into yogurt may have the ability to influence the immune process in humans, specifically via anti-inflammatory properties, particularly for individuals with metabolic disorders (Bordoni et al. 2015). Studies performed on the effects of yogurt on the immune system are described in the following sections.

9.1 HUMAN STUDIES

9.1.1 Cytokine Production

Solis Pereyra et al. (1997) measured the activity of 2'-5' A synthetase (an IFN-γ-inducible protein) in human mononuclear cells in blood following the ingestion of yogurt or milk bacteria. Twenty-four hours after ingestion, the level of 2′-5′ A synthetase of the yogurt-fed subjects was 83% ($p = .002$) higher than that of the milk-fed controls. Moreover, an increase of 2′-5′ A synthetase activity in human blood mononuclear cells was also found in subjects who consumed 10^8 CFU yogurt bacteria/day for 15 days (Solis Pereyra et al. 1997). The same authors reported basal production of IFN-γ in control subjects and showed that IFN production was increased with yogurt consumption. Both yogurt strains seem to be involved in the stimulation of IFN-γ and the induced production of IL-1β and of TNF-α (Solis Pereyra and Lemonnier 1993).

A nutrition intervention with yogurt was conducted on a group of adolescents with anorexia nervosa (DSM IV diagnostic criteria) to assess the effects of feeding yogurt on immunological parameters during patient refeeding. Sixteen healthy adolescents and 16 anorexia nervosa patients consumed 375 g/day of yogurt for 10 weeks, while control groups of 19 healthy adolescents and 14 anorexia nervosa patients consumed 400 mL of milk for the same amount of time. Over the study period, leukocytes and lymphocytes were lower in the anorexic patients than the healthy adolescents. There was significant time and intervention effect for both CD8+ and INF-γ production in the anorexic group and in healthy adolescents. There was a significant increase in CD8+ in both control groups compared with the yogurt intervention groups. There was also a significant increase in INF-γ production in the yogurt anorexic group compared with the control anorexic group. The authors conclude that consuming yogurt during refeeding therapy can have positive effects on immunologic markers that are related to the nutritional status of anorexic nervosa patients (Nova et al. 2006).

A randomized trial evaluated the effect of a conventional yogurt and a probiotic yogurt on cytokine production. For 2 weeks each, young healthy women consumed 100 g, then 200 g of either a conventional yogurt or a probiotic yogurt containing *Lactobacillus casei*. The authors discovered that both conventional and probiotic yogurt stimulated the production of pro-inflammatory cytokines. Indeed, they observed an increase in TNF-α in both groups. A higher production of interleukin (IL)-1β in the conventional yogurt group and of IFN-γ in the probiotic group were also observed. Conventional yogurt was able to enhance the production of pro-inflammatory cytokines (Meyer et al. 2007).

9.1.2 Natural Killer Cell Activity

The effect of consuming 200 g of a conventional yogurt supplemented with lyophilized *L. bulgaricus* and *Streptococcus thermophilus* once a day for 28 days was evaluated on serum IFN-γ levels and on the number of natural killer (NK) cells in the peripheral blood in healthy subjects. Increases in the NK cell subset population and IFN-γ levels in subjects were observed. The authors hypothesized that yogurt bacteria may act on the NK cell subset or that bacteria induce cytokine production by other cell types, which then activate resting NK cells to produce IFN-γ (de Simone et al. 1988).

9.1.3 T and B Lymphocyte Function

Yogurt consumption was evaluated on intestinal immunity in subjects aged 44–85 years old who were undergoing a colonic resection and had signs of immunodeficiency.

Patients consumed 500 g of skimmed yogurt per day for 1 month. Yogurt induced a greater release of IFN-γ with the activation of CD4+ and CD8+ cells. Stimulation by *Lactobacillus* of the B lymphocytes in Peyer's patches appeared to induce increased production of immunoglobulin G (IgG) and of sIgA. In this study, LAB supplementation improved immunity and restored the microbiota in colonic resection subjects (Losacco et al. 1994).

A crossover study performed with healthy subjects evaluated the effects of yogurt bacteria on the production of cytokines by circulating mononuclear cells. Subjects maintained their normal dietary practices for the entire study (2×15-day periods), except that during the first period they were asked to consume at least one yogurt per day and during the second period they were asked not to consume any fermented milk. Blood samples were collected at the end of each period. The consumption of fermented milks significantly increased 2′-5′ A synthetase activity in mononuclear cells, suggesting increased IFN production. To explain these results, an *in vitro* study was performed and showed that mononuclear cells produced IFN-γ in the presence of *S. thermophilus*. It was suggested that *S. thermophilus* may stimulate CD4+ and CD8 lymphocytes and that muramyl dipeptide, a component of the bacterial wall, could explain the part recognized by CD4+ T lymphocytes (Aattouri and Lemonnier 1997).

Meyer et al. (2006) carried out a clinical trial in 33 healthy young women who were asked to consume 100 g of either conventional yogurt (*L. bulgaricus* and *S. thermophilus*) or a probiotic yogurt (*L. casei*) for 14 days. The number of circulating cytotoxic T lymphocytes did not increase significantly in the conventional yogurt group, but the expression of CD69 on T lymphocytes increased, especially on CD8+ and T cells. Conventional yogurt was able to stimulate cellular immune function (Meyer et al. 2006).

9.1.4 Phagocytic Activity

It has been shown in healthy subjects that dietary deprivation of fermented foods for 2 weeks decreases the phagocytic activity of leukocytes. The ingestion of a standard yogurt counteracted the fall in the immune response, although the probiotic product (*L. gasseri* CECT5714 and *L. coryniformis* CECT5711) was more effective (Olivares et al. 2006).

9.2 MECHANISMS OF ACTION

The immunomodulating and antimicrobial activities of yogurt LAB in the gut depend on components produced by the bacteria such as organic acids, carbon dioxide, hydrogen peroxide, bacteriocins, and ethanol that promote a lower pH (Adolfsson et al. 2004). LAB could also compete with pathogens by consuming nutrients and compete for space in the gut. Moreover, the immunostimulatory activity of cultured dairy products has been reported to be mediated by glycopeptides in the bacterial cell wall (Bogdanov et al. 1977). In mice, a mixture of live *L. bulgaricus* and *S. thermophilus* induced plasma IFN-α, β, and γ production, whereas heat-killed bacteria lost their capacity to induce IFN-γ. It was suggested that the molecular integrity of the bacterial wall is necessary to induce IFN-γ production (Solis Pereyra et al. 1997).

LAB's interactions with the mucosal epithelial lining of the gastrointestinal tract and with the immune cells residing in the gut are important mechanisms by which LAB modulates gut immune function (Adolfsson et al. 2004). Interestingly, the action of some probiotics on the gut wall could be explained by a change in the composition of the gut mucus, modulation of the permeability of the gut barrier, and stimulation of the production of some defensins (Antoine 2010). It has been shown in mice that yogurt and LAB could stimulate the systemic immune response (monocyte function and number of immunoglobulin-secreting cells) and the local immune response (IgA secretion into the intestine) (Perdigón et al. 1999, Vitini et al. 2000, de Moreno de LeBlanc et al. 2008).

The influence of yogurt consumption on cytokine production may reflect its effects on systemic immunity (Nova et al. 2007, Meyer et al. 2007). Several studies have demonstrated that the consumption of yogurt increases the production of IFN-γ (Meydani and Ha 2000; Makino et al. 2016). IFN-γ is commonly regarded as the major cytokine of T helper type 1 (Th1)-lymphocytes and has anti-infectious properties. IFN-γ has been shown to enhance the expression of the secretory component, thus playing an important role in increasing external transport of dimeric IgA (Meydani and Ha 2000). The ability of yogurt to stimulate the production of IFN-γ may, however, be strain specific and traditional yogurt strains may enhance immunity when specific strains are selected. For example, the OLL1073R-1 strain of *L. delbrueckii* spp. *bulgaricus* is a robust producer of exopolysaccharides, which have immunostimulatory properties (Makino et al. 2016).

The ability of LAB to survive in the gastrointestinal tract can influence the immunogenicity of the bacteria (Meydani and Ha 2000). It is thought that the cell integrity of yogurt bacteria is necessary to observe any immunomodulation effects following yogurt consumption (Solis Pereyra et al. 1997). However, some studies have shown no difference in antigenicity between viable and nonviable bacteria (Hatcher and Lambrecht 1993). Traditional and probiotic yogurt bacteria are transient in the gut and a regular intake seems to be necessary to provide a sustainable benefit to the host's defense (Antoine 2010).

In addition to bacteria, yogurt contains other nonbacterial components, produced during fermentation, which can contribute to immunogenicity. Peptides and free fatty acids have been shown to enhance the immune response (Pihlanto and Korhonen 2003). Milk components such as whey protein, calcium and vitamins, and trace elements can also influence the immune system (Meydani and Ha 2000).

9.3 CONCLUSIONS

- Human studies evaluating the immunostimulatory/immunomodulatory effects of yogurt consumption have focused on indicators of the immune response, such as peripheral blood mononuclear cell cytokine production, NK cell activity, lymphocyte function, and phagocytic activity.
- The influence of yogurt consumption on the production of some cytokines such as IFN-γ reflects its potential effects on systemic immunity and may help promote anti-infective mechanisms such as macrophage or NK cell activity.

- Yogurt bacteria are transient in the gut and a regular intake could be necessary to provide a sustainable benefit on host defense. Further studies would be useful to determine the dose of yogurt that is required to observe an effect.
- There is a need for fundamental and applied research to establish the relation between *S. thermophilus*, *L. bulgaricus*, and other nonbacterial components of yogurt and their interaction with the microbiota, epithelium, and immune system. Bacteria cell wall components, end products of bacterial metabolism, or milk proteins might be of interest in immune system modulation (Meydani and Ha 2000). Furthermore, strain-specific immunomodulatory properties of traditional yogurt cultures should also be identified.

REFERENCES

Aattouri, N., and D. Lemonnier. 1997. Production of interferon induced by *Streptococcus thermophilus*: Role of CD4+ and CD8+ lymphocytes. *J Nutr Biochem* 8 (1):25–31.

Adolfsson, O., S. N. Meydani, and R. M. Russell. 2004. Yogurt and gut function. *Am J Clin Nutr* 80 (2):245–56.

Antoine, J. M. 2010. Probiotics: Beneficial factors of the defence system. *Proc Nutr Soc* 69 (3):429–33.

Bogdanov, I. G., V. T. Velichkov, A. I. Gurevich, P. G. Dalev, and M. N. Kolosov. 1977. Antitumor effect of glycopeptides from the cell wall of Lactobacillus bulgaricus. *Biull Eksp Biol Med* 84 (12):709–12.

Bordoni, A., F. Danesi, D. Dardevet, D. Dupont, A. S. Fernandez, D. Gille, C. N. Dos Santos et al. 2015. Dairy products and inflammation: A review of the clinical evidence. *Crit Rev Food Sci Nutr* 264. Online only. doi:10.1080/10408398.2014.967385

De Moreno de LeBlanc, A., S. Chaves, E. Carmuega, R. Weill, J. Antóine, and G. Perdigón. 2008. Effect of long-term continuous consumption of fermented milk containing probiotic bacteria on mucosal immunity and the activity of peritoneal macrophages. *Immunobiology* 213 (2):97–108.

De Moreno de Leblanc, A., and G. Perdigón. 2004. Yogurt feeding inhibits promotion and progression of experimental colorectal cancer. *Med Sci Monit* 10 (4):BR96–104.

De Simone, C., L. Baldinelli, S. Di Fabio, S. Tzantzoglou, E. Jirillo, B. Bianchi-Salvadori, and R. Vesely. 1988. Lactobacilli feeding increases NK cells and gamma-IFN levels in humans. In *Dietetics in the 90s: Role of the Dietitian/Nutritionist*. Ed. M. F. Moyal, 177–80. Paris: John Libbey Eurotext.

Hatcher, G. E., and R. S. Lambrecht. 1993. Augmentation of macrophage phagocytic activity by cell-free extracts of selected lactic acid-producing bacteria. *J Dairy Sci* 76 (9):2485–92.

Losacco, T., G. De Leo, C. Punzo, N. M. Pellegrino, V. Neri, G. D'Eredita, G. Di Ciaula, and M. V. Pitzalis. 1994. Immune evaluations in cancer patients after colorectal resection. *G Chir* 15 (10):429–32.

Makino, S., A. Sato, A. Goto, M. Nakamura, M. Ogawa, Y. Chiba, J. Hemmi, H. Kano, K. Takeda, K. Okumura, and Y. Asami. 2016. Enhanced natural killer cell activation by exopolysaccharides derived from yogurt fermented with *Lactobacillus delbrueckii* ssp. *bulgaricus* OLL1073R-1. *J Dairy Sci* 99 (2):915–23.

Meydani, S. N., and W. K. Ha. 2000. Immunologic effects of yogurt. *Am J Clin Nutr* 71 (4):861–72.

Meyer, A. L., I. Elmadfa, I. Herbacek, and M. Micksche. 2007. Probiotic, as well as conventional yogurt, can enhance the stimulated production of proinflammatory cytokines. *J Hum Nutr Diet* 20:590–98.

Meyer, A. L., M. Micksche, I. Herbacek, and I. Elmadfa. 2006. Daily intake of probiotic as well as conventional yogurt has a stimulating effect on cellular immunity in young healthy women. *Ann Nutr Metab* 50 (3):282–89.

Nova, E., O. Toro, P. Varela, I. López-Vidriero, G. Morandé, and A. Marcos. 2006. Effects of a nutritional intervention with yogurt on lymphocyte subsets and cytokine production capacity in anorexia nervosa patients. *Eur J Nutr* 45 (4):225–33.

Nova, E., J. Wärnberg, S. Gómez-Martínez, L. E. Díaz, J. Romeo, and A. Marcos. 2007. Immunomodulatory effects of probiotics in different stages of life. *Br J Nutr* 98 (Suppl 1):S90–95.

Olivares, M., M. Paz Díaz-Ropero, N. Gómez, S. Sierra, F. Lara-Villoslada, R. Martín, J. Miguel Rodríguez, and J. Xaus. 2006. Dietary deprivation of fermented foods causes a fall in innate immune response. Lactic acid bacteria can counteract the immunological effect of this deprivation. *J Dairy Res* 73 (4):492–98.

Perdigón, G., E. Vintiñi, S. Alvarez, M. Medina, and M. Medici. 1999. Study of the possible mechanisms involved in the mucosal immune system activation by lactic acid bacteria. *J Dairy Sci* 82 (6):1108–14.

Pihlanto, A., and H. Korhonen. 2003. Bioactive peptides and proteins. *Adv Food Nutr Res* 47:175–276.

Plaisancié, P., J. Claustre, M. Estienne, G. Henry, R. Boutrou, A. Paquet, and J. Léonil. 2013. A novel bioactive peptide from yoghurts modulates expression of the gel-forming MUC2 mucin as well as population of goblet cells and Paneth cells along the small intestine. *J Nutr Biochem* 24 (1):213–21.

Solis Pereyra, B., N. Aattouri, and D. Lemonnier. 1997. Role of food in the stimulation of cytokine production. *Am J Clin Nutr* 66 (2):521S–25S.

Solis Pereyra, B., and D. Lemonnier. 1993. Induction of human cytokines by bacteria used in dairy foods. *Nutr Res* 13 (10):1127–40.

Vitini, E., S. Alvarez, M. Medina, M. Medici, M. V. de Budeguer, and G. Perdigón. 2000. Gut mucosal immunostimulation by lactic acid bacteria. *Biocell* 24 (3):223–32.

10 Cancer

Cancer represents a large group of diseases. One defining feature of cancer is the rapid proliferation of abnormal cells, which can invade any part of the body. Tobacco and alcohol use, unhealthy diet, and physical inactivity are major cancer risk factors worldwide (Stewart and Wild 2014). Until now, much of the population-based studies investigating the potential impact of dairy product consumption on cancer risk have assessed the effects of milk, total dairy, or calcium intake. The following sections will focus on the relationship between yogurt and some of the most common types of cancer for which diet is a risk factor: colon cancer and breast cancer (de Moreno de LeBlanc et al. 2007). Moreover, since the World Cancer Research Fund and American Institute for Cancer Research (WCRF/AICR) report concluded that there was a probable association between diets that are high in calcium and an increased risk of prostate cancer (Lampe 2011), it appears important to review the potential impact of yogurt consumption on prostate cancer.

10.1 COLORECTAL CANCER

Colorectal cancer (CRC) is very common in the developed world. It has been estimated that over 70% of colon cancers in men are preventable by a combination of dietary and lifestyle changes (Pala et al. 2011). Many studies have suggested that dairy product consumption may have a protective effect against the risk of CRC (Huncharek et al. 2009, Park et al. 2007). More than a century ago, it was suggested that lactic acid bacteria (LAB) present in yogurt and other fermented dairy products had a protective effect against CRC (Pala et al. 2011). In the 1980s, epidemiological studies began to demonstrate evidence of the potential protective properties of yogurt on CRC (Jain 1998). In 2007, a systematic review prepared by the WCRF concluded that evidence from human epidemiological studies regarding fermented dairy products and CRC was too limited to draw conclusions and the associations remained inconclusive (WCRF 2007, Wiseman 2008).

Since the 2007 WCRF/AICR report, a number of additional studies have been published and the state of evidence has been updated in a rigorous meta-analysis. This meta-analysis showed that milk and total dairy products, but not cheese or other dairy products, were associated with a reduction in CRC risk. However, the authors state that because of the few studies that were reported on other specific types of dairy products such as yogurt, this study may have had limited statistical power to detect associations with these products (Aune et al. 2012). A later meta-analysis of 15 studies, however, confirmed that nonfermented milk was associated with a lower risk of CRC. Based on seven studies, no associations between CRC and cheese or fermented milks were found (Ralston et al. 2014). In the following sections, studies examining the association between yogurt and CRC are described in more detail.

10.1.1 Observational Studies

10.1.1.1 Case-Control Studies

A large population-based case-control study was performed in California and included patients diagnosed with invasive adenocarcinomas. Interviews consisted of a diet recall of a reference year, 2 years before their cancer was diagnosed. A 30-year life-events calendar was also completed to include nondietary factors in the analysis. After adjustment for nutrients and nondietary risk factors, a protective effect of yogurt consumption was found against CRC. Interestingly, total calories were associated with excess risk throughout the colon and the calcium intake was associated with a significantly decreased risk (Peters et al. 1992).

In the Netherlands, a case-control study was carried out in 3,111 subjects, including 443 CRC patients. A semiquantitative food frequency questionnaire on food and beverage intake over the preceding year was self-administered. In the cohort, yogurt accounted for 39% of the total dairy product intake. The investigators concluded that the data did not support a protective role for yogurt or fermented dairy products on the risk of CRC. The median daily intake corresponded to quite a high consumption in this population compared with the United States. The limitations of the study included a short follow-up of 3.3 years, which may have been too short to reach definitive conclusions (Kampman et al. 1994b). Moreover, the potential presence of lactose malabsorbers, combined with the relatively high level of dairy product intake in the studied population, could have contributed to mask a potential protective effect of fermented dairy products, since lactose malabsorption has been proposed to induce colonic adaptation to undigested lactose and lower the risk of colon cancer (Boutron et al. 1996).

Senesse et al. (2002) performed a case-control study in subjects with small adenoma ($n=154$), large adenoma ($n=208$), or with polyp-free controls ($n=427$) in France. The consumption of animal fat was associated with an increased risk of large adenomas, whereas yogurt intake was associated with a lower risk ($p=.02$). Yogurt was consumed by less than 75% of the subjects. Other types of foods (but not yogurt) showed effects on small adenomas, suggesting that diet could have an influence on different stages of carcinogenesis (Senesse et al. 2002).

The relationship between the daily consumption of specific food groups and the development of CRC was investigated in Madrid in 196 patients with diagnosed CRC. Patients were compared with 196 controls matched by age, sex, and geographical area. All patients completed a questionnaire, giving information on diet and other risk factors for CRC. The results showed a modest inverse association with yogurt consumption (Juarranz Sanz et al. 2004).

Data from a large network of hospital-based case-control studies in Italy was analyzed (1,953 CRC cases and 4,154 controls). There was a modest inverse association between milk and dairy products and CRC and a lack of association with yogurt and cheese. Milk and dairy products were not strong risk modulators for any of the cancers considered in this study (Gallus et al. 2006).

A case-control study was performed in 52 subjects in a Greek population with histologically confirmed advanced colorectal polyps. Data concerning lifestyle and dietary factors was collected using a validated questionnaire. The consumption of yogurt ($p = .024$), cheese, fish, vegetables, and garlic, and physical activity level were significantly and inversely associated with colorectal polyps. Interestingly, increasing age and central obesity were strongly associated with the presence of colorectal polyps (Karagianni et al. 2010).

A large Canadian case-control study performed in new CRC patients aged 20–74 years from Newfoundland, Labrador, and Ontario revealed inverse associations between CRC risk and intakes of total dairy products and milk. In this study, fermented dairy foods such as yogurt and cheese were not significantly related to CRC risk. However, the authors indicated that the intakes of yogurt were too low to expect significant associations to emerge (Sun et al. 2011).

10.1.1.2 Prospective Cohort Studies

A prospective study was performed in the United States to evaluate the effects of calcium intake, vitamin D, and specific dairy products on the incidence of CRC. Food habits were recorded through self-administered semiquantitative food frequency questionnaires. After adjustment for covariates, no significant protective roles of yogurt or milk were found. There was, however, a limited range of fermented dairy product intake and the study population had higher fiber and lower saturated fat intakes than the general population (Kampman et al. 1994a).

Kearney et al. (1996) examined the associations between intakes of calcium, vitamin D, and dairy foods and the risk of incident CRC in 47,935 U.S. males aged 40–75 years. Within this cohort, 203 new cases of colon cancer were reported. The consumption of fermented dairy products (including yogurt, sour cream, cottage cheese, cream cheese, and hard cheese) and milk was not significantly associated with the risk of colon cancer. Calcium and vitamin D were inversely associated with colon cancer risk, but after adjusting for confounding variables the relationship was no longer statistically significant (Kearney et al. 1996).

The relationship between the consumption of milk, milk products, calcium, lactose, and vitamin D and the incidence of CRC was investigated in 9959 men and women aged 15 years or older without a history of cancer at baseline. Seventy-two new cancer cases were detected in the large bowel (38 in the colon and 34 in the rectum) after a 24-year follow-up. Milk and total milk product intake was suggested to be inversely related to colon cancer incidence, whereas the consumption of fermented milk (yogurt, buttermilk, and cultured whole milk) was not associated with the risk of CRC. Calcium intake, mainly provided by fermented milk products, was associated with increased incidences of CRC. However, the authors state that this association was probably not caused by the intake of calcium, but by other undetermined substances in fermented milk products or associated with the consumption of these foods. Interestingly, the intake of lactose showed an inverse relationship with colon cancer. To explain this result, the authors suggested that lactose could favor the growth of LAB, which may have antimutagenic and anticarcinogenic properties, and/or that the unhydrolyzed lactose could have similar beneficial alterations in colonic function as other prebiotics fermented by colonic microbiota. This study showed that a high consumption of milk potentially reduced the risk of colon cancer and that this association did not appear to be due to the intake of calcium or vitamin D, or to specific effects of fermented milk (Jarvinen et al. 2001).

A prospective study analyzed the relationship between diet and CRC mortality in men and women (40–79 years old) enrolled in the Japan Collaborative Cohort Study. Yogurt intake was inversely associated with male rectal cancer mortality (p for trend = .04). However, due to the small sample size and the limited precision of the food frequency questionnaire, further investigation would be needed to confirm this association (Kojima et al. 2004).

Intakes of calcium and vitamin D in relation to CRC risk were assessed in a large prospective cohort followed for 10 years from the U.S. Women's Health Study. In this cohort, dairy products accounted for 53% and 39% of dietary calcium and vitamin D intakes, respectively. Intakes of total calcium and vitamin D were not associated with the risk of CRC. Moreover, no associations were observed between CRC risk and the intake of specific dairy products; yogurt, fermented milk products, low-fat dairy, high-fat dairy, milk, or cheese (Lin et al. 2005).

The effect of dairy products, calcium, vitamin D, and phosphorus intake on the adenoma–carcinoma sequence was investigated in the French *Etude Epidémiologique auprès des femmes de la MGEN*–European Prospective Investigation into Cancer and Nutrition (E3N-EPIC) prospective study. The diet was assessed using a self-administered questionnaire completed at baseline. There was a trend of a decreased risk of both adenoma (p trend = .04) and cancer (p trend = .08) with an increased calcium intake. Increasing the consumption of total dairy products decreased the relative risk of adenoma. No specific effects of any dairy products (yogurt, milk, cottage cheese, or cheese) were observed on colorectal tumor risk, except for a protective effect of high milk consumption on CRC. Phosphorus intake decreased the risk of adenoma, but no effect of vitamin D was observed (Kesse et al. 2005).

A prospective study from the Cohort of Swedish Men examined the relationships between the intakes of calcium and dairy foods and the risk of CRC during a mean follow-up of 6.7 years (449 incident cases of CRC). A high consumption of dairy foods and calcium were both associated with a lower risk of CRC. There was no significant association between yogurt or cheese consumption with CRC risk. The authors state that a potential explanation for the lack of significant association with yogurt and cheese may be that these foods are not important sources of dietary calcium intake in Sweden (Larsson et al. 2006).

Prospective cohort data from the Jichi Medical School Cohort Study in Japan was used to examine the relationship between dairy product intake and various cancers. Almost 6% of the cohort consumed yogurt daily; no relationships between yogurt intake and colon, stomach, lung, pancreas, bile duct, other cancers, or total cancers were found (Matsumoto et al. 2007).

A prospective study was performed to test the specific effect of yogurt on CRC. Participants from the EPIC–Italy cohort (14,178 men and 31,063 women) were followed for 12 years and 289 incident cases of CRC were diagnosed. Participants completed a dietary questionnaire, which included specific questions on yogurt intake. Yogurt intake was significantly associated with a decreased CRC risk in this cohort. This association was stronger in men. The authors stated that this was the first prospective cohort study to find a clear relation between increased yogurt consumption and lowered CRC incidence (Pala et al. 2011).

Cancer

The associations between intakes of specific dairy products and dietary calcium with CRC risk were investigated by the EPIC study (477,122 men and women; dietary questionnaires administered at baseline; 11 years of follow-up; 4,513 incident cases of CRC). The authors observed an inverse association between CRC risk and dietary calcium and total milk consumption, which did not differ according to the fat content of milk. Moreover, inverse associations were observed for yogurt and cheese in categorical models. However, these associations were nonsignificant in linear models (Murphy et al. 2013). In another cohort of 3,859 adults from the EPIC study, prediagnostic dairy intakes were analyzed and intakes of total dairy, milk, yogurt, and cheese were not associated with CRC-specific deaths. These findings indicated that while dairy products may be inversely associated with CRC risk, they are not likely to be associated with CRC survival (Dik et al. 2014).

10.1.1.3 Meta-Analyses

A pooled analysis of 10 cohort studies that included 534,536 individuals, among whom 4,992 incident cases of CRC were diagnosed following 6–16 years of follow-up (1976–1998), revealed a weak association between yogurt intake and CRC risk that was not significant. Because the consumption of yogurt was relatively low in most of the cohort studies investigated, the authors suggested that this study had limited ability to detect an association. A higher consumption of milk and calcium was associated with a lower risk of CRC (Cho et al. 2004).

10.1.2 CLINICAL STUDIES

Bartram et al. (1994) examined 12 healthy volunteers for the effect of yogurt consumption on the fecal bacterial flora and on various risk indexes for colon carcinogenesis (stool weight and pH, fecal concentrations of short-chain fatty acids, neutral sterols, bile salts, mean oral–anal transit time, and several immune parameters). No effects were observed. However, subjects consumed yogurt for only 3 weeks. The authors postulated that, considering the great stability of the human flora, a longer study involving more subjects would likely be necessary to observe possible changes in CRC markers (Bartram et al. 1994)

10.1.3 MECHANISMS OF ACTION

The administration of fermented products could modulate the microbiota, stimulate intestinal immune cells, and maintain a regulated immune response, all of which are useful against intestinal inflammation and offer protection against colon cancer (de Moreno de Leblanc and Perdigon 2010). It has been shown that LAB may protect against cancer by binding mutagens, lowering the pH of the colon lumen, reducing inflammation, and inhibiting bacterial enzymes that form carcinogens from procarcinogens in the gastrointestinal tract (Pala et al. 2011). The potential pathways by which LAB protects against some cancers are illustrated in Figure 10.1. The fermentation of *Lactobacillus bulgaricus* and *Streptococcus thermophilus* can also produce bioactive compounds with antimutagenic activity (Jain 1998).

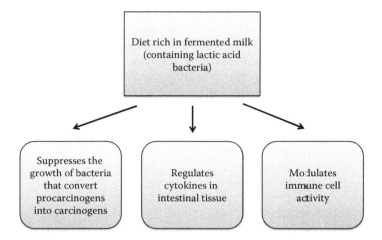

FIGURE 10.1 Possible mechanisms by which yogurt LAB can act on colon and breast cancer. (Adapted from de Moreno de LeBlanc *Br J Nutr* 98 (Suppl 1):S105–10, 2007.)

The calcium content of dairy products has also been hypothesized to protect against CRC risk. Calcium may bind pro-inflammatory secondary bile acids and ionize fatty acids, which could reduce cell proliferation and promote cell differentiation (Aune et al. 2012). A meta-analysis based on 15 studies reported that for every 300 mg increase in calcium intake per day, there was an 8% decrease in CRC risk (Keum et al. 2014). In the report from the WCRF/AICR on CRC, it was stated that milk and a high calcium intake probably protect against CRC, while body fatness and abdominal fat are possible promoters of CRC risk (WCRF/AICR 2011).

Other possible protective components of dairy products include conjugated linoleic acid (CLA) and butyric acid, specific peptides and lactoferrin (de Moreno de LeBlanc et al. 2007), and vitamin D in fortified dairy products (Aune et al. 2012). Interestingly, the protective effects of dairy products could be more important for the distal colon (Gallus et al. 2006, Larsson et al. 2006).

10.1.4 Conclusions

- Based on systematic reviews of observational studies, there is a probable association between milk intake and a lower risk of CRC.
- Some epidemiological studies have shown an inverse relationship between yogurt and a reduced risk of CRC, while others did not find any effect of yogurt. No studies have shown negative impacts of yogurt on CRC risk.
- The calcium and LAB content of yogurt, among other constituents, may exert protective effects against CRC risk.

10.2 BREAST CANCER

Breast cancer is the most important women's cancer in the developed world. Due to an increased life expectancy, urbanization, and Western lifestyles, its incidence is increasing in the developing world as well (WHO 2012). The WCRF/AICR concluded that the available evidence is insufficient to establish associations between dairy and meat intake and premenopausal or postmenopausal breast cancer risk. Moreover, a recent analysis of African-American women (1,268 incident breast cancer cases) provides little support for associations of dairy intake or specific types of dairy with breast cancer risk (Genkinger et al. 2013). However, *in vitro* and *in vivo* studies have shown that milk fermented with LAB may have a beneficial effect on breast cancer (de Moreno de LeBlanc et al. 2007). The studies evaluating the effect of yogurt on breast cancer will be discussed in the following sections.

10.2.1 Case-Control Studies

A French case-control study investigated the potential relationship between the risk of breast cancer and the consumption of dairy products in 1010 breast cancer subjects and 1950 controls with nonmalignant disease. An inverse association was found between the frequency of yogurt consumption and the risk of breast cancer. Authors also found that the level of fat in the milk consumed and cheese consumption were positively associated with the risk of breast cancer (Le et al. 1986).

In the Netherlands, results from a case-control study indicated a significantly lower consumption of fermented milk products (predominantly yogurt and buttermilk) among 133 incident breast cancer cases compared with 289 women from municipal population registries in the same area as the hospital population ($p < .01$). No statistically significant differences were observed between breast cancer cases and controls for the daily intake of milk. The authors concluded that these results support the hypothesis that a high consumption of fermented milk products may protect against breast cancer (van't Veer et al. 1989).

In the Netherlands, dietary factors were studied in relation to breast cancer incidence in 133 breast cancer cases and 289 controls. Dietary factors were classified according to their possible effect on intestinal microflora (total fat, fiber, and fermented milk products) or their antioxidant potential (beta-carotene, selenium, and polyunsaturated fatty acids). From the six interactions evaluated, the combination of a high intake of fermented milk products and a high fiber intake was the only one to show synergistic protection against breast cancer. Moreover, authors observed that the combination of a low intake of fat and a high intake of fermented milk products and fiber provided substantial protection against breast cancer (van't Veer et al. 1991).

A case-control study was performed in Uruguay to investigate the relationship between the intakes of milk and dairy products and the risk of breast cancer. Of the 333 women who were interviewed, 111 had breast cancer and 222 were frequency-matched healthy women. The questionnaire included a detailed 120-item food frequency section with a particular emphasis on the types of milk and dairy products. After controlling for potential confounders, skim yogurt and ricotta cheese were associated with a significant decrease in breast cancer incidence, whereas intakes of whole milk, chocolate milk, and Gruyére cheese were associated with a significant increased risk of breast cancer. In this study, the combined intake of low-fat and fermented products was found to be the most protective (Ronco et al. 2002).

In an Italian study consisting of a large network of hospital-based case-control studies, a nonsignificant inverse association was observed between yogurt consumption and breast cancer. Analyses showed that an increment of one portion of yogurt per day was inversely associated with breast cancer risk (Gallus et al. 2006).

10.2.2 Prospective Cohort Studies

No association between yogurt intake and breast cancer (pre- or postmenopausal) was observed in a prospective cohort of 64,904 women from the Norwegian Women and Cancer Study, although yogurt intake averaged only 25 g/day or one portion per week in this population. High intakes of white cheese (≥ 25 g/day) were associated with a 50% reduction in risk of premenopausal breast cancer ($p = .02$) (Hjartåker et al. 2010).

In the large prospective Black Women's Health Study, 1,268 incident breast cancer cases were identified among 52,062 women over 12 years of follow-up. There was a nonsignificant, modest inverse association between yogurt consumption and the risk of breast cancer. Results did not differ according to menopausal status. Associations with intakes of milk, dietary calcium, and vitamin D were also null. It was concluded that there is little support for associations between dairy intake and breast cancer risk in African-American women (Genkinger et al. 2013).

In an Iranian case-control study, the relationship between the dietary intake of women and their susceptibility to breast cancer was investigated. High-fat milk and high-fat cheese were significantly associated with a greater risk of breast cancer. Whole-fat yogurt was also associated with a risk for breast cancer; however, the relationship lost significance once the model adjusted for body mass index (BMI), age, and education (Mobarakeh et al. 2014).

10.2.3 Reviews

Missmer et al. (2002) pooled primary data from eight prospective cohort studies from North America and Western Europe with 351,041 women, 7,379 of whom were diagnosed with invasive breast cancer within the 15-year follow-up period. There was no significant effect of yogurt consumption on breast cancer risk (Missmer et al. 2002).

A review of the relationship between dairy intake and breast cancer risk was conducted, focusing primarily on the results of cohort and case-control studies (Moorman and Terry 2004). Two studies evaluating the specific effect of yogurt showed that it was inversely and significantly associated with breast cancer risk (Le et al. 1986, Ronco et al. 2002), whereas no significant association was found in two other studies (Matos et al. 1991, Levi et al. 1993). The authors concluded that the available epidemiologic evidence did not support a strong association between the consumption of milk or other dairy products and breast cancer risk.

10.2.4 Mechanisms of Action

Several mechanisms have been proposed to explain how dairy products could influence breast cancer risk. Milk product contaminants, high dietary fat intake, and growth factors such as insulin-like growth factor 1 (IGF-1) have been suggested to promote breast cancer cell growth (Moorman and Terry 2004). Interestingly, a study performed in postmenopausal women has shown that fat from fermented milk products was negatively associated with breast cancer risk ($p = .003$) (Wirfalt et al. 2005). Moreover, there is an 80% reduction in the IGF-1 content of milk following lactic acid fermentation, which suggests a low IGF-1 content in fermented milks and cheeses (L'Agence nationale de sécurité sanitaire alimentation environnement travail 2012).

Studies suggesting that dairy products protect against breast cancer have focused on the anticarcinogenic properties of some of its constituents: calcium, vitamin D, (Bener and El Ayoubi 2012), and CLA (Moorman and Terry 2004). The effects of CLA on breast cancer in humans have been inconsistent (Linos and Willett 2009). Future research on the potential impact of yogurt and dairy products on the incidence of breast cancer should include the specific roles of energy balance and vitamin D in the analyses (Linos and Willett 2007). Moreover, yogurt bacteria may affect immune stimulation, thereby exerting beneficial effects on breast cancer. However, a study failed to show an increase in *ex vivo* cell-mediated immune function in young women with breast cancer following yogurt consumption (Campbell et al. 2000). More studies on specific yogurt strains and yogurt's nutrients are required to clarify a potential link (de Moreno de LeBlanc et al. 2007).

10.2.5 Conclusions

- There is no strong evidence that yogurt has a protective effect on breast cancer. However, some observational studies have suggested a possible beneficial effect of yogurt consumption on breast cancer.
- Retrospective studies evaluating the association between yogurt consumption during childhood and future breast cancer are warranted, given that breast tissue could be particularly sensitive during adolescence to carcinogenic exposure.

10.3 PROSTATE CANCER

Studies have reported that higher intakes of calcium and dairy products, a major source of dietary calcium, increase the risk of prostate cancer (Ahn et al. 2007, Gallus et al. 2006, Kesse et al. 2006). Moreover, the WCRF/AICR report concluded that there was a probable association between diets high in calcium and an increased risk of prostate cancer (Lampe 2011). However, a recent meta-analysis of 45 observational studies did not support any association between dairy product consumption and an increased risk of prostate cancer (Huncharek et al. 2008). Few studies have investigated the effect of specific dairy products on this type of cancer.

10.3.1 Case-Control Studies

The effect of intakes of various foods on the risk of prostate cancer was examined using data from three case-control studies in Canada (617 incident cases of prostate cancer and 636 population controls from Ontario, Québec, and British Columbia).

Controls were frequency matched by age and residence. No appreciable change in prostate cancer risk was observed with higher intakes of yogurt (Jain et al. 1999).

In a case-control study with 1294 patients from 4 regions in Italy, no association was observed between prostate cancer risk and yogurt intake (Bosetti et al. 2004) and another Italian case-control study found a nonsignificant positive association between yogurt intake and prostate cancer risk (Gallus et al. 2006).

10.3.2 Prospective Cohort Studies

In a prospective study from the National Health and Nutrition Examination Epidemiologic Follow-up Study, 131 prostate cancer cases were identified. No significant effect of yogurt consumption (consumer vs. nonconsumer) on prostate cancer risk was observed (Tseng et al. 2005).

A prospective study including 2776 men from the French *Supplémentation en Vitamines et Minéraux Anti-oxydants* (SU.VI.MAX) cohort was conducted to test the association between the risk of prostate cancer and the consumption of dairy products and calcium. Sixty-nine subjects developed prostate cancer during the follow-up period (median: 7.7 years). A high yogurt consumption (>100 g/day) was positively associated with prostate cancer risk, but the relationship was not significant. Specific analysis showed that an increase of one 125 g serving/day of yogurt increased the risk of prostate cancer independently of the calcium content ($p = .02$). Moreover, a higher risk of prostate cancer was observed among subjects with higher dairy products and calcium intakes (Kesse et al. 2006).

A population-based prospective study performed in 43,435 men aged 45–74 years tested the association between dairy products and prostate cancer in Japan, where the intake of these items and the incidence of prostate cancer are low. Total dairy products, milk, and yogurt were significantly associated with a dose-dependent increase in the risk of prostate cancer (multivariate models adjusted for age, area, smoking status, alcohol, marital status, green tea, and genistein) (Kurahashi et al. 2008).

10.3.3 Meta-Analyses

A meta-analysis of 32 studies investigated the association between dairy, calcium, and prostate cancer. Total dairy, total milk, low-fat milk, cheese, total calcium, dietary calcium, and dairy calcium were all positively associated with a greater risk of prostate cancer. In analyses of six cohort studies that investigated yogurt, no associations were found between yogurt and prostate cancer (Aune et al. 2015).

10.3.4 Mechanisms of Action

The increased risk of prostate cancer observed in some studies following the consumption of dairy products has been mostly attributed to calcium and fat content. Calcium could act by suppressing circulating levels of 1,25-hydroxyvitamin D or by increasing IGF-1 levels, which have been shown to be related to the risk of prostate cancer (Kurahashi et al. 2008). Another mechanism is that an increased fat intake might lead to increased testosterone levels and this could influence prostate cancer risk (Gann et al. 1996). The effects of specific saturated fatty acids require more investigation because epidemiologic and laboratory data is sparse (Kurahashi et al. 2008). Some authors have also suggested that increased milk protein–mediated mechanistic target of rapamycin complex 1 (mTORC1) signaling through elevated branched-chain amino acids (BCAAs), and constant exposure to milk estrogens derived from pregnant cows may contribute to the association between high dairy consumption and an increased risk of prostate cancer in Western countries (Melnik et al. 2012). In a prospective cohort study, phosphorus was associated with total, lethal, and high-grade prostate cancer. This association remained significant even after controlling for calcium intake, red meat, and dairy. While phosphorus intake is correlated to dairy intake, its food sources are more varied than in the case of calcium. The mechanism potentially explaining the link between phosphorus and prostate cancer is via the promotion of bone remodeling that occurs with high phosphorus intakes. Prostate cancer is thought to spread to the bone during the remodeling activity and this coincides with an increased risk, particularly in advanced stages of cancer (Wilson et al. 2015).

10.3.5 Conclusions

- Based on systematic reviews and meta-analyses, there is a probable association between diets high in calcium and an increased risk of prostate cancer. There may also be a positive association between dairy food intake and prostate cancer, but findings from meta-analyses are inconsistent.
- Some studies have shown a significant positive association between the consumption of yogurt and prostate cancer risk, while other studies did not confirm such a relationship. The mechanisms underlying the potential associations are not clear, but they may be related to the intake of excess calcium.

REFERENCES

Ahn, J., D. Albanes, U. Peters, A. Schatzkin, U. Lim, M. Freedman, N. Chatterjee, et al. 2007. Dairy products, calcium intake, and risk of prostate cancer in the prostate, lung, colorectal, and ovarian cancer screening trial. *Cancer Epidemiol Biomarkers Prev* 12:2623–30.

Aune, D., R. Lau, D. S. Chan, R. Vieira, D. C. Greenwood, E. Kampman, and T. Norat. 2012. Dairy products and colorectal cancer risk: A systematic review and meta-analysis of cohort studies. *Ann Oncol* 23 (1):37–45.

Aune, D., D. A. Navarro Rosenblatt, D. S. Chan, A. R. Vieira, R. Vieira, D. C. Greenwood, L. J. Vatten, et al. 2015. Dairy products, calcium, and prostate cancer risk: A systematic review and meta-analysis of cohort studies. *Am J Clin Nutr* 101 (1):87–117.

Bartram, H. P., W. Scheppach, S. Gerlach, G. Ruckdeschel, E. Kelber, and H. Kasper. 1994. Does yogurt enriched with *Bifidobacterium longum* affect colonic microbiology and fecal metabolites in health subjects? *Am J Clin Nutr* 59 (2):428–32.

Bener, A., and H. R. El Ayoubi. 2012. The role of vitamin D deficiency and osteoporosis in breast cancer. *Int J Rheum Dis* 15 (6):554–61.

Bosetti, C., S. Micelotta, L. Dal Maso, R. Talamini, M. Montella, E. Negri, E. Conti, et al. 2004. Food groups and risk of prostate cancer in Italy. *Int J Cancer* 110 (3):424–8.

Boutron, M. C., J. Faivre, P. Marteau, C. Couillault, P. Senesse, and V. Quipourt. 1996. Calcium, phosphorus, vitamin D, dairy products and colorectal carcinogenesis: A french case-control study. *Br J Cancer* 74 (1):145–51.

Campbell, C. G., B. P. Chew, L. O. Luedecke, and T. D. Shultz. 2000. Yogurt consumption does not enhance immune function in healthy premenopausal women. *Nutr Cancer* 37 (1):27–35.

Cho, E., S. A. Smith-Warner, D. Spiegelman, W. L. Beeson, P. A. van den Brandt, G. A. Colditz, A. R. Folsom et al. 2004. Dairy foods, calcium, and colorectal cancer: A pooled analysis of 10 cohort studies. *J Natl Cancer Inst* 96 (13):1015–22.

De Moreno de LeBlanc, A., C. Matar, and G. Perdigón. 2007. The application of probiotics in cancer. *Br J Nutr* 98 Suppl 1:S105–10.

De Moreno de Leblanc, A., and G. Perdigón. 2010. The application of probiotic fermented milks in cancer and intestinal inflammation. *Proc Nutr Soc* 69 (3):421–8.

Dik, V. K., N. Murphy, P. D. Siersema, V. Fedirko, M. Jenab, S. Y. Kong, C. P. Hansen et al. 2014. Prediagnostic intake of dairy products and dietary calcium and colorectal cancer survival: Results from the EPIC cohort study. *Cancer Epidemiol Biomarkers Prev* 23 (9):1813–23.

Gallus, S., F. Bravi, R. Talamini, E. Negri, M. Montella, V. Ramazzotti, S. Franceschi, et al. 2006. Milk, dairy products and cancer risk (Italy). *Cancer Causes Control* 17 (4):429–37.

Gann, P. H., C. H. Hennekens, J. Ma, C. Longcope, and M. J. Stampfer. 1996. Prospective study of sex hormone levels and risk of prostate cancer. *J Natl Cancer Inst* 88 (16):1118–26.

Genkinger, J. M., K. H. Makambi, J. R. Palmer, L. Rosenberg, and L. L. Adams-Campbell. 2013. Consumption of dairy and meat in relation to breast cancer risk in the Black Women's Health Study. *Cancer Causes Control* 24 (4):675–84.

Hjartåker, A., M. Thoresen, D. Engeset, and E. Lund. 2010. Dairy consumption and calcium intake and risk of breast cancer in a prospective cohort: The Norwegian Women and Cancer study. *Cancer Causes Control* 21 (11):1875–85.

Huncharek, M., J. Muscat, and B. Kupelnick. 2008. Dairy products, dietary calcium and vitamin D intake as risk factors for prostate cancer: A meta-analysis of 26,769 cases from 45 observational studies. *Nutr Cancer* 60 (4):421–41.

Huncharek, M., J. Muscat, and B. Kupelnick. 2009. Colorectal cancer risk and dietary intake of calcium, vitamin D, and dairy products: A meta-analysis of 26,335 cases from 60 observational studies. *Nutr Cancer* 61 (1):47–69.

Jain, M. G. 1998. Dairy foods, dairy fats, and cancer: A review of epidemiological evidence. *Nutr Res* 18 (5):905–37.

Jain, M. G., G. T. Hislop, G. R. Howe, and P. Ghadirian. 1999. Plant foods, antioxidants, and prostate cancer risk: Findings from case-control studies in Canada. *Nutr Cancer* 34 (2):173–84.

Jarvinen, R., P. Knekt, T. Hakulinen, and A. Aromaa. 2001. Prospective study on milk products, calcium and cancers of the colon and rectum. *Eur J Clin Nutr* 55 (11):1000–7.

Juarranz Sanz, M., T. Soriano Llora, M. E. Calle Purón, D. Martínez Hernández, A. González Navarro, and V. Domínguez Rojas. 2004. Influence of the diet on the development of colorectal cancer in a population of Madrid. *Rev Clin Esp* 204 (7):355–61.

Kampman, E., E. Giovannucci, P. van't Veer, E. Rimm, M. J. Stampfer, G. A. Colditz, F. J. Kok, and W. C. Willett. 1994a. Calcium, vitamin D, dairy foods, and the occurrence of colorectal adenomas among men and women in two prospective studies. *Am J Epidemiol* 139 (1):16–29.

Kampman, E., P. van't Veer, G. J. Hiddink, P. van Aken-Schneijder, F. J. Kok, and R. J. Hermus. 1994b. Fermented dairy products, dietary calcium and colon cancer: A case-control study in The Netherlands. *Int J Cancer* 59 (2):170–6.

Karagianni, V., E. Merikas, F. Georgopoulos, A. Gikas, N. Athanasopoulos, G. Malgarinos, G. Peros, et al. 2010. Risk factors for colorectal polyps: Findings from a Greek case-control study. *Rev Med Chir Soc Med Nat Iasi* 114 (3):662–70.

Kearney, J., E. Giovannucci, E. B. Rimm, A. Ascherio, M. J. Stampfer, G. A. Colditz, A. Wing, et al. 1996. Calcium, vitamin D, and dairy foods and the occurrence of colon cancer in men. *Am J Epidemiol* 143 (9):907–17.

Kesse, E., S. Bertrais, P. Astorg, A. Jaouen, N. Arnault, P. Galan, and S. Hercberg. 2006. Dairy products, calcium and phosphorus intake, and the risk of prostate cancer: Results of the French prospective SU.VI.MAX (Supplementation en Vitamines et Mineraux Antioxydants) study. *Br J Nutr* 95 (3):539–45.

Kesse, E., M.C. Boutron-Ruault, T. Norat, E. Riboli, and F. Clavel-Chapelon. 2005. Dietary calcium, phosphorus, vitamin D, dairy products and the risk of colorectal adenoma and cancer among French women of the E3N-EPIC prospective study. *Int J Cancer* 117:137–44.

Keum, N., D. Aune, D. C. Greenwood, W. Ju, and E. L. Giovannucci. 2014. Calcium intake and colorectal cancer risk: Dose-response meta-analysis of prospective observational studies. *Int J Cancer* 135 (8):1940–48.

Kojima, M., K. Wakai, K. Tamakoshi, S. Tokudome, H. Toyoshima, Y. Watanabe, N. Hayakawa, et al. 2004. Diet and colorectal cancer mortality: Results from the Japan Collaborative Cohort Study. *Nutr Cancer* 50 (1):23–32.

Kurahashi, N., M. Inoue, M. Iwasaki, S. Sasazuki, and A. S. Tsugane. 2008. Dairy product, saturated fatty acid, and calcium intake and prostate cancer in a prospective cohort of Japanese men. *Cancer Epidemiol Biomarkers Prev* 17 (4):930–37.

L'Agence nationale de sécurité sanitaire alimentation environnement travail. 2012. *Étude des liens entre facteurs de croissance, consommation de lait et produits laitiers et cancers*. France: ANSES Éditions.

Lampe, J. W. 2011. Dairy products and cancer. *J Am Coll Nutr* 30 (5 Suppl 1):464S–70S.

Larsson, S. C., L. Bergkvist, J. Rutegard, E. Giovannucci, and A. Wolk. 2006. Calcium and dairy food intakes are inversely associated with colorectal cancer risk in the Cohort of Swedish Men. *Am J Clin Nutr* 83 (3):667–73; quiz 728–29.

Le, M. G., L. H. Moulton, C. Hill, and A. Kramar. 1986. Consumption of dairy produce and alcohol in a case-control study of breast cancer. *J Natl Cancer Inst* 77 (3):633–36.

Levi, F., C. La Vecchia, C. Gulie, and E. Negri. 1993. Dietary factors and breast cancer risk in Vaud, Switzerland. *Nutr Cancer* 19 (3):327–35.

Lin, J., S. M. Zhang, N. R. Cook, J. E. Manson, I. M. Lee, and J. E. Buring. 2005. Intakes of calcium and vitamin D and risk of colorectal cancer in women. *Am J Epidemiol* 161 (8):755–64.

Linos, E., and W. Willett. 2009. Meat, dairy, and breast cancer: Do we have an answer? *Am J Clin Nutr* 90 (3):455–56.

Linos, E., and W. C. Willett. 2007. Diet and breast cancer risk reduction. *J Natl Compr Canc Netw* 5 (8):711–18.

Matos, E. L., M. Khlat, D. I. Loria, M. Vilensky, and D. M. Parkin. 1991. Cancer in migrants to Argentina. *Int J Cancer* 49 (6):805–11.

Matsumoto, M., S. Ishikawa, Y. Nakamura, K. Kayaba, and E. Kajii. 2007. Consumption of dairy products and cancer risks. *Journal of Epidemiology* 17 (2):38–44.

Melnik, B. C., S. M. John, P. Carrera-Bastos, and L. Cordain. 2012. The impact of cow's milk-mediated mTORC1-signaling in the initiation and progression of prostate cancer. *Nutr Metab (Lond)* 9 (1):74.

Missmer, S. A., S. A. Smith-Warner, D. Spiegelman, S. S. Yaun, H. O. Adami, W. L. Beeson, P. A. van den Brandt et al. 2002. Meat and dairy food consumption and breast cancer: A pooled analysis of cohort studies. *Int J Epidemiol* 31 (1):78–85.

Mobarakeh, Z. S., K. Mirzaei, N. Hatmi, M. Ebrahimi, S. Dabiran, and G. Sotoudeh. 2014. Dietary habits contributing to breast cancer risk among Iranian women. *Asian Pac J Cancer Prev* 15 (21):9543–47.

Moorman, P. G., and P. D. Terry. 2004. Consumption of dairy products and the risk of breast cancer: A review of the literature. *Am J Clin Nutr* 80 (1):5–14.

Murphy, N., T. Norat, P. Ferrari, M. Jenab, B. Bueno-de-Mesquita, G. Skeie, A. Olsen, A. Tjønneland et al. 2013. Consumption of dairy products and colorectal cancer in the European Prospective Investigation into Cancer and Nutrition (EPIC). *PLoS One* 8 (9):e72715.

Pala, V., S. Sieri, F. Berrino, P. Vineis, C. Sacerdote, D. Palli, G. Masala et al. 2011. Yogurt consumption and risk of colorectal cancer in the Italian European Prospective Investigation into Cancer and Nutrition cohort. *Int J Cancer* 129 (11):2712–19.

Park, S. Y., S. P. Murphy, L. R. Wilkens, A. M. Nomura, B. E. Henderson, and L. N. Kolonel. 2007. Calcium and vitamin D intake and risk of colorectal cancer: The Multiethnic Cohort Study. *Am J Epidemiol* 165 (7):784–93.

Peters, R. K., M. C. Pike, D. Garabrant, and T. M. Mack. 1992. Diet and colon cancer in Los Angeles County, California. *Cancer Causes Control* 3 (5):457–73.

Ralston, R. A., H. Truby, C. E. Palermo, and K. Z. Walker. 2014. Colorectal cancer and non-fermented milk, solid cheese, and fermented milk consumption: A systematic review and meta-analysis of prospective studies. *Crit Rev Food Sci Nutr* 54 (9):1167–79.

Ronco, A. L., E. De Stéfani, and R. Dáttoli. 2002. Dairy foods and risk of breast cancer: A case-control study in Montevideo, Uruguay. *Eur J Cancer Prev* 11 (5):457–63.

Senesse, P., Boutron-Ruault M. C., Faivre J., Chatelain N., and Belghiti C. 2002. Foods as risk factors for colorectal adenomas: A case-control study in Burgundy (France). *Nutr Cancer* 44 (1):7–15.

Stewart, B. W., and C. P. Wild. 2014. *World Cancer Report 2014*. Lyon, France: WHO.

Sun, Z., P. P. Wang, B. Roebothan, M. Cotterchio, R. Green, S. Buehler, J. Zhao, et al. 2011. Calcium and vitamin D and risk of colorectal cancer: Results from a large population-based case-control study in Newfoundland and Labrador and Ontario. *Can J Public Health* 102 (5):382–89.

Tseng, M., R. A. Breslow, B. I. Graubard, and R. G. Ziegler. 2005. Dairy, calcium, and vitamin D intakes and prostate cancer risk in the National Health and Nutrition Examination Epidemiologic Follow-up Study cohort. *Am J Clin Nutr* 81 (5):1147–54.

van't Veer, P., J. M. Dekker, J. W. Lamers, F. J. Kok, E. G. Schouten, H. A. Brants, F. Sturmans, and R. J. Hermus. 1989. Consumption of fermented milk products and breast cancer: A case-control study in The Netherlands. *Cancer Res* 49 (14):4020–23.

van't Veer, P., E. M. van Leer, A. Rietdijk, F. J. Kok, E. G. Schouten, R. J. Hermus, and F. Sturmans. 1991. Combination of dietary factors in relation to breast-cancer occurrence. *Int J Cancer* 47 (5):649–53.

WCRF. 2007. *Food, Nutrition, Physical Activity and the Prevention of Cancer: A Global Perspective*. Washington, DC: AICR.

WCRF/AICR. 2011. *Continuous Update Project Report Summary. Food, Nutrition, Physical Activity, and the Prevention of Colorectal Cancer*. London: AICR.

WHO. 2012. Cancer; breast cancer: Prevention and control. http://www.who.int/cancer/detection/breastcancer/en/index.html.

Wilson, K. M., I. M. Shui, L. A. Mucci, and E. Giovannucci. 2015. Calcium and phosphorus intake and prostate cancer risk: A 24-y follow-up study. *Am J Clin Nutr* 101 (1):173–83.

Wirfalt, E., I. Mattisson, B. Gullberg, H. Olsson, and G. Berglund. 2005. Fat from different foods show diverging relations with breast cancer risk in postmenopausal women. *Nutr Cancer* 53 (2):135–43.

Wiseman, M. 2008. The second World Cancer Research Fund/American Institute for Cancer Research expert report. Food, nutrition, physical activity, and the prevention of cancer: A global perspective. *Proc Nutr Soc* 67 (3):253–56.

11 Allergy and Atopic Diseases

Atopic diseases arise from aberrant immune responses to environmental allergens (Stone 2003). The atopic diseases of childhood consist of atopic dermatitis, allergic rhinitis, and allergic asthma. The Mediterranean diet has been found to protect against the development of asthma (Nagel et al. 2010, Chatzi and Kogevinas 2009) and atopy in children (Chatzi and Kogevinas 2009). However, epidemiological evidence regarding the association between the intake of dairy foods and allergic disorders has been inconsistent (Miyake et al. 2012). This chapter discusses a few studies that have been carried out in humans regarding the effect of yogurt on atopic diseases.

11.1 ECZEMA AND ATOPIC DERMATITIS

An epidemiological study was performed in 134 Japanese junior high school students to investigate the relationship between fermented milk or fermented soybean food intake and the occurrence of atopic diseases. Regular yogurt and/or fermented milk consumption was associated with a significant reduction in allergy development compared with those who did not frequently consume fermented foods (Enomoto et al. 2006).

Uenishi et al. (2008) investigated whether foods play a role in the irregular aggravation of skin lesions in 69 Japanese children (3–15 years) with atopic dermatitis. In total, 24 types of food items were confirmed to aggravate skin lesions in at least one of the patients examined. Predominant offending foods were chocolate, cheese, and yogurt. Specific immunoglobulin E (IgE) values to challenge test-positive foods were mostly negative, suggesting that food-induced, non-IgE-mediated aggravation of skin lesions occurred in some patients. An improvement of the disease was observed after the exclusion of the offending foods for 3 months. These results suggest that foods play an important role in the irregular aggravation of skin lesions in children (Uenishi et al. 2008). A follow-up study carried out by the same group tested whether tree nut-related foods and fermented foods could aggravate the atopic dermatitis of breast-fed infants through transfer. In 92 exclusively breast-fed Japanese infants with atopic dermatitis, 73% experienced an improvement of skin lesions when mothers avoided tree nut-related foods and aggravations when these foods were reintroduced. The predominant offenders were chocolate, soy sauce, yogurt, and miso soup (as shown by the challenge test to specific foods). The results suggest that tree nut-related foods and fermented foods can be triggers for atopic dermatitis in breast-fed infants. However, only two categories of foods were tested in this study (Uenishi et al. 2011).

The factors determining allergic signs and symptoms in early childhood were investigated in 109 Turkish children (mean age: 31.6 ± 3.5 months). The introduction of cow's milk before 12 months was a significant risk factor for atopy. Smoking during lactation and having an older sibling showed a trend toward an increased risk, while regular yogurt consumption showed a trend toward decreasing the risk for atopy (Ozmert et al. 2009).

Miyake et al. (2010) performed a prospective study to evaluate the association between the maternal consumption of dairy products, calcium, and vitamin D during pregnancy and the risk of eczema and wheeze in 763 Japanese mother–child pairs. The maternal intake of yogurt, total dairy products, milk, cheese, and calcium during pregnancy was not associated with the risk of eczema in the offspring (Miyake et al. 2010).

The impact of the introduction of complementary food in the first year of life and the association with the development of atopic dermatitis was investigated in the 1041 children who participated in the Protection Against Allergy: Study in Rural Environments birth cohort study (five European countries). The introduction of yogurt and the diversity of food introduced in the first year of life significantly reduced the risk for atopic dermatitis (Roduit et al. 2012). The authors discussed the possibility that yogurt bacteria and the increased level in short-chain fatty acids in plasma and fecal samples following yogurt consumption might have played a role in the observed effect.

11.2 ALLERGIC RHINITIS

Van de Water et al. (1999) performed a year-long study in which they gave young adults (20–40 years) and seniors (55–70 years) 200 g/day of live yogurt, pasteurized fermented milk, or no fermented milk. The subjects completed a questionnaire detailing health parameters on a weekly basis. The consumption of live culture groups was significantly associated with a decrease in allergic symptoms in both age groups ($p < .05$). There was little effect on interferon-gamma (IFN-γ) and IgE production, although seniors in the yogurt group had lower levels of total IgE throughout the year. Compared with no yogurt and pasteurized fermented milk, the live yogurt reduced nasal allergies, especially in the young adult population (Van de Water et al. 1999).

Trapp et al. (1993) found a decrease in allergic rhinitis symptoms in individuals consuming live yogurt, compared with subjects consuming a normal diet of pasteurized fermented milk, over a period of 1 year. Clinical improvements were observed in the live-active yogurt group, but were not associated with significant increases in IFN-γ production or decreases in total and allergen-specific IgE (Trapp et al. 1993).

Wheeler et al. (1997) compared the immune parameters of participants who received 16 oz (480 mL) of yogurt versus 16 oz (480 mL) of milk per day in a randomized crossover design. Yogurt containing live bacteria or 2% milk was consumed for 1 month by 20 adults with a history of atopic diseases (rhinoconjunctivitis or asthma). No significant improvements in any of the determined immune parameters (measurements of cellular, humoral, and phagocytic functions) were observed (Wheeler et al. 1997).

The immunological and clinical effects of yogurt and partially skimmed milk consumption were evaluated in subjects with demonstrated allergic rhinopathy and in healthy control subjects. Allergic rhinopathy was evaluated before and after 4 months of treatment. Cultured peripheral blood mononuclear cells in the yogurt-fed group released more IFN-γ and less interleukin 4 (IL-4). Serum IgE remained unaltered. The mucociliary transport time and the symptom score showed a significant improvement after yogurt feeding. In this study, yogurt feeding appeared to improve or prevent allergic recurrences in rhinopathic patients (Aldinucci et al. 2002).

11.3 ALLERGIC ASTHMA

A cross-sectional study involving 1601 young adults assessed whether the food and nutrient intakes of adults with asthma differ from those of adults without asthma. There were no significant associations between the food category *other dairy* (which included yogurt, cheese, and ice cream) and the asthma categories *current asthma*, *doctor-diagnosed asthma*, *bronchial hyperreactivity*, and *atopy*. However, an increased risk was observed for *asthma* with *other dairy* consumption. Whole milk intake showed a protective effect against current asthma, doctor-diagnosed asthma, bronchial hyperreactivity, and atopy. The authors concluded that the intakes of dairy products, soy beverages, apples, and pears, but not of nutrients per se, were positively associated with a range of asthma definitions (Woods et al. 2003).

In Japan, a cross-sectional study involving 472 elementary school children was performed on yogurt and allergic diseases. Positive rates of mite- and grass-specific IgE were higher in the high yogurt-consuming group. The prevalence of asthma in the intermediate consumption group was significantly lower than that in the non-consuming group. The authors concluded that the consumption of fermented milk affects allergic sensitization for some allergens. Furthermore, the development of asthma and the relationship between the level of yogurt consumption and disease development may not be simple (Suzuki et al. 2008).

A prospective study involving 763 Japanese mother–child pairs examined the association between the maternal consumption of dairy products, calcium, and vitamin D during pregnancy and the risk of wheeze and eczema. No association was observed between maternal yogurt consumption during pregnancy and the risk of wheeze in the offspring. However, higher maternal consumptions of total dairy products, milk, cheese, and calcium during pregnancy were significantly related to a decreased risk of wheeze in their offspring (Miyake et al. 2010).

A longitudinal study was performed to examine the relationship between maternal dairy intake during pregnancy and the development of asthma and allergic rhinitis in childhood. Maternal whole-milk and full-fat yogurt intake showed protective associations for child outcomes at 18 months. However, results differed by outcomes examined in early versus late childhood and at the 7-year assessment maternal low-fat yogurt consumption was directly associated with child asthma and allergic rhinitis. The authors stated that the association between low-fat yogurt and later childhood outcomes suggested that compounds specific to this food, such as artificial sweeteners, could be involved (Maslova et al. 2012).

The impact of a Mediterranean diet adherence during pregnancy on wheeze and eczema was evaluated in the first year of life. Analysis by specific dairy products showed that a high milk intake during pregnancy was inversely associated with wheeze in the first year of life, while yogurt and cheese intakes were not associated with the risk of infantile wheeze and eczema in this study (Chatzi et al. 2013).

To examine the relationship between the maternal dietary intake of dairy foods, calcium, and vitamin D during pregnancy and the incidence of allergic disorders in children (23–29 months), 1354 mother–child pairs were studied. There were no associations between yogurt intake and wheeze, eczema, or physician-diagnosed asthma; however, there was a nonsignificant reduced risk with yogurt intake for physician-diagnosed eczema. There was also a significant inverse exposure–response association in the crude and adjusted models trend ($p = .03$ and $p = .01$, respectively). Further analysis, excluding women who had experienced substantial changes in their diet in the month prior to participating in the study, found a significant inverse relationship between yogurt and physician-diagnosed eczema (OR = 0.36 [95% CI, 0.07–0.99; $p = .005$]). A similar relationship was found for calcium. Yogurt intake was moderately and significantly correlated to calcium intake (Pearson correlation coefficient, 0.43, $p < .0001$). An inverse relationship was also found between eczema and total dairy intake, whereas high maternal intakes of vitamin D during pregnancy may increase the risk for infantile eczema (Miyake et al. 2014).

11.4 MECHANISMS OF ACTION

Experimental data and clinical studies showed that the immune system of infants can be stimulated by the endogenous intestinal microbiota (Hauer 2006). Effects of probiotics on atopic diseases such as atopic dermatitis (Lenoir-Wijnkoop et al. 2007) have been observed, but the mechanisms involved in this potential effect need to be defined (Nova et al. 2007). Figure 11.1 illustrates potential mechanisms that may be involved. Fermented milk in particular is thought to improve the gut mucosal barrier and reduce inflammation. The action of lactic acid produced by lactic acid bacteria (LAB) species may relieve skin issues by promoting and regulating the immune system through stimulating the gastrointestinal mucosal barrier, producing beneficial metabolites, and protecting against pathogens (Vaughn and Sivamani 2015).

Low bacterial diversity of the microbiota has also been suggested to be associated with atopic diseases, but its association with atopic dermatitis remains to be clarified (Bisgaard et al. 2011). It is thought that the diversity of the gut microbiota is different in those with allergic disorders. It has also been suggested that a shift between the balance of cytokine Th1 responses to Th2 responses may be responsible for the release of IL-4, IL-5, IL-3, and IgE production and an allergic response. It is possible that the consumption of yogurt bacteria may help activate Th1 responses, which can suppress Th2 responses. As discussed in the chapter on immune responses, yogurt's microorganisms have been shown to modulate the production of IFN-γ. IFN-γ can inhibit IgE synthesis, which plays a role in hypersensitivity reactions (Adolfsson et al. 2004, Michail 2009). Moreover, it has been suggested that short-chain fatty acids secreted after yogurt intake and conjugated linoleic acid may confer benefits to individuals with atopic dermatitis and asthma (Vaughn and Sivamani 2015, Macredmond and Dorscheid 2011, Roduit et al. 2012). Lactic acid produced by yogurt bacteria creates an ideal pH environment, which may enhance the skin barrier by increasing its thickness and promoting the production of pro-collagen 1 (Usuki et al. 2003, Puch et al. 2008).

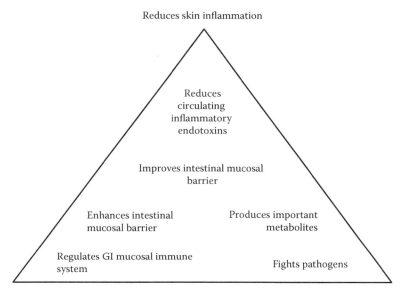

FIGURE 11.1 The potential mechanisms by which lactic acid bacteria may diminish skin inflammation in allergic disorders. (Adapted from Vaughn, A. R., and R. K. Sivamani, *J Altern Complement Med,* 21 (7), 380–385, 2015.)

11.5 CONCLUSIONS

The few studies available on the effects of yogurt on both atopic diseases and respiratory illnesses have shown inconsistent results. The duration of the study, the dose of yogurt used, and variations in genetic and environmental factors that may differ between populations could explain discrepancies between results. Studies performed thus far are not sufficient to draw any conclusions regarding the effect of yogurt, its strains, or its nutrients on allergy and related diseases.

REFERENCES

Adolfsson, O., S. N. Meydani, and R. M. Russell. 2004. Yogurt and gut function. *Am J Clin Nutr* 80 (2):245–56.

Aldinucci, C., L. Bellussi, G. Monciatti, G. C. Passali, L. Salerni, D. Passali, and V. Bocci. 2002. Effects of dietary yoghurt on immunological and clinical parameters of rhinopathic patients. *Eur J Clin Nutr* 56 (12):1155–61.

Bisgaard, H., N. Li, K. Bonnelykke, B. L. Chawes, T. Skov, G. Paludan-Muller, J. Stokholm, et al. 2011. Reduced diversity of the intestinal microbiota during infancy is associated with increased risk of allergic disease at school age. *J Allergy Clin Immunol* 128 (3):646–52 e1–5.

Chatzi, L., R. Garcia, T. Roumeliotaki, M. Basterrechea, H. Begiristain, C. Iñiguez, J. Vioque, et al. 2013. Mediterranean diet adherence during pregnancy and risk of wheeze and eczema in the first year of life: INMA (Spain) and RHEA (Greece) mother-child cohort studies. *Br J Nutr* 110 (11):1–11.

Chatzi, L., and M. Kogevinas. 2009. Prenatal and childhood Mediterranean diet and the development of asthma and allergies in children. *Public Health Nutr* 12 (9A):1629–34.

Enomoto, T., K. Shimizu, and S. Shimazu. 2006. Suppression of allergy development by habitual intake of fermented milk foods, evidence from an epidemiological study. *Arerugi* 55 (11):1394–99.

Hauer, A. 2006. Probiotics in allergic diseases of childhood. *MMW Fortschr Med* 148 (35–36):34–36.

Lenoir-Wijnkoop, I., M. E. Sanders, M. D. Cabana, E. Caglar, G. Corthier, N. Rayes, P. M. Sherman, et al. 2007. Probiotic and prebiotic influence beyond the intestinal tract. *Nutr Rev* 65 (11):469–89.

Macredmond, R., and D. R. Dorscheid. 2011. Conjugated linoleic acid (CLA): Is it time to supplement asthma therapy? *Pulm Pharmacol Ther* 24 (5):540–48.

Maslova, E., T. I. Halldorsson, M. Strom, and S. F. Olsen. 2012. Low-fat yoghurt intake in pregnancy associated with increased child asthma and allergic rhinitis risk: A prospective cohort study. *J Nutr Sci* 1 (5):1–11.

Michail, S. 2009. The role of probiotics in allergic diseases. *Allergy Asthma Clin Immunol* 5 (1):5.

Miyake, Y., S. Sasaki, K. Tanaka, and Y. Hirota. 2010. Dairy food, calcium and vitamin D intake in pregnancy, and wheeze and eczema in infants. *Eur Respir J* 35 (6):1228–34.

Miyake, Y., K. Tanaka, H. Okubo, S. Sasaki, and M. Arakawa. 2012. Dairy food, calcium and vitamin D intake and prevalence of allergic disorders in pregnant Japanese women. *Int J Tuberc Lung Dis* 16 (2):255–61.

Miyake, Y., K. Tanaka, H. Okubo, S. Sasaki, and M. Arakawa. 2014. Maternal consumption of dairy products, calcium, and vitamin D during pregnancy and infantile allergic disorders. *Ann Allergy, Asthma Immunol* 113 (1):82–87.

Nagel, G., G. Weinmayr, A. Kleiner, L. Garcia-Marcos, and D. P. Strachan. 2010. Effect of diet on asthma and allergic sensitisation in the International Study on Allergies and Asthma in Childhood (ISAAC) Phase Two. *Thorax* 65 (6):516–22.

Nova, E., J. Wärnberg, S. Gómez-Martínez, L. E. Díaz, J. Romeo, and A. Marcos. 2007. Immunomodulatory effects of probiotics in different stages of life. *Br J Nutr* 98 (Suppl 1):S90–95.

Ozmert, E. N., E. Kale-Cekinmez, K. Yurdakok, and B. E. Sekerel. 2009. Determinants of allergic signs and symptoms in 24–48-month-old Turkish children. *Turk J Pediatr* 51 (2):103–109.

Puch, F., S. Samson-Villeger, D. Guyonnet, J.-L. Blachon, A. V. Rawlings, and T. Lassel. 2008. Consumption of functional fermented milk containing borage oil, green tea and vitamin E enhances skin barrier function. *Exp Dermatol* 17 (8):668–74.

Roduit, C., R. Frei, G. Loss, G. Buchele, J. Weber, M. Depner, S. Loeliger, et al. 2012. Development of atopic dermatitis according to age of onset and association with early-life exposures. *J Allergy Clin Immunol* 130 (1):130–6 e5.

Stone, K. D. 2003. Atopic diseases of childhood. *Curr Opin Pediatr* 15 (5):495–511.

Suzuki, Y., Y. Mashita, H. Inoue, M. Funamizu, A. Haneda, N. Shimojo, Y. Kawano, et al. 2008. Relationship between allergy and fermented milk intake in school children. *Arerugi* 57 (1):37–45.

Trapp, C. L., C. C. Chang, G. M. Halpern, C. L. Keen, and M. E. Gershwin. 1993. The influence of chronic yogurt consumption on populations of young and elderly adults. *Int J Immunother* 9 (1):53–64.

Uenishi, T., H. Sugiura, T. Tanaka, and M. Uehara. 2008. Role of foods in irregular aggravation of skin lesions in children with atopic dermatitis. *J Dermatol* 35 (7):407–12.

Uenishi, T., H. Sugiura, T. Tanaka, and M. Uehara. 2011. Aggravation of atopic dermatitis in breast-fed infants by tree nut-related foods and fermented foods in breast milk. *J Dermatol* 38 (2):140–45.

Usuki, A., A. Ohashi, H. Sato, Y. Ochiai, M. Ichihashi, and Y. Funasaka. 2003. The inhibitory effect of glycolic acid and lactic acid on melanin synthesis in melanoma cells. *Exp Dermatol* 12:43–50.

Van de Water, J., C. L. Keen, and M. E. Gershwin. 1999. The influence of chronic yogurt consumption on immunity. *J Nutr* 129 (7 Suppl):1492S–5S.

Vaughn, A. R., and R. K. Sivamani. 2015. Effects of fermented dairy products on skin: A systematic review. *J Altern Complement Med* 21 (7):380–85.

Wheeler, J. G., M. L. Bogle, S. J. Shema, M. A. Shirrell, K. C. Stine, A. J. Pittler, A. W. Burks, et al. 1997. Impact of dietary yogurt on immune function. *Am J Med Sci* 313 (2):120–23.

Woods, R. K., E. H. Walters, J. M. Raven, R. Wolfe, P. D. Ireland, F. C. Thien, and M. J. Abramson. 2003. Food and nutrient intakes and asthma risk in young adults. *Am J Clin Nutr* 78 (3):414–21.

12 Bone Mineralization and Osteoporosis

A combination of endogenous (genetic and hormonal) and exogenous (nutrition and physical activity) factors influence skeletal development during growth, bone maintenance during adulthood, and bone resorption during aging (Cadogan et al. 1997, Rizzoli et al. 2010). Figure 12.1 describes the factors that affect the development and loss of peak bone mass. Genetics account for 60%–80% of the peak bone mass variance (Rizzoli et al. 2010). Moreover, dietary calcium predicts 10%–15% of skeletal calcium retention during adolescence (Weaver 2008). Peak bone mass is usually achieved by age 30. Therefore, consuming the recommended doses of calcium and vitamin D in adolescence and young adulthood will ensure peak bone mass development (IOM 1997, Heaney et al. 2000).

However, even in developed countries, average calcium, vitamin D, and dairy product intakes are often less than the recommended levels (see Chapter 2.2). Yogurt and dairy products not only contain calcium and vitamin D (in fortified yogurts), but also other important nutrients for bone health, including protein, phosphorus, magnesium, sodium, potassium, vitamin B12, and zinc (Sunyecz 2008, Price et al. 2012). In older people, osteoporosis and the subsequent risk of bone fracture have become a major public health problem both in developed and developing countries and they occur most commonly in postmenopausal women (Harvey et al. 2010). Osteoporosis causes more than 8.9 million fractures annually worldwide, of which more than 4.5 million occur in Europe and in the Americas (WHO 2007). Moreover, osteoporosis is not only a major cause of fractures, but it is also one of the main diseases that cause people to become bedridden (WHO 2007). Osteoporosis is defined on the basis of bone mass density and is characterized by the presence of fragility fractures (Kanis 1994). According to the World Health Organization, osteoporosis is defined as a bone mass density that lies 2.5 standard deviations or more below the average value for young healthy adults (a T-score of <-2.5 SD) as measured by dual-energy x-ray absorptiometry (DEXA) (Kanis 1994, WHO 2007). In elderly people, bone loss and fracture risk could be accelerated by insufficient dietary intake and physiological changes, such as changes to the ability to absorb calcium or a decrease in cutaneous vitamin D biosynthesis (Moschonis and Manios 2006, Moschonis et al. 2011). A decrease in estrogen production after menopause results in an increase in bone resorption and a decrease in calcium absorption (Breslau 1994).

To prevent osteoporosis, the International Osteoporosis Foundation has recommended that children, adolescents, and adults maintain adequate intakes of calcium and vitamin D (International Osteoporosis Foundation 2015). Physicians should highlight proper nutrition and supplementation in calcium and vitamin D at pertinent times (Sunyecz 2008). Interestingly, it has been shown that improving dairy product

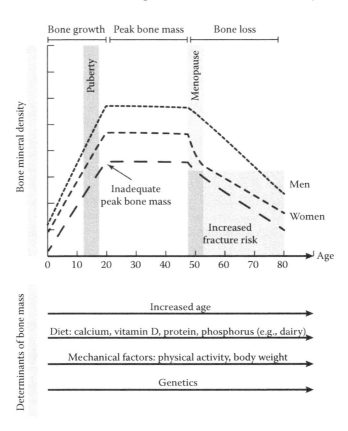

FIGURE 12.1 Determinants of peak bone mass. (Adapted from Heaney, R. P. et al., *Osteoporosis International*, 11 (12), 985–1009, 2000.)

consumption is likely to decrease the societal burden of hip fractures associated with a low calcium intake (Lotters et al. 2013).

Very high levels of calcium supplementation have been associated with increased risks of kidney stones and cardiovascular events, particularly myocardial infarction (Celotti and Bignamini 1999, Bolland et al. 2011). However, a systematic review on calcium supplementation and incident kidney stone risk demonstrated that most of the studies have shown no increase in kidney stone risk with a high calcium intake (from supplements or from diet) (Heaney 2008). While the negative impacts of high supplemental calcium intake are fairly known, it is not clear whether dietary sources of calcium have the potential to exert the same negative impacts as those seen by Bolland et al. (2011). Fortified dairy products are thought to be better than calcium supplements alone and a daily consumption of three servings of dairy is recommended to meet the adequate intakes for bone health (Rizzoli 2014). Increasing dairy product intake to 3–4 servings/day could result in a 20% reduction in hip fractures in the United States (McCarron and Heaney 2004). Fortified dairy products, including yogurts, may result in more favorable changes in biochemical indexes of bone mass than treatments using just calcium supplements (Manios et al. 2007). The importance of calcium in the formation and maintenance of healthy bone is well accepted (Heaney et al. 2002, Rizzoli 2014, Rizzoli et al. 2010). A claim of calcium and the maintenance of normal bone has been approved by the European Food Safety Authority (EFSA Panel of Dietetic Products 2009). Dairy products offer an excellent source of dietary calcium, protein, vitamin D, potassium, and phosphorus, nutrients which are essential to bone mass accrual and maintenance. A significant positive association between dairy product intake and bone mineral content exists (Rizzoli 2014). Reviews studying the effect of calcium on bone quality concluded that dairy product consumption is at least as good as the effects observed with calcium supplements. A significant proportion of studies have targeted childhood and adolescence to assess the effect of calcium and dairy product consumption on bone health, since these periods coincide with bone growth (Heaney 2000, Heaney and Weaver 2005). Heaney et al. (2002) analyzed the relationship between calcium intake and bone health in 139 papers. The author concluded that a very large body of evidence establishes that high calcium intakes increase bone gain during growth, retard age-related bone loss, and reduce osteoporotic fracture risk. However, there are weaknesses in the methods used to estimate long-term calcium intake. Furthermore, there is multifactorial complexity associated with osteoporotic responses to interventions (Heaney et al. 2000). Following this review, more than 100 additional studies have been published on the subject and the proportions of positive and null studies remain at about 75%–80% and 20%–25%, respectively (Heaney 2009).

A meta-analysis examining the effects of dairy products on bone mineral content in children has shown that calcium and dairy products are significantly associated with an increased total body and lumbar bone mineral content in children (Huncharek et al. 2008). Moreover, the inhibition of bone turnover by milk consumption was observed in postmenopausal women (Bonjour et al. 2008). The evidence regarding the utility and the dose of calcium and vitamin D supplements or dairy products to prevent or delay bone loss in adults has been reviewed and challenged by some authors (Lee and Majka 2006, Jackson et al. 2006, Roux et al. 2008, Lanou et al. 2005, Lanou 2009, Spangler et al. 2011, Rabenda et al. 2011). There are many questions about the limitations of these studies. Furthermore, the preventive effects of dairy products against osteoporosis in later life, while highly probable, are not yet fully established (Heaney 2000, Fenton and Hanley 2006, Heaney 2009, Lappe and Heaney 2012). The following sections will discuss the few studies available on the specific effects of yogurt on bone health and osteoporosis.

12.1 STUDIES IN CHILDREN AND ADOLESCENTS

The effect of yogurt supplementation on the growth of 403 Chinese preschool children (3–5 years) whose height for age and/or weight for age were less than the reference level was evaluated. Children in the treatment group consumed 125 g of yogurt 5 days per week for 10 months and the control group received no supplementation. In the yogurt intervention group, the intake of calcium, zinc, and vitamin B2 was significantly higher than that of the control group. The researchers observed that the bone mineral density in children consuming yogurt was significantly higher that of the control group after 9 months of intervention (He et al. 2005).

Uenishi performed a study with 38,719 high school students (14,996 males and 23,723 females) in Japan to measure the effects of dairy product intake on bone mineralization in adolescents. Milk intake (R2 = 2.8%, $p < .0001$) and yogurt intake (R2 = 0.1%, $p < .0001$) were independently associated with the bone strength as measured by quantitative ultrasound (Uenishi 2006).

12.2 STUDIES IN OLDER ADULTS

12.2.1 CROSS-SECTIONAL AND CASE-CONTROL STUDIES

Southeast Asians are particularly at risk of osteoporosis (Malhotra and Mithal 2008). Interestingly, following a pilot case-control study in 100 subjects with a first hip fracture in three hospitals across India, yogurt was identified as a protective food for hip fractures. Other variables that also demonstrated protective effects included milk, increased activity, exercise, increased body mass index (BMI), calcium and vitamin supplements, almonds, fish, and paneer. Tea and other caffeinated beverages were significant risk factors (Jha et al. 2010).

Although osteoporosis is more common in women, it remains a significant health concern among men. A study performed in 592 healthy Moroccan men identified some determinants associated with low bone mineral density. The prevalence of osteoporosis and osteopenia were 8.7% and 52.8% in this population, respectively. The consumptions of milk, coffee, soft drinks or alcohol, cheese, and yogurt were evaluated. Yogurt was not associated with osteopenia or osteoporosis. In multiple regression analyses, only age, BMI, and high coffee consumption were independently associated with osteoporotic status. The authors concluded that a low BMI and aging were the main risk factors associated with osteoporosis in Moroccan men (El Maghraoui et al. 2010).

In a small sample of 170 women (32–59 years) from northeastern Poland, bone mineral density was not associated with yogurt intake, other dairy products, or dietary calcium. However, regular bone mineral density was characterized by a cluster of factors, including a younger age, a nonmenopausal status, a high consumption of dairy products during adulthood, and a high consumption of dairy products during childhood and adolescence (Wadolowska et al. 2013).

In a cross section of 135 women (22–65 years) from Kosovo, hip bone mineral density was examined in relation to dairy product and calcium intakes. Yogurt and other dairy products were not associated with hip bone mineral density, but high total dietary calcium intake was associated with a higher hip bone mineral density. The study was limited to a very small sample size and it did not adjust for known or potential confounders (e.g., age) (Bahtiri et al. 2014).

The Geelong Osteoporosis Study in Australia observed a higher risk of proximal humerus fractures in older men who also had intakes of milk. In women, proximal humerus fractures were associated with lower intakes of nonmilk dairy products (yogurt and cheese). This cohort, however, was small and relatively few ($n = 72$) proximal humerus fractures were observed (Holloway et al. 2015).

12.2.2 Prospective Studies

A prospective study with 12 years of follow-up was performed with a cohort of adults (mean age 55 years) from the Framingham Heart Study Offspring Cohort to assess the association between different types of dairy products and bone mineral density at the femoral neck, trochanter, and spine, as well as the incident hip fracture. Subjects with a high yogurt intake (>4 servings/week) had a higher trochanter-bone mineral density compared with those with no intake ($p = .03$). Yogurt intake showed a weak protective trend for hip fracture. No other dairy groups showed a significant association with hip fracture; however, the incidence of hip fractures was very low ($n = 43$) and there was little power for detection (Sahni et al. 2013).

A cohort of 534 elderly Australian women (80–90 years old) from the Calcium Intake Fracture Outcome Study (CAIFOS) Aged Extension Study was followed for 10 years. Their dairy consumption (milk, yogurt, and cheese) and various measures of bone health were assessed over the follow-up period. There was a significantly higher appendicular bone mineralization and skeletal muscle mass among respondents with the highest tertile of dairy intake (>2.2 servings/day) compared with the lower tertile of dairy intake (<1.5 servings/day). In the group with highest tertile of dairy intake, yogurt consumption was approximately 0.57 servings/day, where one serving was equivalent to 200 g. Results from this study suggested that yogurt consumption may play an important role in contributing to total dairy intake for bone health even when it is consumed in small to moderate quantities (Radavelli-Bagatini et al. 2014).

A group of 764 elderly men and women (68–96 years old) from the Framingham Heart Study Offspring Cohort were followed from 1988–1989 to 2008 for hip fractures and dietary data was collected at baseline. In this study, no associations between total dairy, milk, yogurt, cheese, cream and milk, and yogurt and hip fractures were found. The study concluded that other mechanisms in addition to dairy intake may explain hip fracture risk. However, a major limitation was that dietary intake was only available at baseline, when the population was significantly younger (48–77), and may not reflect the actual dairy consumption over the course of the follow-up (Sahni et al. 2014).

A prospective study examined mortality and fractures in a large Swedish cohort of 61,433 women and 45,339 men who were followed for a mean of 20.1 years and found that a high consumption of milk increased the risk of fractures, whereas there was a 10%–15% decreased risk of hip fractures for every serving of fermented milk (yogurt and other soured milk products). The author made a clear warning that the results should be interpreted with caution due to the possibility of residual confounding and the observational nature of the study (Michaelsson et al. 2014). Nevertheless, the findings of this study were heavily criticized by fellow researchers (Bonneux 2014, Hill 2014, Hettinga 2014). For example, one group of authors cited statistical problems with the study, such as not controlling for osteoporosis status; women with osteoporosis tend to have to increase their milk intake (Labos and Brophy 2014).

A study conducted with a cohort of community-dwelling older adults from the Study on Nutrition and Cardiovascular Risk in Spain found that the consumption of seven or more servings of low-fat milk and yogurt per week was significantly associated with a lower incidence of frailty (OR = 52; 95% CI = 0.29–0.90; $p = .03$) compared with the intake of less than one serving per week. The authors also observed that this relationship was not apparent for whole milk and yogurt (OR = 1.53; 95% CI = 0.90–2.60; $p = .10$) (Lana et al. 2015).

12.2.3 CLINICAL STUDIES

The impact of adding three servings of yogurt per day to the habitual diet was on the excretion of N-telepeptide, a marker of bone resorption, was evaluated in postmenopausal women with low calcium intakes. The comparison group was given three servings per day of a nutritionally poor snack. After 7–10 days of the intervention, yogurt consumption led to a significant reduction in the bone resorption marker N-telepeptide compared with the nutritionally poor snack group (Heaney et al. 2002).

12.2.4 SYSTEMATIC REVIEWS

A systematic review conducted on dietary calcium and fracture risk found no association between the two. Furthermore, 25 out of the 28 cohort studies identified that examined milk and fracture risk found neutral associations and 3 out of the 28 found inverse associations (Bolland et al. 2015). The Michaelsson et al. (2014) milk study, however, was not included in the review. The authors of the review conclude that dietary calcium is not associated with fracture risk and that increasing calcium intake through supplements or diet should not be recommended a preventive measure (Bolland et al. 2015). Nevertheless, among at-risk populations, higher levels of vitamin D and calcium fortification may provide an increased protection against bone fragility. For example, the daily intake of 125 g of a yogurt fortified with 10 µg vitamin D3 and 800 mg calcium has been shown to provide a greater degree of protection from accelerated bone resorption in elderly women who are institutionalized (Bonjour et al. 2013) and living in community-dwelling home settings compared with a nonfortified yogurt (Bonjour et al. 2015). The consumption of a standard portion of commercial fortified yogurt providing 200 µg vitamin D and 400 mg of calcium is thought to be a cost-effective strategy to prevent osteoporotic fractures in all women with low bone mineral densities, as well as all adults in the general population over the age of 70 (Ethgen et al. 2015).

12.3 MECHANISMS OF ACTION

Dietary intake is important to supply the materials needed for bone synthesis (Heaney 2000). Yogurt and dairy products contain high amounts of calcium and phosphorus per unit of energy compared with other typical foods in an adult diet, which are the main constituents of bone mineral (along with protein). Bone contains about 99% and 80% of the body's entire supply of Ca and P, respectively, and, interestingly, the bone mass ratio of Ca:P is about 2.2, close to that measured in human milk (Heaney 2000, Bonjour 2011). Calcium intake, its turnover, and its rate of absorption and excretion determine its availability for growth and bone development (Lanou et al.

2005). In postmenopausal women, high calcium intakes reduce the elevated bone remodeling that follows menopause in women by suppressing parathyroid hormone (PTH) secretion (Heaney 2009).

Vitamin D supports calcium absorption and thereby maintains the level of calcium and phosphorus in the blood. Moreover, vitamin D stimulates osteoclast formation, differentiation, and bone resorption. The immunoregulatory mechanisms by which vitamin D mediates muscle function may also have a positive impact on bone health (Laird et al. 2010). The maintenance of bone strength is dependent on the maintenance of muscle mass, which exerts a trophic effect on bone by applying force during muscle contractions (Surdykowski et al. 2010). Vitamin D has been shown to increase insulin-like growth factor 2 (IGF-2) production and to upregulate insulin-like growth factor binding protein (IGFBP) 5 messenger RNA (mRNA), which is important in bone growth (Heaney 2009).

Dietary protein could also stimulate IGF-1 production (Conigrave et al. 2008). Moreover, research supports the notion that protein may play an important role in the maintenance of bone health by other mechanisms, for example via calcium absorption (Gueguen and Pointillart 2000) and muscle strength and mass. Calcium intake may influence the effect of dietary protein on the skeleton (Dawson-Hughes and Harris 2002). Human studies have shown the beneficial effects of milk protein on bone metabolism and density (Kumegawa 2006). Casein phosphopeptide and lactoferrin could play a beneficial role on bone health (Uenishi 2006). Lactoperoxidase has been identified as the predominant inhibitor of osteoclastogenesis in milk basic protein (Morita et al. 2011). More studies are necessary to verify the preventive effect of an adequate protein intake on osteoporosis in different populations (Kim et al. 2013).

Potassium, magnesium, zinc, vitamin A, and vitamin C are other essential nutrients that are vital to bone health (WHO 2007). In the United States, a diet low in dairy products will most of the time be low in one or more of the nutrients needed for healthy bones (Heaney 2009). Additional properties of yogurt potentially explaining its protective benefits against hip fractures are based on the increased bioavailability of calcium and vitamin D in yogurt through mechanisms that include the reduced lactose content, increasing digestibility; the reduced pH of small intestine; and the bacterial culture modulation of gut microbiota (Rizzoli 2014).

12.4 CONCLUSIONS

- The importance of calcium in the development and maintenance of healthy bone is well accepted. However, there are concerns over high levels of calcium intake, but excess calcium from food sources is rare.
- Although literature supporting the beneficial effects of dairy products on bone health and osteoporosis prevention is abundant, it remains inconsistent.
- Given that yogurt is an excellent source of calcium and other nutrients that promote bone health, the regular intake of yogurt as well as other dairy products during adolescence and young adulthood could have positive effects on bone mineral mass gain.

- The public health burden of hip fractures associated with a low calcium intake is likely to be improved by dairy consumption, of which yogurt may play an important role.

REFERENCES

Bahtiri, E., H. Islami, R. Hoxha, H. Q. Bytyqi, F. Sermaxhaj, and E. Halimi. 2014. Calcium and dairy products consumption and association with total hip bone mineral density in women from Kosovo. *Med Arch* 68 (4):259–62.

Bolland, M. J., A. Grey, A. Avenell, G. D. Gamble, and I. R. Reid. 2011. Calcium supplements with or without vitamin D and risk of cardiovascular events: Reanalysis of the Women's Health Initiative limited access dataset and meta-analysis. *BMJ* 342:d2040.

Bolland, M. J., W. Leung, V. Tai, S. Bastin, G. D. Gamble, A. Grey, and I. R. Reid. 2015. Calcium intake and risk of fracture: Systematic review. *BMJ* 351:h4580.

Bonjour, J. P. 2011. Calcium and phosphate: A duet of ions playing for bone health. *J Am Coll Nutr* 30 (5 Suppl 1):438S–48S.

Bonjour, J. P., V. Benoit, S. Atkin, and S. Walrand. 2015. Fortification of yogurts with vitamin D and calcium enhances the inhibition of serum parathyroid hormone and bone resorption markers: A double blind randomized controlled trial in women over 60 living in a community dwelling home. *J Nutr Health Aging* 19 (5):563–69.

Bonjour, J. P., V. Benoit, F. Payen, and M. Kraenzlin. 2013. Consumption of yogurts fortified in vitamin D and calcium reduces serum parathyroid hormone and markers of bone resorption: A double-blind randomized controlled trial in institutionalized elderly women. *J Clin Endocrinol Metab* 98 (7):2915–21.

Bonjour, J. P., M. Brandolini-Bunlon, Y. Boirie, F. Morel-Laporte, V. Braesco, M. C. Bertiere, and J. C. Souberbielle. 2008. Inhibition of bone turnover by milk intake in postmenopausal women. *Br J Nutr* 100 (4):866–74.

Bonneux, L. 2014. Unaccounted sex differences undermine association between milk intake and risk of mortality and fractures. *BMJ* 349:7012.

Breslau, N. A. 1994. Calcium, estrogen, and progestin in the treatment of osteoporosis. *Rheum Dis Clin North Am* 20 (3):691–716.

Cadogan, J., R. Eastell, N. Jones, and M. E. Barker. 1997. Milk intake and bone mineral acquisition in adolescent girls: Randomised, controlled intervention trial. *BMJ* 315 (7118):1255–60.

Celotti, F., and A. Bignamini. 1999. Dietary calcium and mineral/vitamin supplementation: A controversial problem. *J Int Med Res* 27 (1):1–14.

Conigrave, A. D., E. M. Brown, and R. Rizzoli. 2008. Dietary protein and bone health: Roles of amino acid-sensing receptors in the control of calcium metabolism and bone homeostasis. *Annu Rev Nutr* 28:131–55.

Dawson-Hughes, B., and S. S. Harris. 2002. Calcium intake influences the association of protein intake with rates of bone loss in elderly men and women. *Am J Clin Nutr* 75 (4):773–79.

EFSA Panel of Dietetic Products, Nutrition and Allergies. 2009. Scientific opinion on the substantiation of health claims related to calcium and maintenance of bones and teeth (ID 224, 230, 231, 354, 3099), muscle function and neurotransmission (ID 226, 227, 230, 235), blood coagulation (ID 230, 236), energy-yielding metabolism (ID 234), function of digestive enzymes (ID 355), and maintenance of normal blood pressure (ID 225, 385, 1419) pursuant to Article 13(1) of Regulation (EC) no 1924/20061. *EFSA J* 7 (9):1210.

El Maghraoui, A., M. Ghazi, S. Gassim, I. Ghozlani, A. Mounach, A. Rezqi, and M. Dehhaoui. 2010. Risk factors of osteoporosis in healthy Moroccan men. *BMC Musculoskelet Disord* 11:148.

Ethgen, O., M. Hiligsmann, N. Burlet, and J. Y. Reginster. 2015. Cost-effectiveness of personalized supplementation with vitamin D-rich dairy products in the prevention of osteoporotic fractures. *Osteoporos Int* 27 (1): 301–28.

Fenton, T. R., and D. A. Hanley. 2006. Calcium, dairy products, and bone health in children and young adults: An inaccurate conclusion. *Pediatrics* 117 (1):259–60; author reply 260–61.

Gueguen, L., and A. Pointillart. 2000. The bioavailability of dietary calcium. *J Am Coll Nutr* 19 (2 Suppl):119S–36S.

Harvey, N., E. Dennison, and C. Cooper. 2010. Osteoporosis: Impact on health and economics. *Nat Rev Rheumatol* 6 (2):99–105.

He, M., Y. X. Yang, H. Han, J. H. Men, L. H. Bian, and G. D. Wang. 2005. Effects of yogurt supplementation on the growth of preschool children in Beijing suburbs. *Biomed Environ Sci* 18 (3):192–97.

Heaney, R. P. 2000. Calcium, dairy products and osteoporosis. *J Am Coll Nutr* 19 (2 Suppl):83S–99S.

Heaney, R. P. 2008. Calcium supplementation and incident kidney stone risk: A systematic review. *J Am Coll Nutr* 27 (5):519–27.

Heaney, R. P. 2009. Dairy and bone health. *J Am Coll Nutr* 28 (Suppl 1):82S–90S.

Heaney, R. P., S. Abrams, B. Dawson-Hughes, A. Looker, R. Marcus, V. Matkovic, and C. Weaver. 2000. Peak bone mass. *Osteoporos Int* 11 (12):985–1009.

Heaney, R. P., K. Rafferty, and M. S. Dowell. 2002. Effect of yogurt on a urinary marker of bone resorption in postmenopausal women. *J Am Diet Assoc* 102 (11):1672–74.

Heaney, R. P., and C. M. Weaver. 2005. Newer perspectives on calcium nutrition and bone quality. *J Am Coll Nutr* 24 (6 Suppl):574S–81S.

Hettinga, K. 2014. Study used wrong assumption about galactose content of fermented dairy products. *BMJ* 349:g7000.

Hill, T. R. 2014. Vitamin D status, bone fracture, and mortality. *BMJ* 349:g6995.

Holloway, K. L., G. Bucki-Smith, A. G. Morse, S. L. Brennan-Olsen, M. A. Kotowicz, D. J. Moloney, K. M. Sanders, et al. 2015. Humeral fractures in south-eastern Australia: Epidemiology and risk factors. *Calcif Tissue Int* 97 (5):453–65.

Huncharek, M., J. Muscat, and B. Kupelnick. 2008. Impact of dairy products and dietary calcium on bone-mineral content in children: Results of a meta-analysis. *Bone* 43 (2):312–21.

International Osteoporosis Foundation. 2015. Osteoporosis & musculoskeletal disorders: Osteoporosis—prevention. International Osteoporosis Foundation Accessed March 15. http://www.iofbonehealth.org/preventing-osteoporosis.

IOM. 1997. *Dietary Reference Intakes: Calcium, Phosphorus, Magnesium, Vitamin D and Fluoride*. Edited by Food and Nutrition Board. Washington, DC: National Academy Press.

Jackson, R. D., A. Z. LaCroix, M. Gass, R. B. Wallace, J. Robbins, C. E. Lewis, T. Bassford, et al. 2006. Calcium plus vitamin D supplementation and the risk of fractures. *N Engl J Med* 354 (7):669–83.

Jha, R. M., A. Mithal, N. Malhotra, and E. M. Brown. 2010. Pilot case-control investigation of risk factors for hip fractures in the urban Indian population. *BMC Musculoskelet Disord* 11:49.

Kanis, J. A. 1994. Assessment of fracture risk and its application to screening for postmenopausal osteoporosis: Synopsis of a WHO report. WHO Study Group. *Osteoporos Int* 4 (6):368–81.

Kim, J., B. Kim, H. Lee, H. Choi, and C. Won. 2013. The relationship between prevalence of osteoporosis and proportion of daily protein intake. *Korean J Fam Med* 34 (1):43–48.

Kumegawa, M. 2006. Prevention of osteoporosis by foods and dietary supplements. Bone reinforcement factor in milk: milk basic protein (MBP). *Clin Calcium* 16 (10):1624–31.

Labos, C., and J. Brophy. 2014. Statistical problems with study on milk intake and mortality and fractures. *BMJ* 349:g6991.

Laird, E., M. Ward, E. McSorley, J. J. Strain, and J. Wallace. 2010. Vitamin D and bone health: Potential mechanisms. *Nutrients* 2 (7):693–724.

Lana, A., F. Rodriguez-Artalejo, and E. Lopez-Garcia. 2015. Dairy consumption and risk of frailty in older adults: A prospective cohort study. *J Am Geriatr Soc* 63 (9):1852–60.

Lanou, A. J. 2009. Should dairy be recommended as part of a healthy vegetarian diet? Counterpoint. *Am J Clin Nutr* 89 (5):1638S–42S.

Lanou, A. J., S. E. Berkow, and N. D. Barnard. 2005. Calcium, dairy products, and bone health in children and young adults: A reevaluation of the evidence. *Pediatrics* 115 (3):736–43.

Lappe, J. M., and R. P. Heaney. 2012. Why randomized controlled trials of calcium and vitamin D sometimes fail. *Dermatoendocrinol* 4 (2):95–100.

Lee, C., and D. S. Majka. 2006. Is calcium and vitamin D supplementation overrated? *J Am Diet Assoc* 106 (7):1032–34.

Lotters, F. J., I. Lenoir-Wijnkoop, P. Fardellone, R. Rizzoli, E. Rocher, and M. J. Poley. 2013. Dairy foods and osteoporosis: An example of assessing the health-economic impact of food products. *Osteoporos Int* 24 (1):139–50.

Malhotra, N., and A. Mithal. 2008. Osteoporosis in Indians. *Indian J Med Res* 127 (3):263–68.

Manios, Y., G. Moschonis, G. Trovas, and G. P. Lyritis. 2007. Changes in biochemical indexes of bone metabolism and bone mineral density after a 12-mo dietary intervention program: The postmenopausal health study. *Am J Clin Nutr* 86 (3):781–89.

McCarron, D. A., and R. P. Heaney. 2004. Estimated healthcare savings associated with adequate dairy food intake. *Am J Hypertens* 17 (1):88–97.

Michaelsson, K., A. Wolk, S. Langenskiold, S. Basu, E. Warensjo Lemming, H. Melhus, and L. Byberg. 2014. Milk intake and risk of mortality and fractures in women and men: Cohort studies. *BMJ* 349:g6015.

Morita, Y., A. Ono, A. Serizawa, K. Yogo, N. Ishida-Kitagawa, T. Takeya, and T. Ogawa. 2011. Purification and identification of lactoperoxidase in milk basic proteins as an inhibitor of osteoclastogenesis. *J Dairy Sci* 94 (5):2270–79.

Moschonis, G., S. Kanellakis, N. Papaioannou, A. Schaafsma, and Y. Manios. 2011. Possible site-specific effect of an intervention combining nutrition and lifestyle counselling with consumption of fortified dairy products on bone mass: The Postmenopausal Health Study II. *J Bone Miner Metab* 29 (4):501–506.

Moschonis, G., and Y. Manios. 2006. Skeletal site-dependent response of bone mineral density and quantitative ultrasound parameters following a 12-month dietary intervention using dairy products fortified with calcium and vitamin D: The Postmenopausal Health Study. *Br J Nutr* 96 (6):1140–48.

Price, C. T., J. R. Langford, and F. A. Liporace. 2012. Essential nutrients for bone health and a review of their availability in the average North American diet. *Open Orthop J* 6:143–49.

Rabenda, V., O. Bruyère, and J. Y. Reginster. 2011. Relationship between bone mineral density changes and risk of fractures among patients receiving calcium with or without vitamin D supplementation: A meta-regression. *Osteoporos Int* 22 (3):893–901.

Radavelli-Bagatini, S., K. Zhu, J. R. Lewis, and R. L. Prince. 2014. Dairy food intake, peripheral bone structure, and muscle mass in elderly ambulatory women. *J Bone Miner Res* 29 (7):1691–700.

Rizzoli, R. 2014. Dairy products, yogurts, and bone health. *Am J Clin Nutr* 99 (5):1256S–62S.

Rizzoli, R., M. L. Bianchi, M. Garabedian, H. A. McKay, and L. A. Moreno. 2010. Maximizing bone mineral mass gain during growth for the prevention of fractures in the adolescents and the elderly. *Bone* 46 (2):294–305.

Roux, C., H. A. Bischoff-Ferrari, S. E. Papapoulos, A. E. de Papp, J. A. West, and R. Bouillon. 2008. New insights into the role of vitamin D and calcium in osteoporosis management: An expert roundtable discussion. *Curr Med Res Opin* 24 (5):1363–70.

Sahni, S., K. M. Mangano, K. L. Tucker, D. P. Kiel, V. A. Casey, and M. T. Hannan. 2014. Protective association of milk intake on the risk of hip fracture: Results from the Framingham Original Cohort. *J Bone Miner Res* 29 (8):1756–62.

Sahni, S., K. L. Tucker, D. P. Kiel, L. Quach, V. A. Casey, and M. T. Hannan. 2013. Milk and yogurt consumption are linked with higher bone mineral density but not with hip fracture: The Framingham Offspring Study. *Arch Osteoporos* 8 (1–2):119.

Spangler, M., B. B. Phillips, M. B. Ross, and K. G. Moores. 2011. Calcium supplementation in postmenopausal women to reduce the risk of osteoporotic fractures. *Am J Health Syst Pharm* 68 (4):309–18.

Sunyecz, J. A. 2008. The use of calcium and vitamin D in the management of osteoporosis. *Ther Clin Risk Manag* 4 (4):827–36.

Surdykowski, A. K., A. M. Kenny, K. L. Insogna, and J. E. Kerstetter. 2010. Optimizing bone health in older adults: The importance of dietary protein. *Aging health* 6 (3):345–57.

Uenishi, K. 2006. Prevention of osteoporosis by foods and dietary supplements. Prevention of osteoporosis by milk and dairy products. *Clin Calcium* 16 (10):1606–14.

Wadolowska, L., K. Sobas, J. W. Szczepanska, M. A. Slowinska, M. Czlapka-Matyasik, and E. Niedzwiedzka. 2013. Dairy products, dietary calcium and bone health: Possibility of prevention of osteoporosis in women: The Polish experience. *Nutrients* 5 (7):2684–707.

Weaver, C. M. 2008. The role of nutrition on optimizing peak bone mass. *Asia Pac J Clin Nutr* 17 (Suppl 1):135–37.

WHO. 2007. WHO Scientific Group on the Assessment of Osteoporosis at Primary Healthcare Level. Brussels: WHO.

General Conclusion

The compilation of literature presented in this book characterizes yogurt as a dairy food that is rich in high-quality proteins, vitamins, and minerals, as well as functional peptides, lipids, and lactic acid bacteria. The combination of these nutrients and ferments creates a food matrix that may confer beneficial properties to this dairy product, which contribute to differentiating it from its base ingredient, milk. The role of yogurt as part of a balanced diet is evidenced by its inclusion by health authorities in food-based guidelines across the globe and regular yogurt consumption contributes to the intake of key micronutrients such as calcium and potassium, which are often consumed in suboptimal quantities (Webb et al. 2014). Based on yogurt's nutrient composition and according to numerous nutrient profiling tools, it scores highly as a nutrient-dense food. Sweetened whole-fat yogurt, however, is often given a lower nutrient density score due its saturated fat and added sugar content, even though it is rich in nutrients. Yogurt's nutrient profile makes it a very attractive dairy food that can be promoted as part of a balanced diet; a single 125 g portion of low-fat fruit yogurt can provide significant proportions of recommended dietary allowances for calcium, phosphorus, and vitamin B12. Furthermore, yogurt is a food that has been consistently identified within healthy dietary patterns among diverse populations (Camilleri et al. 2013, Cormier et al. 2016, Kashino et al. 2015), and its intake is often associated with healthy lifestyle factors such as physical activity (D'Addezio et al. 2015). These associations make yogurt a potential indicator for both healthy diets and healthy lifestyles. With regard to the effects of yogurt consumption on cardiometabolic diseases and other health conditions, the summary of evidence presented in this compilation indicates that:

- The benefits of yogurt consumption on lactose digestion have been established. However, more research is needed to investigate the effects of yogurt on other digestive ailments (e.g., diarrhea).
- There is consistent epidemiological evidence that yogurt consumption reduces type 2 diabetes (T2D) risk, as revealed by multiple meta-analyses of numerous large, high-quality prospective cohort studies. There is little known about any mechanisms responsible for the beneficial associations seen in observational studies.
- Based on individual observational studies, there is promising evidence for yogurt consumption with regard to weight maintenance and reduced adiposity, although more research is needed. In particular, the impacts of replacing high-fat, high-energy snacks with yogurt and the intake of yogurt components (e.g., calcium) on energy balance warrant further investigation.
- There is growing but still insufficient evidence on the relationships between yogurt consumption and hypertension and cardiovascular diseases. Future studies investigating such relationships need to distinguish yogurt from other fermented milks and from other low-fat (or whole-fat) dairy products

to build a consistent, evidence-based case for the cardiovascular benefits of yogurt. A better understanding of the bioactive components in yogurt that may act on blood pressure and the cardiovascular system is also needed.
- Current evidence for the impact of yogurt consumption on metabolic syndrome is mixed and future studies need to use more consistent diagnostic criteria and to compare similar age groups.
- No direct evidence links yogurt consumption to improved bone health or a reduced risk of osteoporosis; however, yogurt is a source of dietary nutrients that are important for bone mass development and maintenance (e.g., protein and calcium).
- There is inconsistent or inadequate evidence to link yogurt consumption to the protection of colorectal and breast cancers, or to the increased risk of prostate cancer.
- There is insufficient evidence to draw any clear conclusions on the relationships between yogurt and immune reactions, or allergy and atopic disease.

Overall, regular yogurt intake appears to provide sustainable health benefits to consumers, but further studies are needed to identify the components that are responsible for the health effects of yogurt and the underlying mechanisms of action. Further research needs to be conducted to fill research gaps and strengthen the quality of information by (1) studying children and adolescent populations; (2) conducting meta-analyses of prospective cohort studies; (3) conducting long-term, well-designed randomized controlled trials; and (4) elucidating potential mechanisms related to appetite control, energy expenditure, and the regulation of metabolism (e.g., adipose tissue and glucose). Randomized controlled trials and animal studies are especially needed to better understand the beneficial associations seen in observational studies, to determine whether a causal relationship exists between yogurt consumption and the reduced risk of certain cardiometabolic diseases (e.g., T2D), and to identify which mechanisms are implicated. Additionally, studies examining the eating behaviors of yogurt consumers would give a better understanding of the associations between yogurt consumers and their improved diet quality, healthier lifestyles, and differences from nonconsumers. Considering the importance of food variety in a balanced diet and the physiological needs of individuals, additional studies would be useful to determine the dose and type of yogurt required to exert a significant impact on disease prevention.

REFERENCES

Camilleri, G. M., E. O. Verger, J. F. Huneau, F. Carpentier, C. Dubuisson, and F. Mariotti. 2013. Plant and animal protein intakes are differently associated with nutrient adequacy of the diet of French adults. *J Nutr* 143 (9):1466–73.

Cormier, H., É. Thifault, V. Garneau, A. Tremblay, V. Drapeau, L. Pérusse, and M. C. Vohl. 2016. Association between yogurt consumption, dietary patterns, and cardio-metabolic risk factors. *Eur J Nutr* 55 (2):577–87.

D'Addezio, L., L. Mistura, S. Sette, and A. Turrini. 2015. Sociodemographic and lifestyle characteristics of yogurt consumers in Italy: Results from the INRAN-SCAI 2005–06 survey. *Med J Nutr Metab* 8:119–29.

Kashino, I., A. Nanri, K. Kurotani, S. Akter, K. Yasuda, M. Sato, H. Hayabuchi, et al. 2015. Association of dietary patterns with serum adipokines among Japanese: A cross-sectional study. *Nutr J* 14:58.

Webb, D., S. M. Donovan, and S. N. Meydani. 2014. The role of yogurt in improving the quality of the American diet and meeting dietary guidelines. *Nutr Rev* 72 (3):180–89.

Index

2010 Dietary Guidelines for Americans, 117

A

ACE, *see* Angiotensin-converting-enzyme (ACE)
Acquired lactase deficiency, 116
Acute diarrhea, 122, 123–124
Adaptive/acquired immune system, 139
Adolescents
    cardiovascular diseases in, 91
    and children
        bone mineralization and osteoporosis in, 169–170
        type 2 diabetes in, 68
        weight and obesity in, 46–51
    metabolic syndrome in, 104–105
Adults, 126
    antibiotic-associated diarrhea in, 126
    bone mineralization and osteoporosis in, 170–172
        clinical studies, 172
        cross-sectional and case-control studies, 170
        prospective studies, 171–172
        systematic reviews, 172
    cardiovascular diseases in, 91–95
        clinical studies, 93–94
        cross-sectional studies, 91–92
        meta-analyses and systematic reviews, 94–95
        prospective studies, 92–93
    hypertension in, 81–84
        cross-sectional studies, 81
        meta-analyses and reviews
        prospective studies
    metabolic syndrome in, 105–108
        cross-sectional studies, 105–106
        prospective cohort studies, 106–108
    type 2 diabetes in, 68–71
        cross-sectional studies, 68
        meta-analyses and systematic reviews, 70–71
        prospective cohort studies, 68–70
    weight and obesity in, 51–56
        clinical studies, 55
        cross-sectional studies, 51–52
        prospective studies, 52–55
        reviews, 55–56
AICR, *see* American Institute for Cancer Research (AICR)
Allergic asthma, 161–162
Allergic rhinitis, and rhinopathy, 160–161
Allergy, and atopic diseases, 159–163
    allergic asthma, 161–162
    allergic rhinitis, 160–161
    eczema and dermatitis, 159–160
    mechanisms of action, 162–163
Alpha-lactalbumin, 57
Alpha-Tocopherol, Beta-Carotene Cancer Prevention Study, 92
American Heart Association, 106
American Institute for Cancer Research (AICR), 145, 150, 151, 153
Angiotensin-converting-enzyme (ACE), 84–85
Antibiotic-associated diarrhea, 125–126
    studies in adults, 126
    studies in children, 125–126
Atopic dermatitis, 159–160
ATTICA study, 68
Australian Diabetes, Obesity and Lifestyle Study (AusDiab), 70

B

Bacteria, on cholesterol, 96–97
The Bald Soprano, xv
B cells, 139
Bioactive peptides, 7–8
Bioavailability, 12–13
Biological quality, 5
Body mass index (BMI), 46
Bone mineralization, and osteoporosis, 167–180
    mechanisms of action, 172–173
    studies in children and adolescents, 169–170
    studies in older adults, 170–172
        clinical studies, 172
        cross-sectional and case-control studies, 170
        prospective studies, 171–172
        systematic reviews, 172
Brazilian Longitudinal Study of Adult Health, 106
Breast cancer, 150–153
    case-control studies, 151–152
    mechanisms of action, 152–153
    prospective cohort studies, 152
    reviews, 152
Breath hydrogen, 118

C

CAIFOS, *see* Calcium Intake Fracture Outcome Study (CAIFOS)
Calcium, 11, 12, 26, 32–33, 72, 82, 85–86, 108, 117, 147, 148, 150, 169
Calcium Intake Fracture Outcome Study (CAIFOS), 171
Calcium supplementation, 167–168
Cancer, 145–155
    breast, 150–153
        case-control studies, 151–152
        mechanisms of action, 152–153
        prospective cohort studies, 152
        reviews, 152
    colorectal, 145–150
        clinical studies, 149
        mechanisms of action, 149
        observational studies, 146–149
    prostate, 153–155
        case-control studies, 153–154
        mechanisms of action, 154–155
        meta-analyses, 154
        prospective cohort studies, 154
Carasso, Isaac, xiii
Carbohydrates, 3–5
CARDIA, *see* Coronary Artery Risk Development in Young Adults (CARDIA)
Cardiovascular diseases (CVD), 9, 89–97
    mechanisms of action, 95–97
        effect of bacteria on cholesterol, 96–97
        effect of lipids and other nutrients, 95–96
    studies in adolescents, 91
    studies in adults, 91–95
        clinical studies, 93–94
        cross-sectional studies, 91–92
        meta-analyses and systematic reviews, 94–95
        prospective studies, 92–93
Cardiovascular Health Study, 74
Casein, and whey, 5–7
CCA-IMT, *see* Common carotid artery intima-media thickness (CCA-IMT)
CD4+, 141
CD8+, 140
CHD, *see* Coronary heart disease (CHD)
Children
    and adolescents
        bone mineralization and osteoporosis in, 169–170
        type 2 diabetes in, 68
        weight and obesity in, 46–51
    antibiotic-associated diarrhea in, 125–126

Cholesterol, 96–97
CLA, *see* Conjugated linoleic acid (CLA)
Codex Alimentarius, xi, xxi
Colon cancer, 147
Colorectal cancer (CRC), 145–150
    clinical studies, 149
    mechanisms of action, 149
    observational studies, 146–149
        case-control studies, 146–147
        meta-analyses, 149
        prospective cohort studies, 147–149
Colorectal polyps, 146–147
Common carotid artery intima-media thickness (CCA-IMT), 92
Congenital lactase deficiency, 113, 116
Conjugated linoleic acid (CLA), 9, 58, 153
Coronary Artery Risk Development in Young Adults (CARDIA), 69, 82, 106
Coronary heart disease (CHD), 89, 92–93, 95
CRC, *see* Colorectal cancer (CRC)
Cure de Yaourt, xiii
CVD, *see* Cardiovascular diseases (CVD)
Cytokine production, 139–140

D

Dairy, and yogurt
    consumption, 26–28
    food-based dietary guidelines for, 23–25
Dairy products, 33, 34, 169
Dairy proteins, and peptides, 84–85
DASH, *see* Dietary Approaches to Stop Hypertension (DASH)
DESIR, *see* Epidemiological Study in the Insulin Resistance Syndrome (DESIR)
Deukmedjian, Aram, xiii
DGAC, *see* Dietary Guidelines Advisory Committee (DGAC)
DGAI, *see* Dietary Guidelines Adherence Index (DGAI)
Diarrhea, 122–127
    antibiotic-associated, 125–126
        studies in adults, 126
        studies in children, 125–126c
    mechanisms of action, 126–127
    treatment of acute, 123–124
    treatment of persistent, 124–125
Dietary Approaches to Stop Hypertension (DASH), 81
Dietary Guidelines Adherence Index (DGAI), 106
Dietary Guidelines Advisory Committee (DGAC), 71, 81
Dietary patterns, 34–35
Dose–response analysis, 71
DSM Food Specialities, xv

Index

E

E3N, *see* Etude Epidémiologique auprès des femmes de la MGEN (E3N)
Eczema, 159–160
EFSA, *see* European Food Safety Authority (EFSA)
EPIC, *see* European Prospective Investigation into Cancer and Nutrition (EPIC)
Epidemiological Study in the Insulin Resistance Syndrome (DESIR), 103
Etude Epidémiologique auprès des femmes de la MGEN (E3N), 148
European Food Safety Authority (EFSA), 119–120, 169
European Prospective Investigation into Cancer and Nutrition (EPIC), 69, 70, 83, 93, 148, 149
Exopolysaccharides, 5

F

Fatty acids, 73–75
Fermentation, and ferments, xxi, 75
Fermented milk, xii, xiii
Food processing, and lactic fermentation, 7–9, 10, 11–12, 14
    digestion and generation of bioactive peptides, 7–8
    interaction with minerals, 8–9
Food Standards Agency, 28
Fortified dairy products, 168–169
Framingham Heart Study Offspring Cohort, 54, 65, 83, 106, 171
François I, King, xiii
Fresh yogurt, 119
Fruit-containing yogurt, 5

G

GALT, *see* Gut-associated lymphoid tissue (GALT)
Geelong Osteoporosis Study, 170
German Nutrition Society, 23
Glycemic load, 72–73
Glycomacropeptide (GMP), 57
Grigorov, Stamen, xiii
Gut-associated lymphoid tissue (GALT), 139
Gut health, yogurt and, 113–131
    lactose deficiency, malabsorption, and intolerance, 113–122
        mechanisms of action, 120–122
        studies in adults, 118–120
        studies in children, 117–118
    microbiota, 128
    treatment of diarrhea, 122–127
        acute, 123–124
        antibiotic-associated, 125–126
        mechanisms of action, 126–127
        persistent, 124–125
        viability of yogurt bacteria, 128–131
Gut microbiota, 58

H

HDL, *see* High-density lipoprotein (HDL)
Healthy Eating Index, 30
Healthy Lifestyle in Europe by Nutrition in Adolescence (HELENA), 51, 91
Helper T cells, 139
High-density lipoprotein (HDL), 89, 93, 94, 103, 106
Homeostatic model assessment (HOMA), 68
Hoorn Study, 68, 83, 105
Human studies, 139–143
    cytokine production, 139–140
    natural killer cell activity, 140
    phagocytic activity, 141
    T and B lymphocyte function, 140–141
Hypertension, 81–86
    mechanisms of action, 84–86
        effect of Ca, K, Mg, and lipids, 85–86
        effect of dairy proteins and peptides, 84–85
    studies in adults, 81–84
        cross-sectional studies, 81
        meta-analyses and reviews, 83–84
        prospective studies, 82–83
Hypolactasia, *see* Primary lactase deficiency

I

IDF, *see* International Diabetes Federation (IDF)
IFN-γ, *see* Interferon-gamma (IFN-γ)
IgE, *see* Immunoglobulin E (IgE)
IGF-1, *see* Insulin-like growth factor 1 (IGF-1)
IHD, *see* Ischemic heart disease (IHD)
Immune responses, 139–155
    human studies, 139–143
        cytokine production, 139–140
        natural killer cell activity, 140
        phagocytic activity, 141
        T and B lymphocyte function, 140–141
    mechanisms of action, 141–142
Immunoglobulin E (IgE), 160, 162
INFOGENE, 52
Insulin-like growth factor 1 (IGF-1), 153
Interferon-gamma (IFN-γ), 140, 141, 142, 162
International Diabetes Federation (IDF), 65, 103
International Osteoporosis Foundation, 167
IOM, *see* U.S. Institute of Medicine (IOM)
Ionesco, Eugène, xv

IPP, *see* Isoleucine-proline-proline (IPP)
Ischemic heart disease (IHD), 92
Isoleucine-proline-proline (IPP), 84

J

Japan Collaborative Cohort Study, 148
Japan Public Health Center-based Prospective Study, 69
Jichi Medical School Cohort Study, 148

K

Korean National Health and Nutrition Examination Study, 52

L

LAB, *see* Lactic acid bacteria (LAB)
Lactic acid bacteria (LAB), 14–15, 72, 127, 139, 142
Lactic fermentation, food processing and, xii, 7–9, 10, 11–12, 14
    digestion and generation of bioactive peptides, 7–8
    interaction with minerals, 8–9
Lactobacillus acidophilus, 129
Lactobacillus bulgaricus, xiii, 7, 128, 129–130
Lactobacillus delbrueckii, xxi
Lactoferrin, 7
Lactose, 3, 12
Lactose deficiency, and intolerance, 113–122
    mechanisms of action, 120–122
        activity of yogurt bacteria, 120–121
        colonic processing of lactose and adaptation, 121
        physical properties, 121
    studies in adults, 118–120
    studies in children, 117–118
LDL, *see* Low-density lipoprotein (LDL)
Lifestyle, and sociodemographic factors, 35–36
LIM, *see* Nutrients to Limit (LIM)
Lipids, 9–10
    effect of Ca, K, Mg, and, 85–86
    food processing and lactic fermentation, 10
    and other nutrients, 95–96
    yogurt, 57–58
Low-density lipoprotein (LDL), 89, 93, 94, 95
Lymphocytes, 139

M

Malmo Diet and Cancer study, 74
Metabolic syndrome (MetS), 103–109
    mechanisms of action, 108
    studies in adolescents, 104–105
    studies in adults, 105–108
        cross-sectional studies, 105–106
        prospective cohort studies, 106–108
Metchnikoff, Elie, xiii
MetS, *see* Metabolic syndrome (MetS)
Micro-, and macronutrients, 56–58
Microbiota, 128
Milk, xi–xii
Milk proteins, 5, 7
Minerals, 10–13
    bioavailability, 12–13
    food processing and lactic fermentation, 11–12
Monounsaturated fatty acids (MUFA), 9
MUFA, *see* Monounsaturated fatty acids (MUFA)

N

National Cholesterol Education Program, 106
National Diet and Nutrition Survey, 27
National Health and Nutrition Examination Survey (NHANES), 51, 68, 105–106, 154
National Heart, Lung, and Blood Institute, 106
National Institute of Nutrition, 23
National Institutes of Health (NIH), 113, 117
Natural killer (NK) cells, 140
Netherlands Cohort Study (NLCS), 92
NHANES, *see* National Health and Nutrition Exam Survey (NHANES)
NIH, *see* National Institutes of Health (NIH)
NK, *see* Natural killer (NK) cells
NLCS, *see* Netherlands Cohort Study (NLCS)
NRF9.3, *see* Nutrient Rich Food score (NRF9.3)
N-telepeptide, 172
Nutrient adequacy, 30–34
Nutrient Adequacy Score for Individual Foods (SAIN), 28, 30
Nutrient density, 28–30
Nutrient Rich Food score (NRF9.3), 28, 30
Nutrients to Limit (LIM), 28, 30
Nutrition Evidence Library, 81

O

Observation of Cardiovascular Risk Factors in Luxembourg, 52
OCTT, *see* Orocecal transit time (OCTT)
Ofcom, *see* Office of Communications (Ofcom)
Office of Communications (Ofcom), 28, 30
Orocecal transit time (OCTT), 119, 121
Osmotic diarrhea, 122
Osteoporosis, *see* Bone mineralization, and osteoporosis

P

PANDiet, *see* Probability of Adequate Nutrient Intake (PANDiet)

Pasteur, Louis, xiii
Pasteurized yogurt, 118
PCR, see Polymerase chain reaction (PCR) technique
Peptides, 73
Persistent diarrhea, 122, 124–125
Phagocytic activity, 141
Phosphopeptides, 12
Phosphorus, 11, 155
Plain yogurt, 31–32
Polymerase chain reaction (PCR) technique, 130
Polyunsaturated fatty acids (PUFA), 9
PREDIMED, see Prevención con Dieta Mediterránea (PREDIMED)
Prevención con Dieta Mediterránea (PREDIMED), 70, 83, 95, 107–108
Primary lactase deficiency, 116
Probability of Adequate Nutrient Intake (PANDiet), 34
Prostate cancer, 153–155
    case-control studies, 153–154
    mechanisms of action, 154–155
    meta-analyses, 154
    prospective cohort studies, 154
Proteins, 5–9, 73
    biological quality, 5
    casein and whey, 5–7
    food processing and lactic fermentation, 7–9
        digestion and generation of bioactive peptides, 7–8
        interaction with minerals, 8–9
PUFA, see Polyunsaturated fatty acids (PUFA)

R

RDA, see Recommended dietary allowance (RDA)
Reaven, G. M., 103
Recommended dietary allowance (RDA), 23, 26

S

SAIN, see Nutrient Adequacy Score for Individual Foods (SAIN)
Satiety, 56, 57
Saturated fatty acids (SFAs), 9, 74, 89, 90, 96
SCFA, see Short-chain fatty acids (SCFA)
Secondary hypolactasia, see Acquired lactase deficiency
Secretory diarrhea, 122
Seguimiento Universidad de Navarra (SUN), 36, 54, 107
SFAs, see Saturated fatty acids (SFAs)
Short-chain fatty acids (SCFA), 96–97
Société parisienne du Yaourt Danone, xiii
Starter cultures, 14–15
Streptococcus thermophilus, xxi, 7, 10, 120, 128, 129–130

SUN, see Seguimiento Universidad de Navarra (SUN)
Supplementation en Vitamines et Mineraux Antioxidants (SU.VI.MAX), 53, 154
Swedish Malmö Diet and Cancer, 92
Sweetened yogurt, 5, 179
Sydney Childhood Eye Study, 91

T

T2D, see Type 2 diabetes (T2D)
T and B lymphocyte function, 140–141
Tehran Lipid and Glucose Study (TLGS), 81, 104
TG, see Triglycerides (TG)
Third Generation cohort, 106
TLGS, see Tehran Lipid and Glucose Study (TLGS)
Trans-palmitoleate, 74
T regulatory cells, 139
Triglycerides (TG), 103, 106
Type 2 diabetes (T2D), 65–76
    mechanisms of action, 71–75
        fatty acids, 73–75
        fermentation and ferments, 75
        glycemic load, 72–73
        proteins, 73
        vitamins and minerals, 72
    studies in adults, 68–71
        cross-sectional studies, 68
        meta-analyses and systematic reviews, 70–71
        prospective cohort studies, 68–70
    studies in children and adolescents, 68

U

USDA, see U.S. Department of Agriculture (USDA)
U.S. Department of Agriculture (USDA), 32, 81
U.S. Institute of Medicine (IOM), 26
U.S. Women's Health Study, 148

V

Valine-proline-proline (VPP), 84
Viscosity, 58
Vitamin B12, 14
Vitamin D, 13–14, 26, 72, 82, 117, 147, 148, 173
Vitamins, 13–14
    food processing and lactic fermentation, 14
    and minerals, 72
VPP, see Valine-proline-proline (VPP)

W

WCRF, see World Cancer Research Fund (WCRF)

Weight management, and obesity, 45–59
    mechanisms of action, 56–58
        gut microbiota, 58
        micro- and macronutrients, 56–58
        studies on satiety, 56
        viscosity, 58
    studies in adults, 51–56
        clinical studies, 55
        cross-sectional studies, 51–52
        prospective studies, 52–55
        reviews, 55–56
    studies in children and adolescents, 46–51
Whey proteins, 57
WHO, *see* World Health Organization (WHO)
Whole-fat yogurts, 32
World Cancer Research Fund (WCRF), 145, 150, 151, 153
World Gastroenterology Organization, 123
World Health Organization (WHO), 122, 123, 167

Y

Yogurt, xii, xiv–xv, xxi
    bacteria
        activity of, 120–121
        viability of, 128–131
    composition, 3–17
        carbohydrates, 3–5
        lipids, 9–10
        matrix, 15–16
        minerals, 10–13
        proteins, 5–9
        starter cultures, 14–15
        vitamins, 13–14
    consumption, 23–37
        dairy and, consumption, 26–28
        dietary patterns, 34–35
        food-based dietary guidelines for dairy and, 23–25
        lifestyle and sociodemographic factors, 35–36
        nutrient adequacy, 30–34
        nutrient density, 28–30
    and gut health, 113–131
        lactose deficiency, malabsorption, and intolerance, 113–122
        microbiota, 128
        treatment of diarrhea, 122–127
        viability of yogurt bacteria, 128–131
    and health, xiii
    origin, xi

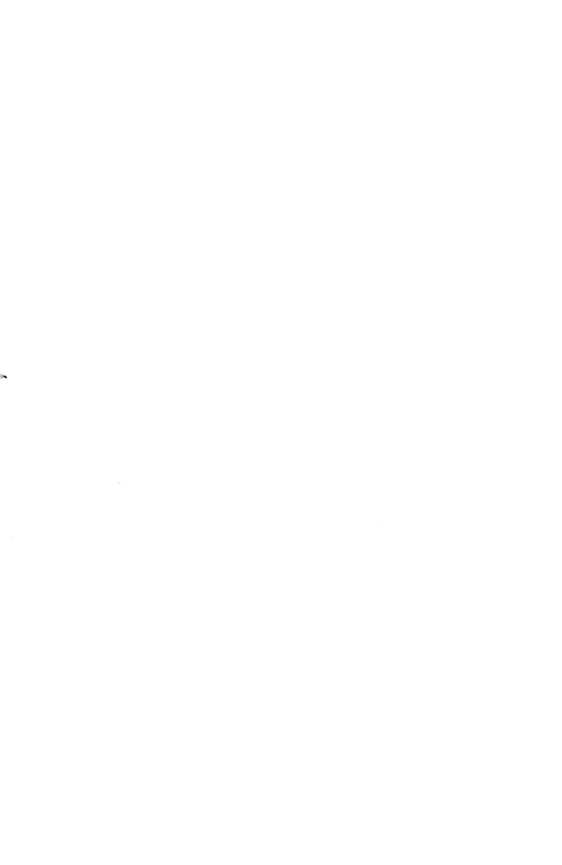